HEAD
AND
NECK
CANCER

Wiley Series on
CANCER INVESTIGATION AND MANAGEMENT

Series Editors

Professor J.M.A. Whitehouse *and* Dr. C.J. Williams
CRC Medical Oncology Unit, University of Southampton, UK

and

Professor G.P. Canellos
*Harvard Medical School and Dana-Farber Cancer Institute,
Boston, USA*

Volume 1

Breast Cancer: Diagnosis and Management
Gianni Bonadonna
*Istituto Nazionale per lo Studio e la Cura dei Tumori,
Milan, Italy*

Volume 2

Head and Neck Cancer
Robert E. Wittes
*Memorial Sloan-Kettering Cancer Center,
New York, USA*

Volume 3

Cancer of the Female Reproductive System
Christopher J. Williams *and* J. Michael Whitehouse
*CRC Medical Oncology Unit,
University of Southampton, UK
(in preparation)*

CANCER INVESTIGATION AND MANAGEMENT

Volume 2

HEAD
AND
NECK
CANCER

EDITED BY

ROBERT E. WITTES
Division of Cancer Treatment,
National Cancer Institute,
Bethesda, Maryland, USA

A Wiley Medical Publication

JOHN WILEY & SONS
Chichester · New York · Brisbane · Toronto · Singapore

Library of Congress Cataloging in Publication Data:
Main entry under title:

Head and neck cancer.

   (Wiley series on cancer investigation and management;
v. 2) (A Wiley medical publication)
   Includes index.
   1. Head—Cancer. 2. Neck—Cancer.
I. Wittes, Robert E. II. Series. III. Series: Wiley medical
publication. [DNLM: 1. Head and Neck Neoplasms.
W1 WI53H v.22 / WE 707 H43171]
RC280.H4H383   1985   616.99′491   84-15351
ISBN 0 471 10539 2

British Library Cataloguing in Publication Data:

Wittes, Robert E.
  Head and neck cancer.—(Cancer investigation and
  management)—(Wiley medical publication)
  1. Head—Cancer 2. Neck—Cancer
  I. Title II. Series
  616.99′491   RC280.H4

  ISBN 0 471 10539 2

Typeset by MHL Typesetting Limited, Coventry
Printed at The Bath Press, Avon

Contents

A. EPIDEMIOLOGY

B. STAGING

C. TREATMENT AND PREVENTION

Series Preface

The exciting but increasingly frenetic search for information with which to establish facts, may for future historians characterize the twentieth century. Unfortunately, like some vast panorama where despite its reality every perspective is different, appreciations change and established facts become fiction; sometimes only to emerge again as fact. The field of cancer has proved a fertile substrate and literature on every topic has proliferated at a rate which reflects the interest and enthusiasm of student, researcher, teacher and clinician alike. Unfortunately, the sheer volume of information available, disseminated as it is throughout many different and disparate publications, means that a genuine appreciation of current thinking has become increasingly hard to obtain. Experts in a particular topic become less easy to find as understanding becomes more complex and information more voluminous.

In editing this series we have these problems very much in mind, and so have approached leading experts with a request that they and others of their choice set out to reflect the 'current understanding' relating to the management of tumours of different organs. Detection and staging of cancer is one of the foundations on which we base our current treatments and we have used this as an approach to cancer as a whole. Each volume reviews clinical and experimental ways of detecting tumour and discusses their impact on the management of cancer.

In an attempt to give a balanced view of current thinking, the more controversial aspects are separated from dogma and established practice has been subjected to review. There is no value in seeking the opinion of a critical mind only to muzzle his views. Each author has therefore been free to roam over his topic within the confines of his brief. We anticipate that each volume will provide a digest, collectively distilled by the topic editor, of interest to the specialist and non-specialist clinician alike. While some chapters may perhaps serve primarily as reference works, they and their companions are intended as informative reading. Gaps there will certainly be, since it is left to textbooks to provide comprehensive documentation.

J.M.A. Whitehouse
C.J. Williams
G.P. Canellos

Preface

No group of neoplasms presents greater difficulties to the physician than the squamous cancers of the upper aerodigestive tract. The need to maximize a patient's chance of cure and at the same time preserve quality of life is a formidable challenge. A team approach is clearly necessary; surgeons from several subspecialties, diagnostic and therapeutic radiologists, general internists and medical oncologists, nurses, dentists, maxillofacial prosthodontists, nutritionists, speech therapists, social workers, and psychiatrists all have important roles.

The volume is not an attempt at another textbook but is rather a description of selected areas of particular current interest. Probably as a consequence of the editor's personal bias, treatment receives the most attention. We have emphasized particularly the increasing study of combined modality therapy, the coming of age of chemotherapy as an investigational modality, and various aspects of developmental radiotherapy. A survey of clinical immunology as it relates to natural history and treatment, the role of nutritional intervention, pathogenesis and treatment of hypercalcaemia, the use of lasers, and the potential of hyperthermia are all dealt with in individual chapters. Major issues in clinical trials methodology are the focus of a separate section. Since the role of environmental carcinogens is so clearly established for most squamous head and neck cancers, we have included critical surveys of their epidemiology. Finally, progress in our ability to culture human cancer cells in both colony-forming assays and as cell lines will make possible a deeper understanding of the biology of these cancers.

I am very grateful to William Soper for compiling the index and for valuable editorial assistance. Mary Jane Mathews and Candia Hench contributed their expert secretarial assistance. I also thank the editorial staff at John Wiley for their help and, above all, their patience.

List of Contributors

G.A. ALEXANDER — Division of Cancer Treatment, National Cancer Institute, Bethesda, Maryland, USA

M. AL-SARRAF — Department of Oncology, Wayne State University School of Medicine, Detroit, Michigan, USA

B.M. BERGAD — Department of Epidemiology and Preventive Medicine, Memorial Sloan–Kettering Cancer Center, New York, USA

N.M. BLEEHEN — MRC Unit of Clinical Oncology and Radiotherapeutics, Cambridge, UK

S.E. BUSH — St Joseph Hospital, Albuquerque, New Mexico, USA

T.E. CAREY — Departments of Otorhinolaryngology and Microbiology/Immunology, University of Michigan School of Medicine, Ann Arbor, Michigan, USA

R.R. CONNELLY — Division of Cancer Cause and Prevention, National Cancer Institute, Bethesda, Maryland, USA

J.M. DALY — Department of Surgery, Memorial Sloan–Kettering Cancer Center, New York, USA

M. EISENBERGER — Division of Cancer Treatment, National Cancer Institute, Bethesda, Maryland, USA

K.K. FU — Department of Radiation Oncology, University of California Hospital, San Francisco, California, USA

T.W. GRIFFIN — Radiation Oncology Department, University of Washington Hospital, Seattle, Washington, USA

B.E. HEARNE — Department of Surgery, Memorial Sloan–Kettering Cancer Center, New York, USA

E.Y. HILAL — Mercy Hospital, Pittsburgh, Pennsylvania, USA

D.D. VON HOFF — Department of Medicine, University of Texas Health Science Center, San Antonio, Texas, USA

P.H. LEVINE — Division of Cancer Cause and Prevention, National Cancer Institute, Bethesda, Maryland, USA

R.W. MAKUCH — Biometric Research Branch, National Cancer Institute, Bethesda, Maryland, USA

J.E. MARKS — Division of Radiation Oncology, Mallinckrodt Institute of Radiology, St Louis, Missouri, USA

D.E. MATTOX — Department of Surgery, University of Texas Health Science Center, San Antonio, Texas, USA

F.L. MEYSKENS — Department of Internal Medicine and Cancer Center, University of Arizona, Tucson, Arizona

J.H. OGURA — Department of Otolaryngology, Washington University School of Medicine, St Louis, Missouri, USA

C.M. PINSKY   Memorial Sloan – Kettering Cancer Center, New York, USA

D.A. PISTENMAA   Division of Cancer Treatment, National Cancer Institute, Bethesda, Maryland, USA

J. POSADA   Division of Cancer Treatment, National Cancer Institute, Bethesda, Maryland, USA

D. SCHOTTENFELD   Department of Epidemiology and Preventive Medicine, Memorial Sloan – Kettering Cancer Center, New York, USA

P. SELLERS   Department of Surgery, Memorial Sloan – Kettering Cancer Center, New York, USA

S.M. SHAPSHAY   Department of Otolaryngology, Lahey Clinical Medical Center, Burlington, Massachusetts, USA

W. SOPER   Division of Cancer Treatment, National Cancer Institute, Bethesda, Maryland, USA

A.F. STEWART   Yale University School of Medicine, New Haven, Connecticut, USA

S.E. THAWLEY   Department of Otolaryngology, Washington University School of Medicine, St Louis, Missouri, USA

B. VIKRAM   Department of Radiation Therapy, Memorial Sloan – Kettering Cancer Center, New York, USA

R.E. WITTES   Division of Cancer Treatment, National Cancer Institute, Bethesda, Maryland, USA

S.D.J. YEH   Memorial Sloan – Kettering Cancer Center, New York, USA

A
EPIDEMIOLOGY

Chapter 1

Epidemiology of Cancers of the Oral Cavity, Pharynx, and Larynx

David Schottenfeld and
Barbara M. Bergad
Department of Epidemiology and Preventive Medicine, Memorial Sloan – Kettering Cancer Center, New York, USA

INTRODUCTION

The ultimate goal of epidemiology is disease prevention. Close examination of incidence patterns and established risk factors facilitate research and intervention strategies designed for ultimately reducing cancer morbidity and mortality.

The American Cancer Society has estimated that 27 000 new cases of buccal cavity and pharyngeal cancer, and 11 000 new cases of laryngeal cancer will occur in the United States in 1983; the corresponding numbers of deaths were estimated to be 9150 and 3700, respectively.[1]

DEMOGRAPHIC PATTERNS

Buccal Cavity and Pharynx

Incidence

Cancers of the buccal cavity and pharynx accounted for 3.4% of all incident malignant neoplasms in the United States, after excluding basal and squamous cell carcinomas of the skin. The most frequently diagnosed primary sites in the buccal cavity and pharynx were tongue, lip, and gum (Table 1.1). A high-risk mucosal region extends backward

TABLE 1.1 AVERAGE ANNUAL AGE-ADJUSTED (1970 UNITED STATES STANDARD) INCIDENCE RATES PER 100 000 POPULATION FOR BUCCAL CAVITY AND PHARYNX CANCER BY SEX AND PRIMARY SITE, SEER PROGRAMME, 1973–77

Primary site	Total	Male	Female
Buccal cavity and pharynx	11.2	17.4	6.2
Tongue	2.0	3.0	1.2
Lip	1.9	3.9	0.3
Gum	1.8	2.4	1.4
Floor of mouth	1.3	2.0	0.7
Tonsil	1.1	1.6	0.7
Hypopharynx	1.0	1.7	0.4
Major salivary gland	0.9	1.1	0.8
Nasopharynx	0.6	0.9	0.3
Oropharynx	0.3	0.5	0.1

from the anterior floor of the mouth, over both lingual–alveolar sulci and lateral margins of the anterior two-thirds of the tongue, and then finally reaches the anterior tonsillar pillar and retromolar trigone complex.[2]

More than 90% of oropharyngeal cancers occurred in patients over 45 years of age, The average annual age-adjusted incidence per 100 000 population, based upon the SEER data for 1973–77, was 19.3 in black males, 16.8 in white males, 7.0 in black females, and 6.0 in white females. Under age 45, the incidence in men was about double that in women. With increasing age the rate of increase accelerated more in men, so that by age 70 the incidence became almost four times greater in men.

Long-term incidence patterns are not available for the United States, but may be inferred from population cancer registries. In Connecticut, over a 25-year period, buccal cavity and pharyngeal cancer incidence decreased in males from 17.9 to 16.8 per 100 000 and increased in females from 3.6 to 5.3 per 100 000 (Table 1.2).

TABLE 1.2   AGE-ADJUSTED (1950 UNITED
STATES STANDARD) INCIDENCE
RATES PER 100 000 POPULATION
FOR BUCCAL CAVITY AND
PHARYNX CANCER BY SEX AND
YEAR OF DIAGNOSIS,
CONNECTICUT, 1950–74

| | Buccal Cavity | | Pharynx | |
Period	Male	Female	Male	Female
1950–54	13.3	2.8	4.6	0.8
1955–59	13.4	2.7	5.1	0.9
1960–64	14.0	3.1	5.3	1.1
1965–69	11.7	3.1	5.2	1.2
1970–74	11.8	4.0	5.0	1.3

Mortality

A survey of mortality in the United States from 1950 to 1969 revealed contrasting patterns for men and women.[3] Mortality among men was elevated in the northeast, around large metropolitan areas. Mortality predominated in lower socioeconomic groups. In women, the southeastern excess of oral cancer occurred in the rural white population, in which snuff-dipping was a relatively common habit.[4]

The secular trend for age-adjusted mortality in the United States, 1950–79, demonstrated the predominance in non-white males since 1965. By 1979 buccal cavity and pharynx cancer mortality in non-white males was 1.7 times greater than in white males. During a period of 30 years, age-adjusted mortality decreased slightly in white males but increased relatively by 84% in non-white males (Table 1.3).[5]

TABLE 1.3   AGE-ADJUSTED (1970 STANDARD
POPULATION) MORTALITY RATES
PER 100 000 POPULATION FOR
BUCCAL CAVITY AND PHARYNX
CANCER BY SEX AND RACE,
UNITED STATES, 1950–79

| | Male | | Female | |
Year	White	Non-white	White	Non-white
1950	6.6	4.9	1.5	2.0
1955	6.2	4.8	1.5	1.6
1960	5.9	5.2	1.6	2.0
1965	5.7	6.3	1.5	1.9
1970	5.9	7.3	1.8	2.1
1975	5.5	8.2	1.9	2.1
1979	5.2	9.0	1.9	2.4

From McKay *et al.*[5]

Data regarding patient survival have not been available on the same scale as data on mortality covering the entire United States population, or on incidence covering selected geographic areas in the United States. Mortality trends reflect both incidence and survival trends. If both incidence and mortality for a specific cancer site remain unchanged or change proportionately over a period of years, no major change in survival should be anticipated. The trend in 5-year relative survival will be influenced by the temporal trend for the percentage of cases localized at the time of diagnosis and/or by the impact of evolving methods of treatment. In general, for each of the subsites within the oral cavity and pharynx, survival was more favourable in the

TABLE 1.4   TRENDS IN 5-YEAR RELATIVE SURVIVAL* FOR BUCCAL CAVITY SUBSITES AND PHARYNX CANCERS IN WHITE MALES (WM) AND FEMALES (WF), 1955–59 AND 1965–69†

| | 5-Year relative survival (%) | | | |
| | 1955–59 | | 1965–69 | |
Site	WM	WF	WM	WF
Lip	88	97‡	84	85‡
Tongue	27	47	32	44
Floor of mouth	43	46‡	42	47
Pharynx	23	29	21	30

* The relative survival rate is the ratio of the observed survival rate to the expected survival rate for persons from the general population who are similar to the patient group with respect to age, race, sex, and calendar year of observation.
† From End Results Program, National Cancer Institute (1976).
‡ Rate has standard error between 5% and 10%.

TABLE 1.5   AGE-ADJUSTED INCIDENCE RATES PER 100 000 POPULATION FOR ORAL CAVITY AND PHARYNX CANCER IN SELECTED POPULATIONS THROUGHOUT THE WORLD BY RANK ORDER, SEX, AND MALE TO FEMALE RATIO, 1968–72*

Country	Male	Female	M/F Ratio
Bombay, India	33.2	12.1	2.7
Puerto Rico	25.9	6.9	3.8
Sao Paulo, Brazil	24.3	4.8	5.1
Singapore (Indian)	22.1	25.5	0.9
Quebec, Canada	15.3	3.7	4.2
Geneva, Switzerland	14.2	3.0	4.7
Connecticut	13.1	4.4	3.0
Detroit, Michigan (White)	11.3	3.8	3.0
Detroit, Michigan (Black)	11.2	4.1	2.7
Hamburg, Federal Republic	9.0	3.3	2.7
Israel (All Jews)	7.4	3.4	2.2
Israel (Non-Jews)	7.1	1.3	5.5
Singapore (Chinese)	6.9	1.7	4.1
Singapore (Malay)	6.0	1.6	3.8
Ibadan, Nigeria	4.2	3.2	1.3

* From Waterhouse *et al.*[7]

women (Table 1.4). This was partially explained by differences observed in the extent of disease at the time of initial diagnosis. For example, the striking contrast in survival for carcinoma of the tongue was reflected in the percentage of women with localized disease (50–55%) as compared with the men (37–43%).[6]

International Patterns

Cancer of the oral cavity showed marked geographic differences, being common among men where alcohol and tobacco consumption were high (e.g. in France, where the age-adjusted mortality was 2.5–3.0 times the United States rate in men) or where betel quid chewing and 'bidi' smoking were frequent (e.g. India). Among men and women in Bombay, cancer of the oral cavity and hypopharynx accounted for 50% of all cancers (Table 1.5).[7] Carcinoma of the tongue, hypopharynx, and oesophagus were attributed partially to smoking of an uncured form of tobacco ('bidi'), which was dried in the sun and rolled in a dried leaf of temburni or banana. Cancer of the roof of the mouth was relatively common where reverse smoking of the lighted end of a slow-burning cheroot was practised (e.g. Sardinia,

Venezuela, Panama, and India). In Visakhapatnam, East India, almost three-quarters of the oral and pharyngeal cancers in women occurred on the hard palate.[8]

Larynx

Incidence

Cancer of the larynx represented approximately 2% of all incident cancers in the United States. The incidence of laryngeal cancer increased significantly in men between ages 35 and 74. The disease rarely affected persons under age 35, and occurred particularly in the interval 60–74 years. Any apparent decline in cross-sectional incidence among males after age 75 may have represented a birth cohort rather than an age phenomenon, because men born before the year 1900 did not smoke as heavily as men born after 1900.[9] The incidence in women peaked during the interval 55–64 years, after which there was a marked increase in the age-specific male/female incidence ratio. The decline in risk in women after age 65 years almost certainly reflected a cohort phenomenon, as the habit of smoking in

TABLE 1.6   AGE-ADJUSTED (1950 UNITED
STATES STANDARD) INCIDENCE
RATES PER 100 000 POPULATION
FOR LARYNX CANCER BY SEX AND
YEAR OF DIAGNOSIS
CONNECTICUT, 1950–74

Year	Male	Female
1950–54	6.1	0.3
1955–59	6.2	0.6
1960–64	8.6	0.7
1965–69	8.6	1.0
1970–74	8.6	1.2

Includes intrinsic and extrinsic larynx, and *in situ* cancers.

women followed by at least 20 years the pattern exhibited in men.

The average annual age-adjusted incidence per 100 000 population for laryngeal cancer was 8.6 for males and 1.2 for females between 1970 and 1974. Based upon the Connecticut registry, the age-adjusted incidence during the period 1960–74 has not changed in males, but has almost doubled in females (Table 1.6).

Mortality

Mortality from laryngeal cancer more than doubled in the non-white male during the past 30 years. Concurrently, the rate of increase in lung cancer mortality in the non-white male was even more significant (Table 1.7). Laryngeal cancer mortality in white males and females did not change materially during the same period of time, while lung cancer mor-

tality increased more than 3-fold in white males, and 4-fold in white females.

The mapping of cancer mortality by county in the United States has revealed a number and variety of geographic patterns and clusters. For larynx and lung cancer during the period 1950–69, mortality was increased in the urban areas of the north. Rates were higher among whites when compared with non-whites in the rural south, and higher among non-whites in the urban south and northeast.[3]

International Patterns

International variation in site-specific incidence and mortality has heightened the epidemiological search and recognition of environmental factors that are major determinants of contrasting patterns. Cancer of the larynx varied worldwide, generally predominated in males, while the rates in females tended to persist below 1.0 per 100 000. The magnitude of larynx cancer may not vary in any constant or predictable relationship to the incidence of lung cancer in the same population. Indian men and women were at highest risk for both laryngeal and oral cavity cancer, but were rather low for lung cancer incidence. In the United Kingdom, incidence rates were fairly low in contrast to the high level of lung cancer. The highest laryngeal cancer incidence in males was reported from São Paulo in Brazil (14.1 per

TABLE 1.7   AGE-ADJUSTED (1970 STANDARD POPULATION) MORTALITY RATES PER 100 000
POPULATION FOR LARYNX AND LUNG CANCER BY SEX AND RACE, UNITED STATES,
1950–79

Year	White Male			Non-white Male			White Female			Non-white Female		
	Larynx	Lung	Ratio*	Larynx	Lung	Ratio*	Larynx	Lung	Ratio*	Larynx	Lung	Ratio*
1950	2.6	21.9	8.4	1.8	16.0	8.9	0.3	4.9	16.3	0.4	4.0	10.0
1955	2.7	30.4	11.3	2.3	24.1	10.5	0.2	5.1	25.5	0.4	5.1	12.8
1960	2.7	38.0	14.1	3.1	37.3	12.0	0.2	5.6	28.0	0.4	5.9	14.8
1965	2.7	47.1	17.4	3.2	45.7	14.3	0.3	7.4	24.7	0.4	7.3	18.3
1970	2.9	57.4	19.8	3.4	62.0	18.3	0.3	11.1	37.0	0.5	11.2	22.4
1975	2.7	64.1	23.7	3.9	73.7	18.9	0.4	15.3	38.3	0.6	14.3	23.8
1979	2.7	68.7	25.4	4.0	81.3	20.3	0.4	19.4	48.5	0.5	18.3	36.6

* Ratio of age-adjusted lung cancer mortality to larynx cancer mortality.
From McKay *et al.*[5]

100 000). In Bombay, India, the highest incidence was reported in women (2.6 per 100 000). In the Mediterranean countries and those lying to the east along the same latitude as India, high incidence rates of laryngeal cancer were not generally accompanied by high rates of lung cancer, but were more significantly correlated with elevated oral and oesophageal cancer incidence.[10]

AETIOLOGY

Tobacco

Epidemiological studies have demonstrated that the risk of oral cavity and laryngeal (i.e. both glottis and supraglottis) cancer was increased among cigarette smokers. The degree of exposure over time, as measured by the average daily amount smoked, affected the relative risk of developing cancer in tissues of the respiratory tract and oral cavity (Table 1.8). When compared with non-smokers, a prospective study of United States veterans who smoked 40 or more cigarettes per day indicated that the relative risk of dying of lung cancer was increased almost 24-fold, of laryngeal cancer 32-fold, and of oral cavity cancer more than 12-fold.[11]

Both laboratory and epidemiological studies have demonstrated that exposure to cigar and pipe tobacco smoke may produce cancers particularly of the oral cavity and larynx. Although the risk of lung cancer was less for cigar or pipe smokers than for cigarette smokers, it was significantly higher than for non-smokers (Table 1.9).

Although there has been general acceptance of the tumorigenic properties of tobacco-smoke condensates, or of forms of tobacco that involve combustion, the use of snuff or chewing tobacco may also cause cancers in the

TABLE 1.8   RELATIVE RISKS* OF DEATH FROM BUCCAL CAVITY, LARYNX, AND LUNG CANCER AMONG MEN ACCORDING TO AVERAGE NUMBER OF CIGARETTES SMOKED PER DAY, UNITED STATES VETERANS STUDY†

Current cigarette smokers (no. per day)	Relative risk of death		
	Lung cancer	Larynx cancer	Buccal cavity cancer
1−9	5.5	5.3	2.9
10−20	9.9	9.2	2.9
21−39	17.4	14.8	6.2
40+	23.9	32.1	12.4

* Relative to a risk of 1.0 in men who never smoked regularly
† From Kahn.[11]

TABLE 1.9   RELATIVE RISKS* OF DEATH FROM BUCCAL CAVITY, LARYNX, AND LUNG CANCER AMONG MEN ACCORDING TO CIGAR AND PIPE SMOKING, UNITED STATES VETERANS STUDY†

Smoking type	Relative risk of death		
	Lung cancer	Larynx cancer	Buccal cavity cancer
Cigar only	1.7	10.3	4.1
Pipe only	2.1	—	3.1
Total pipe and cigar	1.7	7.3	4.2

* Relative to a risk of 1.0 in men who never smoked regularly.
† From Kahn.[11]

mouth and pharynx. Winn *et al.*[4] estimated a four-fold increase in the risk of oral cancer among women in North Carolina who dipped snuff. The area of the mouth in contact with the tobacco powder, the gingivobuccal sulcus, was most often affected after prolonged exposure.

Cultural differences in the use of tobacco products have led to variations in the geographic incidence and anatomic location of head and neck cancers. In countries such as India, China, Thailand, Ceylon, Afghanistan, and the Central Republic of the Soviet Union, where the use of snuff and chewing tobacco was quite common, mortality rates for oral and pharyngeal cancer were among the highest in the world. Tobacco chewing by men and women in India, for example, involved mixing a paste or quid of slaked lime (calcium hydroxide), tobacco leaves, betel nuts, and catechu (an astringent powder), wrapping this in dried betel leaves, and placing this mixture in the lower posterior gingivobuccal sulcus or under the anterior two-thirds of the tongue. The physiological effects of chewing such a mixture were curbing of the appetite and increased salivation. Pathological consequences consisted of extensive leukoplakia and, ultimately, epidermoid carcinoma of the gingivobuccal mucosa, tongue, and extrinsic larynx.[12]

There are general principles of tobacco carcinogenesis that apply to tissues in the upper digestive tract, respiratory tract, and urinary tract. These may be summarized as follows:

(1) There is a dose–response relationship, so that the level of exposure (i.e. amount smoked, chewed, or snuffed; amount of particulate phase constituents or 'tar' content of the smoke; depth and mode of inhalation; duration of the habit; use of filtered versus non-filtered cigarettes) determines ultimately the level of risk for developing a tobacco-related cancer.

(2) Smoking cessation reduces the risk at a rate influenced by the amount smoked previously and the duration of the habit. Among heavy, long-term smokers, at least 10–15 years of smoking cessation may be required before the level of excess risk stabilizes and approaches the level manifested by non-smokers of comparable age

(3) The relative risk for developing a specific type of cancer depends mainly on the susceptibility of a tissue to various concentrations of tobacco smoke constituents and their metabolites. Within the oral cavity and extrinsic larynx, direct contact with tobacco smoke and tobacco juice is of aetiological significance. Other organs such as the pancreas and kidney are affected by systemic metabolites of tobacco after metabolic activation in the liver and/or target tissues.

The lighted cigarette generates about 4000 compounds which can be separated into gas and particulate phases. The major tumorigenic activity of tobacco smoke is contained in the particulate matter or 'tar' fraction. The composition of the tobacco smoke is a function of the physical and chemical properties of the leaf or blends of tobacco. The carcinogenic activity of the particulate matter results from a complex mixture of interacting initiators, promoters, and cocarcinogens. The primary initiators are the polynuclear aromatic hydrocarbons and volatile nitrosamines.[13]

Alcohol

The balance of epidemiological evidence supports the view that excessive alcohol consumption increases the risk of incurring epidermoid carcinomas of the oral cavity, pharynx, larynx, and oesophagus. Alcohol and tobacco act synergistically, and are the salient cofactors responsible for at least 75% of upper aerodigestive tract cancer deaths (Table 1.10). The cancer sites for which tobacco and alcohol are major determinants in the United States, occur with greater frequency in men, lower socioeconomic groups, and with increasing urbanization.[14]

TABLE 1.10   ESTIMATION OF CANCER DEATHS ATTRIBUTABLE TO TOBACCO AND/OR ALCOHOL
CONSUMPTION IN THE UNITED STATES, 1983

Type of cancer	Estimated deaths (1983)*		Proportion attributable to use of tobacco and/or alcohol	Number of deaths attributable to use of tobacco and/or alcohol	
	Men	Women		Men	Women
Mouth and pharynx	6 300	2 850	0.75	4 725	2 138
Larynx	3 100	600	0.75	2 325	450
Oesophagus	6 200	2 300	0.75	4 650	1 725
Subtotal	15 600	5 750	0.75	11 700	4 313
All cancer deaths	238 500	201 500	0.30 (Men)† 0.15 (Women)†	71 550†	30 225†

* From American Cancer Society.[1]
† Including Lung, Urinary Bladder and Pancreas (Primarily Tobacco).

The clearest demonstration of the combined effects of tobacco and alcohol on the relative risk for oral and pharyngeal cancer was provided by Rothman and Keller.[15] For each level of exposure to tobacco, the risk increased with the increasing level of daily alcohol exposure. However, joint exposure to tobacco and alcohol resulted in risk ratios that were $2 - 2\frac{1}{2}$ times those expected if the effects of alcohol and tobacco were only additive (Table 1.11). In general, the appreciable cocarcinogenic action of ethanol with tobacco occurred with levels of exposure exceeding 45 ml of ethanol per day. The subsites within the upper aerodigestive tract manifesting a higher degree of correlation with past ethanol rather than tobacco exposure are floor of mouth, supraglottis, hypopharynx, and oesophagus. This has been interpreted by Kissin[16] as suggesting a direct topical rather than systemic action for ethanol.

A patient with a previous epidermoid carcinoma of the upper aero-digestive tract has an increased risk of developing a new epithelial cancer within a subsite of the oral cavity, pharynx, larynx, and oesophagus. In a previously published cohort study, multiple primaries were three times more frequent in patients with cancer of the supraglottis than of the intrinsic larynx.[17] In the group of patients with an antecedent carcinoma of the supraglottis, the relative risk was increased 30-fold for a subsequent cancer of the oral cavity or pharynx, 18-fold for cancer of the oesophagus, and 5-fold for cancer of the lung. These observations were compatible with the patterns of excessive consumption of alcohol and smoking of cigarette, cigar, and pipe tobacco that were demonstrated in these patients.

Epidemiological studies have stimulated interest in the biochemical mechanisms whereby alcohol consumption increases the risk of developing cancer. In animal experiments, prolonged ethanol administration may be injurious to the liver and nervous system, but has not been shown to be carcinogenic. However, human ethanol consumption may include ingestion of by-products or contaminants known to be carcinogenic and present in alcoholic beverages, concomitant exposure to tobacco, and exacerbated nutritional deficiencies.

A variety of carcinogens including nitrosamines, polycyclic hydro-carbons, fusel

TABLE 1.11   RELATIVE RISK FOR ORAL CAVITY CANCER ACCORDING TO LEVEL OF EXPOSURE TO ALCOHOL AND SMOKING*

Alcohol per day (oz.)	Cigarette equivalents per day			
	0	Less than 20	20 – 39	40 or more
None	1.00	1.52	1.43	2.43
< 0.4	1.40	1.67	3.18	3.25
0.4 – 1.5	1.60	4.36	4.46	8.21
> 1.5	2.33	4.13	9.59	15.50

* From Rothman and Keller.[15] Risks are expressed relative to risk of 1.00 for persons who neither smoked nor drank.

oils (i.e. amyl alcohol by-products of fermentation) and other mutagenic compounds have been found in different types of alcoholic drinks.[18] Nitrosodiethylamine, a carcinogen demonstrated experimentally to be organotropic for upper digestive tract tissues such as the oesophagus, has been detected in apple cider distillates at concentrations of 1 to 3 parts per billion. Nitrosodimethylamine was detected in varying amounts in most beers produced all over the world. Even if one or more carcinogens were identified in specific types of alcoholic beverages, the more fundamental pathogenic relationship observed in epidemiological studies appears to be total ethanol intake.[19]

The two most likely mechanisms whereby ethanol may act as a cocarcinogen in the initiation phase of chemical carcinogenesis involve (a) the cytotoxic effects of ethanol and its metabolites, and (b) the inducing effect of chronic ethanol consumption on microsomal enzyme activity. In addition to these rather direct effects of ethanol on target tissues, a multi-stage process may be influenced by various nutritional deficiencies associated with excessive alcohol consumption, or by effects of ethanol on the immune system.[14]

Dietary Factors

A number of nutritional factors are thought to be important as modifiers of carcinogenesis. Nutritional deficiencies are commonly associated with, or exacerbated by, excessive alcohol ingestion. These give rise to altered mucosal integrity, enzyme and metabolic dysfunction, and morphological abnormalities in specific target organs.

Epidemiological studies have suggested that adequate ingestion of vitamin A tended to protect against epithelial tumours in the oral cavity and respiratory tract.[20,21] Vitamin A and its provitamin, beta-carotene, are needed for normal growth and differentiation of epithelial tissues. A deficiency of vitamin A leads to a loss of mucociliary epithelium in the respiratory tract and its replacement by metaplastic squamous epithelium. Vitamin A

and/or its synthetic analogues have been shown to inhibit tumour induction in the respiratory tract, skin, bladder, and mammary gland model tumour systems. Possible mechanisms of action arising from vitamin A deficiency that are under investigation include: (a) metabolic activation and/or DNA binding of the carcinogen during the initiation phase, (b) enhancement of metaplastic epithelial proliferation during the post-initiation phase, and (c) impairment of immune function.[22-24]

The Plummer–Vinson or Paterson–Kelly syndrome has been noted particularly in middle-aged northern Swedish women, who frequently have poor dentition, and was characterized by iron and multiple vitamin deficiencies, achlorhydria, papillary atrophy of the tongue, glossitis, atrophy of the epithelium of the upper alimentary tract, and oesophageal webs or strictures. Women with this syndrome were at increased risk of developing carcinoma of the oral cavity, hypopharynx (postcricoid), and oesophagus. The epithelial changes have been attributed to complex nutritional deficiencies. Tobacco and alcohol were not major aetiological factors in carcinomas of the upper alimentary tract in the Swedish women. Riboflavin deficiency causes similar epithelial lesions in animals, and McCoy[25] has hypothesized that the common link between Plummer–Vinson disease and alcohol consumption may be the role that iron and riboflavin play in respiratory enzyme chemistry and its relationship to rates of metabolic activation of carcinogenic precursors.

Occupational Factors and Laryngeal Cancer

The risk of developing laryngeal cancer in different occupations was investigated in a case–control study using the interview data of the Third National Cancer Survey.[26] The Third National Cancer Survey was a study of all incident cancers in seven cities and two states during the 3-year period 1969–71. A 10% probability sample of these cancer cases was interviewed to obtain more detailed epidemiological information. The relation between laryngeal cancer and employment was studied by industry and specific job category, after controlling for smoking and drinking. Of the 17 industrial categories studied, four industries – transportation equipment, general building, lumber and wood products, and railroad – were associated with relative risks that were increased 2.0 or higher. Of 22 job categories studied, the relative risk was 4.0 or higher among sheet-metal workers, automobile mechanics, miscellaneous mechanics and repairmen, electricians, and grinding wheel operators.

Specific occupational exposure factors linked with laryngeal cancer include asbestos, mustard gas, and isopropyl alcohol. In addition, one or more studies have reported the following occupational exposures or occupations to be associated with laryngeal cancer: nickel, wood dust, grease and oil, leather, paper, textiles, and naphthalene cleaners. In most instances, the number of exposed cases was small, studies are conflicting or require confirmation, and/or did not always control for smoking and drinking.[9]

Mouthwash and Oral Cancer

Recently, regular use of mouthwash has been suggested as a possible risk factor in the development of oral and pharyngeal cancers. In a study of 200 cases, Weaver *et al.*[27] reported that in a small subgroup of non-smoking and non-drinking cases there was a significant excess of users of mouthwash when compared with 50 controls patients. Blot *et al.*[28] as part of a case–control study of women from North Carolina with oral and pharyngeal cancers, noted almost a 2-fold increase in relative risk among users of mouthwash who abstained from tobacco. The estimation of increased risk in this subgroup of non-users of tobacco was based upon only eight cases and 61 controls. There was no consistent trend in terms of frequency of daily use, or whether the mouthwash was taken in full strength or diluted form. Similarly in the study of Wynder

et al.[29] daily mouthwash use was associated with increased risk in women who were non-smokers and non-drinkers, but no dose–response effect was demonstrable in the women, and no effect was observed in the men. It is of course possible that commercial mouthwashes, which contain various flavouring and colouring agents as well as significant amounts of ethanol, may be irritating and injurious to the oral mucosa after prolonged and regular use, but it is not possible at this time to infer any causal significance.

SUMMARY

It is clear that we have the scientific understanding to prevent most human cancers in the upper aerodigestive tract. Exclusion of tobacco and excessive alcohol consumption in the United States should result in a reduction of over 16 000 deaths per year from cancers of the mouth and pharynx, larynx and esophagus. Alternative or additional co-factors, such as deficiency of essential micronutrients and occupational factors, are relatively important in specific subgroups of the population or in different parts of the world. Public apathy and ignorance about the morbidity and mortality attributed to use of tobacco in various forms and excessive chronic use of alcohol should not deter research of effective cancer control interventions.

REFERENCES

1. American Cancer Society: Cancer Statistics (1983). *Cancer*, **33**, 16–17.
2. Moore, C., and Catlin, D. (1967). Anatomic origins and locations of oral cancer. *Am. J. Surg.*, **114**, 510–513.
3. Blot, W.J., and Fraumeni, J.F., Jr. (1977). Geographic patterns of oral cancer in the United States: etiologic implications. *J. Chron. Dis.*, **30**, 745–757.
4. Winn, D.M., Blot, W.J., Shy, C.M., Pickle, L.W., Toledo, A., and Fraumeni, J.F., Jr. (1981). Snuff dipping and oral cancer among women in the southern United States. *N. Engl. J. Med.*, **304**, 745–749.
5. McKay, F.W., Hanson, M.R., and Miller, R.W. (1982). Cancer mortality in the United

States: 1950–1977. *National Cancer Institute Monographs* (No. 59), Washington, DC, US Government Printing Office.

6. Axtell, L.M., Asire, A.J., and Myers, M.H. (1976). *Cancer Patient Survival* (Report No. 5), Washington, DC, US Government Printing Office.

7. Waterhouse, J., Muir, C.S., Correa, P. *et al.* (1976). Cancer incidence in five continents (Vol. III), *IARC Scientific Publication No. 15*, Lyon.

8. Reddy, C.R. (1974). Carcinoma of hard palate in India in relation to reverse smoking of chuttas. *J. Natl. Cancer. Inst.*, **53**, 615–619.

9. Rothman, K.J., Cann, C.I., Flanders, D., and Fried, M.P. (1980). Epidemiology of laryngeal cancer. *Epidemiol. Rev.*, **2**, 195–209.

10. Dunham, L.J., and Bailar, J.C. (1968). World maps of cancer mortality rates and frequency ratios. *J. Natl. Cancer Inst.*, **41**, 155–203.

11. Kahn, H.A. (1966). The Dorn study of smoking and mortality among U.S. veterans: Report on $8\frac{1}{2}$ years of observation. *J. Natl. Cancer Inst.*, **19**, 1–125.

12. Schonland, M., and Bradshaw, E. (1969). Upper alimentary tract cancer in Natal Indians with special reference to the betel chewing habit. *Br. J. Cancer*, **23**, 670–682.

13. Wynder, E.L., and Hoffman, D. (1982). Tobacco, in *Cancer Epidemiology and Prevention* (Eds D. Schottenfeld and J.F. Fraumeni, Jr.), pp. 277–292, Saunders, Philadelphia.

14. Schottenfeld, D. (1979). Alcohol as a co-factor in the etiology of cancer. *Cancer*, **43** (5), 1962–1966.

15. Rothman, K., and Keller, A.Z. (1972). The effect of joint exposure to alcohol and tobacco on risk of cancer of the mouth and pharynx. *J. Chron. Dis.*, **25**, 711–716.

16. Kissin, B. (1975). Epidemiologic investigations of possible biological inter-actions of alcohol and cancer of the head and neck. *Ann. N.Y. Acad. Sci.*, **252**, 374–384.

17. Schottenfeld, D., Gantt, R.C., and Wynder, E.L. (1974). The role of alcohol and tobacco in multiple primary cancers of the upper digestive

system, larynx, and lung: A prospective study. *Prev. Med.*, **3**, 277–293.

18. Lieber, C.S., Garro, A., and Gordon, G.G. (1982). Alcohol as a mutagen, carcinogen, and teratogen, in *Medical Disorders of Alcoholism: Pathogenesis and Treatment* (Ed. C.S. Lieber), pp. 526–550, Saunders, Philadelphia.

19. Tuyns, A.J. (1982). Alcohol, in *Cancer Epidemiology and Prevention* (Eds D. Schottenfeld and J.F. Fraumeni, Jr.), pp. 293–303, Saunders, Philadelphia.

20. Mettlin, C., Graham, S., and Swanson, M. (1979). Vitamin A and lung cancer. *J. Natl. Cancer Inst.*, **62**, 1435–1438.

21. Marshall, J., Graham, S., Mettlin, C., Shedd, D., and Swanson, M. (1982). Diet in the epidemiology of oral cancer. *Nutr. Cancer*, **3**, 145–149.

22. De Luca, L., Maestri, N., Bonanni, F., and Nelson, D. (1972). Maintenance of epithelial cell differentiation. The mode of action of vitamin A. *Cancer*, **30**, 1326–1331.

23. Sporn, M.B. (1977). Retinoids and carcinogenesis. *Nutr. Rev.*, **35**, 65–69.

24. Genta, V.M., Kaufman, D.G., Harris, C.C., Smith, J.M., Sporn, M.B., and Saffiotti, U. (1974). Vitamin A deficiency enhances binding of benzo(a)pyrene to tracheal epithelial DNA. *Nature*, **247**, 48–49.

25. McCoy, G.D. (1978). A biochemical approach to the etiology of alcohol related cancers of the head and neck. *Laryngoscope*, **88**, 59–62.

26. Flanders, W.D., and Rothman, K.J. (1982). Occupational risk for laryngeal cancer. *Am. J. Public Health*, **72**, 369–372.

27. Weaver, A., Fleming, S.M., and Smith, D.B. (1979). Mouthwash and oral cancer: carcinogen or coincidence? *J. Oral Surg.*, **37**, 250–253.

28. Blot, W.J., Winn, D.M., and Fraumeni, J.F., Jr. (1983). Oral cancer and mouthwash. *J. Natl. Cancer Inst.*, **70**, 251–253.

29. Wynder, E.L., Kabat, G., Rosenberg, S., and Levenstein, M. (1983). Oral cancer and mouthwash use. *J. Natl. Cancer Inst.*, **70**, 255–260.

Chapter 2

Epidemiology of Nasopharyngeal Cancer

Paul H. Levine* and
Roger R. Connelly†
* *Clinical Epidemiology Branch, and*
† *Biometry Branch, Division of Cancer
Cause and Prevention, National
Cancer Institute, Bethesda,
Maryland, USA.*

INTRODUCTION

Nasopharyngeal (NP) cancer has become a disease of particular interest in recent years because of the intriguing epidemiologic patterns and laboratory findings which have led to a number of productive multidisciplinary studies on the cause and control of this disease. While it it a relatively rare form of cancer in the US (approximately 1390 new cases and 760 deaths per year), for certain groups, such as teen-age blacks and adult Chinese-Americans,[60,94] it is disproportionately frequent. Control of the disease is not as good as the ratio of deaths to new cases would seem to indicate, primarily because NP cancer deaths are underreported on death certificates.[129] The 5-year survival rate in the general US population following the diagnosis of NP cancer is approximately 30%[8] and the end results in other populations are similar.[22,63,75,78,142,147,158]

As with many forms of cancer, malignancy of the nasopharynx is a heterogeneous collection of diseases, some with unique disease patterns suggesting distinct aetiologies. NP sarcomas, for example, are primarily a disease of white children,[60,94] whereas non-glandular epithelial-derived NP carcinomas have characteristics differentiating them quite markedly from carcinomas in other sites. In the pathological classification of NP cancer developed by the World Health Organization,[144] the term NPC is used solely for this latter form of NP cancer which comprises the vast majority of cases in endemic areas. It is apparent, however, that the percentage of glandular epithelial and non-epithelial tumours is appreciable in some populations,[18,48,141,155] and it is unfortunate that information on the histological types of tumours has been lacking in many studies of NP cancer.

In recent years, population-based findings utilizing more uniform classification criteria have permitted a more critical evaluation of the mortality and incidence patterns in various ethnic groups that are important in determining the relative influence of environmental and genetic factors on the occurrence of this disease. We will discuss these recent findings and present data on NP cancer in the United States obtained from the Surveillance, Epidemiology, and End Results (SEER) Program of the Biometry Branch, National Cancer Institute.[163] The SEER Program, established in 1972, collects cancer incidence data from five states and several metropolitan areas representing approximately 10% of the US population. Some of the laboratory and analytical epidemiological studies suggesting clues to the aetiology of this disease will also be discussed.

NASOPHARYNGEAL CARCINOMA (EPITHELIAL, NON-GLANDULAR)

Demographic Patterns

Studies of NPC incidence in numerous populations have greatly increased our knowledge of the important demographic features of this disease. Although the most useful cancer registry data are obtained when primary site classifications are supplemented by histological classifications,[12,138] it is possible to utilize studies of NP cancer as a whole since NPC is the predominant morphological type.[141]

The most striking characteristic of NPC is its predilection for Chinese, especially those living in the southeastern provinces of China,[31,44,64,100,110,161] or those born there who have migrated to other parts of southeast Asia and beyond.[19,20,71,74,75,116,141] There are significant geographical variations in risk within China.[31,44,64,100,110,161] As shown in Table 2.1, there are also differences among the emigrant Chinese communities; these probably reflect the variations in risk by place of origin in China.

Other populations at elevated risk are Eskimos,[90,91,106,119] Filipinos,[11,109,122] Malays,[7] and some groups near the Mediterranean Sea.[21,105,121,160] Some of these high-risk groups, such as Eskimos, are anthropologically related to Chinese. However, Japanese and Koreans, who are not only anthropologically related but

have similar patterns of living, habitats and cultural heritages, have much lower risk of developing NPC than the Chinese.[116,160]

In most non-Chinese populations of the world, NPC is a rare disease with age-adjusted incidence rates of less than 1 per 100 000.[160] Non-Chinese in Hong Kong, Singapore, and Selangor (Malaysia) are at substantially less risk than the Chinese of those areas,[7,74,141] suggesting that genetics has an effect on the incidence of this disease (see below). The influence of local environmental factors, however, is suggested by the reports that white US males born in southeast Asia[19] and Japanese born in Hawaii[4,95] may be at increased risk compared to native-born US whites and Japanese.

Analyses of death rates for NP cancer (which reflect primarily NPC mortality) among Chinese in the US have revealed a decreasing trend over time[50] and lower rates among US-born Chinese than among the foreign-born.[20,82,83] NP cancer incidence rates among the Chinese in Hawaii have also decreased over time (Table 2.1). However, incidence rates have not decreased among emigrant Chinese in other places (Table 2.1); an apparent increase in rates over time in Hong Kong is probably due to improved case ascertainment (Ho, personal communication). The decreasing trends in risk among the Chinese in Hawaii and the reduced risk for US-born Chinese suggest that environmental factors are important in the development of the disease.

NPC occurs most frequently in males, the sex ratio worldwide being approximately 2 : 1 – 3 : 1.[141,160] The sex ratio for Taiwan mainlanders may be exceptional but the data are conflicting.[26,101] The male predominance in NPC is not dissimilar from that for most other head and neck tumours.[34,146,163] The age distribution, however, is markedly different, NPC occurring at a much younger age than epithelial tumours of other sites.[141] The finding of young-age peaks in some low-, intermediate-, and high-risk populations[9,30,33,45,60,94,135,136,139] suggests that

TABLE 2.1 NASOPHARYNGEAL CANCER CASES AND AVERAGE
ANNUAL AGE-ADJUSTED (WORLD STANDARD)
INCIDENCE RATES PER 100 000 BY SEX AND TIME
PERIOD AMONG CHINESE IN SELECTED POPULATIONS

Geographical area and time period	Ref.	Number of inhabitants	Males		Females	
			Cases	Rate	Cases	Rate
Hong Kong						
1965–69	74	4 500 000	1980	24.3	875	10.2
1974–77	160	4 366 600	2721	32.9	1128	14.4
Singapore						
1968–72	141	1 551 446	517	18.7	212	7.1
1973–77	160	1 680 159	628	19.4	265	7.5
Taiwan*						
1970	101	7 007 401	322	6.9	120	3.4
Shanghai (urban)						
1973–77	57	5 575 669	687	4.5	354	2.2
Malaysia, Selangor						
1968–72	7†	754 348	197	16.8	90	7.3
1973–77	7†	853 239	240	16.5	117	7.2
Malaysia, Sabah						
1969–75	135	140 000	55	18.6	24	8.4
Hawaii						
1960–64	4	38 197	19	17.1	8	7.9
1968–72	4	37 751	15	12.9	8	6.7
1973–76	SEER	46 054	8	7.6	2	1.4
1977–80	SEER	59 841	12	7.2	5	3.7
S.F.-Oakland						
1969–71	TNCS	88 108	24	16.1	7	4.7
1973–76	SEER	97 931	26	11.8	20	9.9
1977–80	SEER	108 884	56	23.4	24	10.5
Los Angeles						
1972–77	160	67 283	16	7.1	8	4.0

SEER = SEER Program, TNCS = Third National Cancer Survey.
* Selected areas of northern and southern Taiwan, December 1969 – May 1971.
† Number of inhabitants and cases from Dr Armstrong, personal communication.

aetiological factors may be different in the young than in the old.

More recent studies have shown that careful pathological classification of NPC biopsies may provide important data relevant to the demography of NPC; interrelationships among histopathological subtype, age, race, sex and prognosis have been observed.[43,94,142] As noted above, NPC refers only to malignant epithelial tumours without glandular differentiation. Although NPC is considered to have its origin from the epithelium lining the surface and crypts of the nasopharynx, there are several types of epithelial cells including stratified squamous epithelium, pseudo-stratified epithelium, and intermediate types of 'transitional' epithelium,[141] any of which could give rise to NPC.[143] It is quite common for a single tumour to have portions with different patterns of cells,[74,131,142] so that it is not necessarily true that the carcinoma cell type reflects the predominant cell type in the area where the tumour arises. In the past the variety of histopathological subtypes has included as many as 14 different terms often having several designations for the same lesion.[43] In an attempt to develop a classification that could serve as a common basis for international studies, the World Health Organization has proposed three major categories of NPC based solely on light microscopy.[140,144]

I. Squamous cell carcinoma – shows definite evidence of squamous differentiation with the prominence of intercellular bridges and/or keratinization; can be (a) well-differentiated, (b) moderately differentiated, and (c) undifferentiated.
II. Non-keratinizing carcinoma – shows evidence of differentiation with a maturation sequence that results in cells in which squamous differentiation is not evident on light microscopy; the tumour cells have well-defined cell margins and show an arrangement that is stratified or pavemented and not syncytial.
III. Undifferentiated carcinoma – tumour cells tend to have oval or round vesicular nuclei and prominent nucleoli; cell margins often are indistinct and the tumour tends to exhibit a syncytial appearance; spindle-shaped tumour cells, some with hyperchromatic nuclei, may be present; the tumour cells are often arranged in irregular and moderately well-defined masses or in strands of loosely connected cells in lymphoid stroma.

Using the WHO classification, Shanmugarathnam *et al.*[142] studied 363 NPC patients in Singapore and related histopathological features to clinical and laboratory findings. They observed a correlation between the amount of lymphocyte infiltration and 3-year survival in the group of patients with non-keratinizing carcinoma, indicating the importance of adding observations regarding the prominence of lymphocytes in the tumour to the basic WHO classiciation.[89]

Another pathological study involving 112 cases of NPC in the United States revealed that young patients (less than 15 years old) of all races, and black NPC patients of all ages, had undifferentiated tumours, whereas keratinizing squamous cell carcinomas were only found in adult white NPC patients.[43] In an attempt to evaluate the implications of pathological features on a larger series of cases, we have analysed data from nearly 1200 cases of NPC registered between 1969 and 1971 by the Third National Cancer Survey and during 1973–80 by the SEER Program.[94,95] These studies lack a uniform histopathological evaluation of cases but the information on histological type reported for each case was sufficient to allow some evaluation of pathological subtypes. Table 2.2 shows our findings based on cases diagnosed during 1973–80. Squamous cell carcinomas were relatively more frequent among whites, whereas lymphoepitheliomas and transitional cell carcinomas (generally analogous to undifferentiated carcinomas in the WHO classification) were relatively less frequent among whites than among other racial groups. This finding is compatible with the earlier pathology-based study using the WHO classification.[43]

Findings from the SEER data analysis regarding the demographic features of NPC in the United States support the earlier findings[43,60,94] that the incidence of NPC among adolescents and young adults is higher among blacks than among whites (Figure 2.1). The well-known phenomenon of a high incidence rate in Chinese-Americans was also found, with age-specific rates reaching a peak of 44 per 100 000 in the fifth decade of life (Figure 2.1).

Regarding survival in NPC, Chinese-Americans showed a significantly higher 5-year survival rate (52%) than either whites (30%) or blacks (16%). Patients under 40 years of age fared better (55% 5-year survival rate) than those 60 years or older (20% 5-year survival rate), a finding similar to that noted by most other investigations of NPC in children and young adults.[13,40,49,79,103,123,154] The histological categories with the best prognosis were lymphoepithelioma (55%) and transitional cell carcinoma (53%) compared to 30% 5-year survival for squamous cell carcinoma.

TABLE 2.2   DISTRIBUTION OF NASOPHARYNGEAL CANCER CASES BY RACE AND HISTOLOGICAL TYPE: SEER DATA, 1973–80

Histological type (ICD-O Code No.)	Total No. (%)	White Anglo No. (%)	Hispanic No. (%)	Chinese No. (%)	Black No. (%)
Total, all types	1005 (100)	629 (100)	25 (100)	167 (100)	83 (100)
NPC:	888 (88)	540 (86)	22 (88)	161 (96)	74 (89)
Carcinoma (801–804)	152 (15)	91 (14)	4 (16)	25 (15)	12 (14)
Squamous cell carcinoma (807)	532 (53)	341 (54)	15 (60)	83 (50)	45 (54)
Lymphoepithelioma (808)	144 (14)	76 (12)	1 (4)	39 (23)	11 (13)
Transitional cell carcinoma (812)	60 (6)	32 (5)	2 (8)	14 (8)	6 (7)
Other histological types:	117 (12)	89 (14)	3 (12)	6 (4)	9 (11)
Malignant neoplasm (800)	14	8	—	2	1
Adenocarcinoma[a]	34	28	2	1	1
Sarcoma[b]	15	12	—	—	2
Lymphoma[c]	40	30	1	2	3
Miscellaneous types[d]	14	11	—	1	2

	Filipino No. (%)	Japanese No. (%)	Hawaiian No. (%)	Other No. (%)	Unknown No. (%)
Total, all types	38 (100)	20 (100)	13 (100)	15 (100)	15 (100)
NPC:	35 (92)	17 (85)	12 (92)	14 (93)	13 (87)
Carcinoma (801–804)	5 (13)	4 (20)	4 (31)	4 (27)	3 (20)
Squamous cell carcinoma (807)	20 (53)	11 (55)	6 (46)	5 (53)	6 (40)
Lymphoepithelioma (808)	6 (16)	1 (5)	2 (15)	4 (27)	4 (27)
Transitional cell carcinoma (812)	4 (11)	1 (5)	—	1 (7)	—
Other histological types:	3 (8)	3 (15)	1 (8)	1 (7)	2 (13)
Malignant neoplasm (800)	1	1	—	—	1
Adenocarcinoma[a]	1	1	—	—	—
Sarcoma[b]	—	—	—	—	1
Lymphoma[c]	1	1	1	1	—
Miscellaneous types[d]	—	—	—	—	—

[a] 805, 814, 820, 821, 826, 831, 843, 848, 855, 894.
[b] 880, 881, 883, 890, 891, 899.
[c] 959, 961–964, 969, 975.
[d] 872, 898, 907, 937, 950.

Environmental Factors

The vast majority of descriptive studies indicate that environmental factors play a major role in the aetiology of NPC. The difficulties in distinguishing the relative contribution of environment and genetics to the patterns of NPC, which will be reviewed later, pose a particular problem in the Chinese, where genetics appears to play an important role in determining susceptibility. Support for environmental influence, however, is provided when groups of very similar genetic backgrounds show different patterns of NPC in different parts of the world. For example, Japanese in Hawaii appear to have higher rates of NPC than those residing in their native land.[95]

18

Head and Neck Cancer

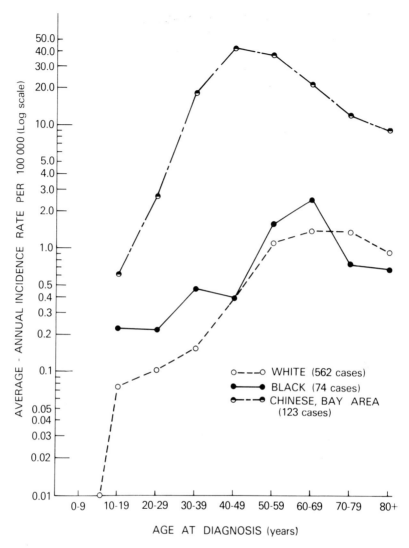

Figure 2.1   Incidence of Nasopharyngeal Carcinoma in the United
States: Seer Data, 1973−80.

The intriguing report of an increased incidence of NPC and related tumours in pigs living in high-incidence NPC areas in China[110,112] also supports the importance of environmental factors but, as with humans, it is difficult to make conclusions from small numbers of cases. While the available data point strongly to environmental factors as major determinants of the patterns of NPC, there is a great deal of controversy regarding the specific environmental agents involved. It is likely that physical, chemical, and biological agents are involved, but each may have a disproportionate influence in different populations.

Among the physical agents under consideration, most epidemiological studies implicate some form of airborne irritants as a major carcinogen in NPC, but the specific irritants differ within the population under study. The historical background for inhalants as a carcinogenic factor has been well reviewed,[74] and was supported by a series of studies from many countries described in a recent symposium on the aetiology and control of NPC.[39] The exposures have been analysed primarily from retrospective studies which have emphasized the evaluation of occupations and personal habits. Regarding occupations, a higher risk of developing NPC has been noted in Chinese chefs, carpenters, painters, bakers, and meat roasters.[164] A striking cluster was reported by Andrews and Michaels,[2,3] who described NPC in three white Canadian bush pilots. The sudden and frequent changes in air pressure in the cabin were postulated to affect the mucus drainage and protection of the nasopharynx, possibly increasing the sensitivity to other carcinogens (all three smoked cigarettes, another suggested risk factor).

Case – control studies, however, have added more concrete support to the hypothesized importance of inhaled irritants in the aetiology of NPC. Henderson *et al.*[65] noted several factors significantly associated with an increased risk of NPC, including occupational exposure to fumes, smoke, and chemicals. The details of chemical exposure were not specified, however, and it is unknown whether direct contact or inhalation was considered to be more important. Exposure to various byproducts of wood and charcoal fires, poor ventilation, and certain religious and cultural habits associated with the inhalation of incense and herbal medicines have been associated with a higher risk to NPC[39] and is suggested as explaining the higher frequency of NPC in the lower socioeconomic groups of Chinese.[58] Several studies have implicated tobacco as also being associated with NPC, an observation relevant to non-Chinese[10,59] as well as Chinese[101,102] populations.

Of interest was that prolonged exposure (whether occupational or non-occupational) appears to be necessary for these factors to be significantly associated with NPC risk. In the study by Henderson *et al.*[65] for example, occupational exposure was important only in those at risk more than 10 years. Cigarette smoking, not evident as a risk factor when only the presence or absence of exposure is evaluated,[65] becomes important when the intensity of smoking is examined, especially in those smoking more than 20 cigarettes a day.[59,101,102] Armstrong *et al.*,[5] investigating the role of occupational exposures in Malaysia, also found a strong dose – response relationship with increasing duration of exposure to dust and smoke.

Frequency of irritation is also possibly relevant to the observation that more NPC patients reported an increased frequency of previous infections of the ear, nose, and throat than matched controls.[58,145] There has been a tendency to discount this observation on the basis of potentially greater attention to minor symptoms by NPC patients than healthy controls (as well as the possibility that some of these symptoms were actually part of the presentation of NPC). An alternative possibility is that there was in fact an increased irritation of the nasopharynx by repeated or chronic infection, perhaps enhanced by certain anatomical features which have been postulated to enhance NP irritation and NP cancer.[41]

Radiation, a physical agent aetiologically linked to several neoplasms, appears unlikely as a contributing factor in NPC. Risk at this site is not increased among atomic bomb survivors.[130] Although medical X-ray therapy has been associated with some head and neck tumours, no cases of NPC have been observed among children exposed to therapeutic irradiation of the tonsils and nasopharynx for various benign conditions[29,137] or those whose scalp was irradiated for tinea capitis.[114,149]

Studies on the role of chemical carcinogens in the aetiology of NPC have focused primarily on the ingestion of salted fish, suggested as an important factor among Chinese,[74,75] Icelanders,[30] and Eskimos.[91] Support for this hypothesis has come from several sources, both epidemiological[5,152,164] and experimental.[77] The strongest epidemiological support comes from a case – control study among

Malaysian Chinese[5] where a dose–response relationship was observed between salted fish consumption and subsequent NPC. Daily consumption of salted fish intake in childhood compared to non-eaters was associated with a relative risk of 17.4, those with less regular salted fish intake having an intermediate risk. The experimental data supporting the aetiological role of salted fish in NPC, while intriguing, is based primarily on indirect evidence from studies involving few animals.[77] Unprocessed salted fish, as consumed by the Chinese in the traditional style, has been shown to have large amounts of nitrites which are converted to carcinogenic nitrosamines.[76] Experimental studies have produced both adenocarcinomas and an undifferentiated carcinoma of the nasal or paranasal sinus cavities in 3 of 20 rats fed salted fish.[77] However, more controlled studies need to be performed before firm conclusions can be reached.

It should be noted that while salted fish could contribute to the high incidence of NPC in some non-Chinese populations, such as Eskimos,[91] or even affect the pattern of NPC in Japanese,[68,72] it is necessary to look for other factors in those groups who do not consume salted fish and do not demonstrate other evidence of excessive exposure to nitrites, such as in Tunisia where the incidence of NPC is high among the young, but where fish is virtually always eaten fresh.

Hirayama and Ito[70] have postulated that herbal medicines could also be involved in the aetiology of NPC and have provided epidemiological and laboratory evidence for the parental plant of croton oil, *Croton tiglium*, and related plants, as a possible aetiological factor in NPC. Their studies demonstrated the geographical similarity between the distribution of *Croton tiglium* in China and the mortality rate for NPC. They further showed that croton oil enhanced the expression of Epstein–Barr virus (EBV) *in vitro* and provided data from a case–control study in Taiwan[102] indicating that there was a synergistic effect of the use of herbal drugs and the effect of EBV as risk factors in NPC.

Of the various infectious agents associated with cases of NPC, only EBV, an oncogenic[148,156] herpes virus known to cause infectious mononucleosis[67] and fatal lymphoproliferative diseases[88,132] in humans, has sufficient clinical and experimental data to be seriously considered as a candidate aetiological agent for NPC as well (for reviews, see Refs 36–38, 47, 85, 86). Of the many sources of data indicating that EBV may cause NPC, the most cogent is the detection of EBV genome in the epithelial tumour cells.[1,35,87,162,167] While EBV genome can frequently be identified in tissue culture cell lines established from normal individuals as well as cancer patients, it is detected directly in fresh human cells only in diseases known to be caused by EBV, such as infectious mononucleosis, or where EBV is suspected as being a probable cause, such as Burkitt's lymphoma and NPC.

Additional data associating EBV with NPC is the antibody pattern, where high titres of a number of EBV antibodies, including IgA antibody to the viral capsid antigen (VCA) and the IgG antibody to the early antigen (EA) complex, are associated with advanced disease, and low titres are associated with limited disease (for a review see Ref. 124). The IgA antibody to VCA, first associated with NPC by the Henles[66] after an initial report of elevated serum IgA levels in NPC patients,[159] has proven to be an important diagnostic tool.[96,125] While IgA anti-VCA is not specific for NPC,[66] a high titre may distinguish NPC from other head and neck tumours;[97] other diseases with elevated IgA antibody levels (particularly chronic lymphocytic leukaemia[125] and infectious mononucleosis[120]) do not pose a diagnostic problem. Elevated IgA anti-VCA levels do occur occasionally in healthy individuals[96,125] but some studies suggest that in high-risk groups to NPC they may even be of predictive value, preceding clinical diagnosis.[73,93,152,165,166] Their most important role at the present time, however, may be in non-endemic areas, such as the Unted States, in the situation where a patient presents with a cervical lymph node suggestive of NPC and no visible primary nasopharyngeal lesion. In that situation an elevated serum IgA anti-VCA level is virtually diagnostic of NPC.[28,96,125]

In endemic areas, serological screening for IgA anti-VCA antibodies to EBV has proven to be extremely useful in the early diagnosis of NPC. In a mass survey of 56 584 persons age 30 years and older in the People's Republic of China, 18 individuals with NPC were found out of 117 Chinese with positive IgA anti-VCA antibody titres to EBV.[165] The overall prevalence of NPC in the six communes surveyed, averaging 32.2 per 100 000 as measured by a clinical mass survey, was found to be 42.0 per 100 000 as a result of the screening for IgA antibody. A subsequent study,[166] applying several EBV-related assays including a more sensitive assay for IgA anti-VCA, was performed on 12 932 residents in Wuzhou City, located in the region included in the earlier study. As expected, a higher rate of IgA anti-VCA positivity was detected in this second study; 13 of the 680 persons examined were found to have NPC, resulting in a significantly higher detection rate of NPC with this more sensitive assay. Studies of the subsequent course of asymptomatic Chinese with elevated IgA anti-VCA antibody titres to EBV are in progress.

Two additional EBV assays of potential clinical importance are the antibody-dependent cellular cytotoxicity (ADCC) test,[127] in which high antibody titres correlate with a good prognosis,[24,126] and the lymphocyte stimulation inhibitor assay,[157] which appears to be the most sensitive indicator of disease activity reported to date.[81] The evidence that this inhibitor of lymphocyte response to EBV is related to IgA and that its removal could be therapeutic,[107] coupled with the potential therapeutic effect of ADCC antibody,[128] suggest that EBV-related serotherapy may be a valuable tool in the treatment of patients with EBV-genome positive NPC, and provides another piece of evidence regarding the causative role of EBV in this tumour.

Genetic Factors

Evidence for a genetic predisposition comes primarily from the high incidence of NPC in Chinese at home and abroad, family studies and laboratory studies of genetic markers. While the marked predilection of NPC for Chinese (and Eskimos, who are anthropologically related) and the occurrence of multiple-case families can be interpreted as supporting environmental aetiologies as well as genetic, the occurrence of unusual family pedigrees[31,74] makes it difficult to ignore the contribution of genetics. In Ho's report,[74] a patient with pathologically documented NPC had 10 children with his wife and concubine. All shared the same household and same lifestyle for at least 3 years, when the concubine left with her three children (Ho, personal communication). NPC subsequently was observed in six of the seven children borne by his wife (two males and four females) but in none of the three borne by his concubine.

A stronger documentation for the role of genetics has been obtained in Singapore where Chinese have the highest incidence of NPC, Indians have the lowest, and Malays are intermediate despite living in similar environments and attending the same schools.[152] A series of laboratory studies on HLA markers in Singapore Chinese NPC patients and controls first demonstrated the presence of an NPC-related HLA antigen[150,153] initially designated Sin-2 and currently designated BW46. Subsequent studies showed that the A2/BW46 haplotype was associated with a significantly higher risk of NPC in Chinese[151] and that HLA types are age-related, BW46 being more frequent in NPC patients age 30 or greater and B17 being more frequent in those less than 30 years old.[23] Survival also proved to be associated with HLA antigens, B13 (particularly when coupled with A2) being more frequent in long-term (>5 years) survivors and B17 being less frequent in 5-year survivors.[23] The association between HLA antigens and the risk of developing NPC has recently been reported in initial studies from mainland China.[152]

While the A and B HLA loci are the most striking assays indicating a genetic component to the aetiology of NPC, a number of other genetic markers have also been investigated. Kirk *et al.* evaluated 25 genetically controlled red-cell enzyme and five serum protein systems in 200 Chinese NPC patients and controls, showing variations in 11 systems between study groups and a significant difference between NPC patients and controls employing a multivariate analysis.[84] Recent studies by Chan *et al.*[23,25] indicate HLA-D typing may provide additional data not reflected in earlier HLA studies on genetic susceptibility.[150,151,153] The application of these laboratory assays to non-Chinese has not been systematically attempted.

MALIGNANT TUMOURS OF GLANDULAR EPITHELIUM (ADENO CARCINOMAS, ADENOID CYSTIC CARCINOMAS, AND OTHER TUMOURS OF THE SALIVARY GLAND TYPE)

As noted above, the WHO classification considers adenocarcinomas and other glandular tumours in the nasopharynx separately from those tumours termed NPC. The relative frequency of these tumours in the nasopharynx is typically under 3% in most populations but has reached 7% in some series of US cases.[141] In the SEER data for 1973–80 (Table 2.2), 34 of 1005 NP cancers (3%) were of this general type; 13 were adenoid cystic carcinomas and 8 were adenocarcinomas that were not subclassified. Of the 13 other glandular tumours, no specific type occurred more than twice. The age distribution of these 34 NP adenocarcinomas was not different from that of NPC but the male/female sex ratio (0.8 : 1) was different. In particular, 12 of the 13 cases of adenoid cystic carcinoma developed in women.

There is very little in the literature that provides aetiological hypotheses on adenocar-cinoma of the nasopharynx, probably related to the relatively low incidence of the disease. Based on the strong association of adenocarcinoma of the nasal cavity and sinuses in woodworkers, however, Mould and Bakowski[115] explored 18 registries in the United Kingdom and, finding 58 adenocarcinomas in the 2302 cases of NP cancer, noted that the most frequent occupational group for the 35 males was the woodworkers (six cases). This occupational tie between adenocarcinoma of the nasopharynx and adenocarcinoma of the nasal cavity and sinuses suggests the possibility of common aetiological relationships.

MALIGNANT LYMPHOMAS

The epidemiology of nasopharyngeal lymphoma is more difficult to define for two reasons: (1) their frequency of occurrence is lost in studies where all extranodal lymphomas are grouped with the more common nodal lymphomas, and (2) data on the pathology of these tumours using any of the more modern histopathological classifications are scarce. From several series where the pathology of all forms of NP cancer was reviewed, however, it appears that the relative frequency of NP lymphoma is particularly high in Japanese and Europeans.[18,155] Sugano *et al.*,[155] evaluating tumours of the upper respiratory tract in 2413 Japanese patients, not only noted a high frequency (33 of 121, or 27%) of NP lymphoma but this site was the most common source of lymphoma in the entire upper respiratory tract with the exception of the palatine tonsil. In a US study of nonepithelial tumours involving the nasal cavity, paranasal sinuses and nasopharynx,[52] lymphoma was the single most common type of malignancy.[55]

In the SEER data for 1973–80 (Table 2.2), 40 of 1005 NP cancers (4%) were non-Hodgkin's lymphoma. The male/female sex ratio for these cases (1.1 : 1) was lower and the median age (63 years) was higher than for NPC cases in this series (2.3 : 1 and 57 years, respectively). The 5-year survival rate for these lymphoma patients was 48%, somewhat better than the rate of 34% for the NPC patients in this series. Extranodal lymphomas at many sites have as good or better prognosis than other cancers of the same organ.[51]

SARCOMAS

As noted in previous reports,[60,94] sarcomas in the nasopharynx are rare but they are the most common NP cancer of preadolescent white children in the US. In the SEER data for 1973–80 (Table 2.2), 15 of 1005 NP cancers (1.5%) were sarcomas; there were 9 embryonal rhabdomyosarcomas, 1 fibrosarcoma, 1 fibrous histiocytoma (malignant), 1 rhabdomyosarcoma, 1 mesenchymoma (malignant), and 2 sarcomas that were not subclassified. Of the 9 embryonal rhabdomyosarcomas, 7 were diagnosed at ages 4–8 years and 1 each at 13 and 15 years, an age distribution that reflects the two peaks seen in a large series of childhood cases.[99,113] That 7 of the 9 NP embryonal rhabdomyosarcomas occurred among girls is not surprising; fatal rhabdomyosarcomas among US children were more frequent among boys than girls at all anatomical sites with one exception – those of the oronasopharynx region.[111]

Six of the 9 patients with embryonal rhabdomyosarcoma were still alive 2–8 years after diagnosis. The relatively favourable prognosis in this small series is comparable to that reported in the recent literature.[42,133] The 9 patients with embryonal rhabdomyosarcoma had a better prognosis than the other 6 sarcoma patients, 5 of whom died within 26 months following diagnosis. In other studies the prognosis for fibrosarcomas appears to be relatively good compared to other soft-tissue sarcomas in the nasopharynx and surrounding area.[53,54] There is some evidence that NP fibrosarcomas develop in previously irradiated angiofibromas.[27]

Studies of childhood rhabdomyosarcomas have identified a familial syndrome of soft-tissue sarcomas and other neoplasms (particularly breast cancer) affecting children and young adults.[99] Familial occurrences of cancer usually suggest that genetic susceptibility or environmental influences, or both, are responsible for such aggregates. Unlike most other malignancies with an age peak in early childhood, rhabdomyosarcoma is not associated with specific congenital malformations[99] and only in multiple neurofibromatosis is rhabdomyosarcoma a part of a defined genetic disorder.[108] The findings of a small case–control study suggest that environmental factors may play an important role in the aetiology of childhood rhabdomyosarcoma.[61]

MISCELLANEOUS MALIGNANT TUMOURS

Several types of tumours other than those previously mentioned can arise in the nasopharynx. In the SEER data for 1973–80 (Table 2.2), 14 of 1005 NP cancers (1.4%) fell into this category; there were 6 malignant melanomas, 4 chordomas, 2 neuroblastomas, 1 carcinosarcoma, and 1 embryonal carcinoma. There were 3 patients who had survived 5 years or more: 2 with malignant melanoma and 1 with chordoma.

DISCUSSION

The variety of cell types that are found in NP cancer, variations in classification, and the relative inaccessibility of the nasopharynx to direct visualization have caused some problems in epidemiological studies on NP cancer. It is apparent from the data cited above that differences exist in patterns of NP cancer in endemic and non-endemic regions, with more undifferentiated NPC and relatively less lymphomas in endemic areas, for example, but with all of the difficulties inherent in pathological classification, precise data on specific subtypes of NP cancer are not always readily available. The pathological problems are also compounded by anatomical and coding problems, with separation of pharyngeal tumours into nasopharynx, oropharynx, and hypopharynx frequently ignored, particularly in mortality data. Furthermore, variations in codes for subsites between different registries or over periods of time can hinder epidemiological studies dramatically. An example of the compounding problems encountered is illustrated by Enterline and Marsh,[46] who examined the carcinogenic effect of nickel on the upper respiratory tract. The coding and pathological vagaries which could have allowed cases to be classified as nasal, sinonasal, nasopharyngeal, or bone cancer emphasize the importance of establishing uniform methodology and requiring large numbers of patients in any epidemiological studies of the upper respiratory tract.

Since most cases of NP cancer in all populations are epithelial non-glandular carcinomas, referred to by WHO as NPC, non-pathology-based studies that report incidence and mortality data on NP cancer actually reflect the pattern of NPC. It is apparent that both genetic and environmental factors affect the incidence of NPC, and it is often difficult to distinguish the relative influence of these factors, even in endemic areas. The predilection of NPC for Chinese, regardless of place of residence, is striking. The risk for NPC in northern Chinese is significantly less than in southern Chinese,[44,100] however, and whether the observed predilection related to place of origin and dialect group[31] is due to cultural habits or genetic differences resulting from limited community mobility has thus far been unresolved. Laboratory assays apparently detecting genetic markers[84,150–153] are now being evaluated in China and the comparison of results obtained in northern and southeastern provinces may help to resolve the issue.

Among the demographic features that provide aetiological clues are the constancy of the sex ratio in most populations. The 2 : 1 – 3 : 1 male predominance has been found in virtually all studies. An equal male/female incidence has been reported for Taiwan Mainlanders,[101] but this was based on small numbers of female cases; the sex ratio was 2.4 : 1 for Mainlanders based on death rates for the years 1968 – 76.[26] The predilection of NPC for males, while

similar to that of most head and neck tumours, is not as high as that of the lip or oropharynx,[34,146,163] cancer sites related to cigarette smoking. This information would tend to emphasize the importance of factors other than tobacco as potential carcinogenic agents for NPC.

Other demographic features, such as the appearance of NPC in certain populations at an early age[9,30,33,45,60,94,135,136,139] and the increased frequency in certain racial/ethnic groups depending on place of residence[4,19,95] suggests groups upon which studies of environmental factors should concentrate; several such studies are in progress.

In part because of the relatively high frequency of one form of NP cancer, nonglandular epithelial carcinoma (NPC), there has been great progress in the evaluation of aetiological factors in this disease. The epidemiological studies noted above strongly implicate environmental and genetic factors in the most commom form of the disease, undifferentiated NPC in the Chinese, but environmental factors also appear to be prominent in non-Chinese as well. There is considerable evidence that physical, chemical and infectious agents are able to interact as cocarcinogens, the Epstein – Barr virus (EBV) being the most common denominator in all parts of the world.

Among the inhaled irritants most directly in contact with the nasopharynx that have thus far been implicated in epidemiological studies, inhaled smoke, which includes products of burnt wood and charcoal[74,75] as well as cigarettes,[10,59,101] leads the list. It is of interest that heavy exposure (as with smoking and lung cancer) seems to increase the risk both in regard to occupational exposure[5,65,164] and personal habits, such as cigarette smoking.[10,59,101] As noted above, however, the relatively low male/female ratio as compared to other head and neck carcinomas where cigarette smoking has a well-defined aetiologic relationship emphasizes the importance of other factors in the causation of NPC.

With potential chemical carcinogens, such

as nitrosamines, a heavy exposure may be necessary to increase the risk.[5] Among the potential ingested carcinogens, recent studies have focused on the possible importance of salted fish, particularly in Chinese,[5,164] with experimental studies emphasizing the particular carcinogenic potential of nitrosamines.[77]

The impressive dose–response relationship and the association with intake at an early age in life reported by Armstrong *et al.*[5] justify the concern about the carcinogenic activity in selected populations but also demonstrate the difficulty in identifying specific carcinogens with malignancies occurring after long latent periods. The interrelationship of heavy salted fish intake and nutritional deficiencies in lower socioeconomic groups has made it difficult to determine whether any one determinant alone is sufficient to result in NPC, but the evidence associating similar dietary habits with gastric cancer in Japanese[62,69] strengthens the potential importance of diet as a cofactor in NPC. The study of time trends in various high-risk groups may be revealing since crude salt, which has a high nitrite content, is being replaced in many areas by sodium chloride; furthermore, improved access to refrigeration is associated with decreased salt intake in many NPC-prone populations. The importance of factors other than nitrosamines from salted fish is illustrated by the relatively high incidence of NPC in Tunisians and young black Americans, who do not share the dietary patterns of the Chinese but who may have key nutritional deficiencies in early childhood.

Emphasizing the opportunity for local carcinogenic factors to vary in different high-risk groups, Hirayama and Ito have suggested that plant extracts with tumour-promoting activity, possibly acting through demonstrated *in vitro* activation of EBV,[70] could be contributing to the pattern of NPC since these plants are found in high-incidence NPC areas of China and the extracts are frequently used to treat food poisoning, acute gastroenteritis, bacterial dysentery, or constipation. Ho[74] had earlier noted the presence of NPC in Chinese for cen-

turies and the apparent relationship to cultural factors, an observation compatible with a number of environmental carcinogens.

The possible role of EBV, which is more difficult to prove because it cannot be removed from the environment as readily as the other postulated carcinogens, is based on strong but indirect data. Most compelling in the aetiological link between EBV and NPC is that, unlike all of the other postulated carcinogens, the association between EBV and the more undifferentiated forms of NPC is not only regular but international; the virus is detected in morphologically similar tumours in all continents and all races where the technology has been applied. The relevant issue still unresolved is whether the relationship between EBV and undifferentiated carcinoma can be interpreted as a means of classifying NPC into different diseases. At the present time this appears unwise, not only because of the frequent appearance of multiple morphological patterns in the same tumour but also the reports of EBV genome in occasional well-differentiated NPCs; such reports appear to be too frequent to attribute them solely to pathological misclassification. There are well-known and perhaps insurmountable obstacles to proving that EBV causes NPC or any other human tumour, but regardless of its role in causation, the importance of EBV-related assays in the diagnosis[96,125] and possibly the control of NPC,[24,81,117,126,157] has been well documented.

In regard to the histological classification of NPC, this topic has important ramifications because of the correlation of histopathology with a number of biological parameters, including survival, demographic features (especially age and racial/ethnic group) and the Epstein–Barr virus. The WHO classification[144] has been recommended as a basis for international comparisons,[152] but the relationship between lymphocyte infiltration and survival in one group of NPC patients[142] supports the argument that the degree of lymphocyte involvement should be noted.[89] Because of the mixed patterns occasionally seen in NPC biopsies,[131,152] there has been considerable discussion as to whether tumours should be classified as to the predominant pattern or the most undifferentiated portion of the tumour. While this discussion may affect epidemiological studies, it also underscores the likelihood that NPC is one entity with a spectrum of host responses possibly affecting the morphology of the tumour, perhaps analogous to the spectrum from lymphocyte predominance to lymphocyte depletion in Hodgkin's disease Therefore, in spite of the serologically and biochemically stronger relationship between EBV and both non-keratinizing and undifferentiated carcinoma, it is premature to conclude that morphology can be related to aetiological factors rather than the biology of host response. More pressing is the need to develop uniform histological classification among pathologists to provide improved comparisons of different populations.

The epidemiological patterns observed in NPC are compatible with the interaction of multiple factors. A number of studies indicate the influence of socioeconomics on the incidence of NPC, higher rates being attributed to lower socioeconomic groups in Hong Kong,[58] Malaysia,[5,6] and the US.[60] In different populations this could indirectly reflect the impact of poor ventilation in the home, reinfection with EBV, the use of herbal medicines, vitamin deficiencies, dietary carcinogens, or certain occupations. Since essentially all of the non-viral carcinogens which are currently suspected of causing NPC in high-risk populations[152] are unlikely to be involved in other groups, such as young blacks in the United States or young Tunisians, other factors need to be sought. The development of case–control studies, with appropriate selection of controls and standardized pathological review, is a problem requiring international attention and cooperation. In Tunisia, for example, where a young age-incidence peak and a moderately high overall incidence rate are apparent,[45] attention could be paid to evaluating the role of EBV and other environmental factors, particularly since genetics

has thus far been shown to have less impact than in Singapore.[14]

The role of genetics, suggested most strongly by an excellent series of laboratory reports on histocompatibility antigens,[23,25,150,151,153] thus far has been documented most strongly in the Chinese. While the detailed pedigree reported by Ho[74] supports a greater effect of genetics than environment on the subsequent occurrence of NPC, other cancer families reported in Chinese[74] could reflect the influence of either genetics or environmental factors. Furthermore, the occurrence of multiple cases of NPC in non-Chinese families,[16,56,92,118] where laboratory markers have not demonstrated genetic susceptibility, and the coincidence of NPC and Burkitt's lymphoma, two diseases associated with EBV, in the same families,[17,80,98] emphasizes the importance of carefully investigating such families for aetiological clues.[15]

In the search for laboratory markers of genetic susceptibility, high-incidence groups are more likely to provide positive associations, if they are present, but close attention must be given to the development of appropriate reagents, the testing of large numbers of individuals, and the division of study cases into subgroups (such as the different Chinese dialect groups in Singapore) before any conclusions can be reached. The equivocal data in Tunisia, for example, should be pursued with more appropriate panels of typing sera, larger numbers of patients, and attention to the ethnic subgroups seen in Tunisia.

The availability of more sophisticated technology applicable to the detection of cancer of the nasopharynx[32,134] should result in more useful epidemiological data if cancer detection is accompanied by more uniform histopathological classification. Newer laboratory techniques able to distinguish undifferentiated carcinomas from lymphomas[104] and to detect subclinical cases of NPC,[165,166] should also lead to more reliable incidence data. The continuation of international cooperation on the study of NPC,[39] hopefully with consideration of other nasopharyngeal malignancies as well, should eventually provide data relevant to the control of these diseases and of malignancies in other sites in the head and neck area.

ACKNOWLEDGEMENT

The authors thank Drs J.F. Fraumeni, Jr, R.W. Miller, and K. Shanmugaratnam for their helpful comments, and Ms Nancy Pointek and Mrs Jeannie C. Williams for their invaluable assistance with preparation of the manuscript.

REFERENCES

1. Anderson-Anvret, M., Forsby, N., Klein, G., Henle, W., and Bjorklund, A. (1979). Relationship between the Epstein–Barr virus genome and nasopharyngeal carcinoma in Caucasian patients. *Int. J. Cancer*, **24**, 762–767.

2. Andrews, P.A.J., and Michaels, L. (1968). Nasopharyngeal cancer in Canadian bush pilots. *Lancet*, **2**, 85–87.

3. Andrews, P.A.J., and Michaels, L. (1968). Aviator's cancer. *Lancet*, **2**, 640.

4. Armstrong, R.W. (1977). Nasopharyngeal carcinoma: opportunities for international collaborative research in Malaysia and Hawaii. *Natl. Cancer Inst. Monogr.*, **47**, 135–141.

5. Armstrong, R.W., Armstrong, M.J., Yu, M.C., and Henderson, B.E. (1983). Salted fish and inhalants as risk factors for nasopharyngeal carcinoma. *Cancer Res.*, **43**, 2967–2970.

6. Armstrong, R.W., Kannan Kutty, M., and Armstrong, M.J. (1978). Self-specific environments associated with nasopharyngeal carcinoma in Selangor, Malaysia. *Soc. Sci. Med.*, **12D**, 149–156.

7. Armstrong, R.W., Kannan Kutty, M., Dharmalingam, S.K., and Ponnudurai, J.R. (1979). Incidence of nasopharyngeal carcinoma in Malaysia, 1968–1977. *Br. J. Cancer*, **40**, 557–567.

8. Axtell, L.M., Asire, A.J., and Myers, M.H. (Eds) (1976). *Cancer Patient Survival, Report No. 5*, DHEW Publ. No. (NIH) 77–992, NIH, Bethesda.

9. Balakrishnan, V. (1975). An additional younger-age peak for cancer of the nasopharynx. *Int. J. Cancer*, **15**, 651–657.

10. Balakrishnan, V., Gangadaran, P., and Nagaraj-Rao, D. (1976). Some epidemiological aspects of nasopharyngeal cancer. In *Liver Cancer: Cancer Problems in Asian Countries* (Eds K. Shanmugaratnam, R. Nambiar, K.K. Tan, and L.K.C. Chan). Singapore Cancer Society, Singapore (1976), pp. 268–274.

11. Basa, G.F., Hirayama, T., and Cruz-Basa, A.G. (1977). Cancer epidemiology in the Philippines. *Natl. Cancer Inst. Monogr.*, **47**, 45–56.

12. Berg, J.W. (1982). Morphologic classification of human cancer. In *Cancer Epidemiology and Prevention* (Eds D. Schottenfeld, and J.F. Fraumeni, Jr.), Saunders, Philadelphia, pp. 74–89.

13. Berry, M.P., Smith, C.R., Brown, T.C., Jenkin, R.D.T., and Rider, W.D. (1980). Nasopharyngeal carcinoma in the young. *Int. J. Radiat. Oncol. Biol. Phys.*, **6**, 415–421.

14. Betuel, H., Camoun, M., Colombani, J., Day, N.E., Ellouz, R., and de-The, G. (1975). The relationship between nasopharyngeal carcinoma and the HL-A system among Tunisians. *Int. J. Cancer*, **16**, 249–254.

15. Blattner, W.A. (1977). Family studies: the interdisciplinary approach. In *Genetics of Human Cancer* (Eds J.J. Mulvihill, R.W. Miller, and J.F. Fraumeni, Jr), Raven Press, New York, pp. 269–280.

16. Brown, T.M., Heath, C.W., Lang, R.M., Lee, S.K., and Whalley, B.W. (1976). Nasopharyngeal cancer in Bermuda. *Cancer*, **37**, 1464–1468.

17. Brubaker, G., Levin, A.G., Steel, C.M., Creasy, G., Cameron, H.M., and Linsell, C.A. (1980). Multiple cases of Burkitt's lymphoma and other neoplasms in families in the North Mara district of Tanzania. *Int. J. Cancer*, **26**, 165–170.

18. Brugere, J., Sancho-Garnier, H., Point, D., and Schwaab, G. (1978). Epidemiology of malignant tumors of the nasopharynx in France: retrospective and prospective studies. In *Nasopharyngeal Carcinoma: Etiology and Control* (Eds G. de-The, and Y. Ito), IARC Sci. Publ. No. 20, IARC, Lyon, pp. 241–249.

19. Buell, P. (1973). Race and place in the etiology of nasopharyngeal cancer: a study based on California death certificates. *Int. J. Cancer*, **11**, 268–271.

20. Buell, P. (1974). The effect of migration on the risk of nasopharyngeal cancer among Chinese. *Cancer Res.*, **34**, 1189–1191.

21. Cammoun, M., Hoerner, G.V., and Mourali, N. (1974). Tumors of the nasopharynx in

Tunisia: an anatomic and clinical study based on 143 cases. *Cancer*, **33**, 184–192.

22. Cancer Registry of Norway (1980). *Survival of cancer patients. Cases diagnosed in Norway 1968–1975.* Norwegian Cancer Society, Oslo.

23. Chan, S.H., Day, N.E., Khor, T.H., Kunaratnam, N., and Chia, K.B. (1981). HLA markers in the development and prognosis of NPC in Chinese. In *Nasopharyngeal Carcinoma* (Eds E. Grundmann, G.R.F. Krueger, and D.V. Ablashi), Gustav Fischer Verlag, Stuttgart, pp. 208–211.

24. Chan, S.H., Levine, P.H., de-The, G., Mulroney, S.E., Lavoue, M.F., Glen, S.P.P., Goh, E.H., Khor, T.H., and Connelly, R.R. (1979). A comparison of the prognostic value of antibody-dependent lymphocyte cytotoxicity and other EBV antibody assays in Chinese patients with nasopharyngeal carcinoma. *Int. J. Cancer*, **23**, 181–185.

25. Chan, S.H., Wee, G.B., Kunaratnam, N., Chia, K.B., and Day, N.E. (1983). HLA locus B and DR antigen association in Chinese NPC patients and controls. In *Nasopharyngeal Carcinoma, Current Concepts* (Eds U. Prasad, D.V. Ablashi, P.H. Levine, and G.R. Pearson), University of Malaya Press, Kuala Lumpur, pp. 307–312.

26. Chen, K.P., Wu, H.Y., Yeh, C.C., and Cheng, Y.J. (1979). *Color Atlas of Cancer Mortality by Administrative and Other Classified Districts in Taiwan Area: 1968–1976*, Natl. Sci. Council, Taipei.

27. Chen, K.T.K., and Bauer, F.W. (1982). Sarcomatous transformation of nasopharyngeal angiofibroma. *Cancer*, **49**, 369–371.

28. Coates, H.L., Pearson, G.R., Neel, H.B., III, Weiland, L.H., and Devine, K.D. (1978). An immunologic basis for detection of occult primary malignancies of the head and neck. *Cancer*, **41**, 912–918.

29. Colman, M., Kirsch, M., and Creditor, M. (1978). Tumors associated with medical X-ray therapy exposure in childhood. In *Late Biological Effects of Ionizing Radiation*, vol. 1, Int. Atomic Energy Agency, Vienna, pp. 167–180.

30. Cooper, M.A., and Hallgrimsson, J. (1981). Tumors in Iceland. 4. Tumors of the upper respiratory tract and ear. A histological classification and some etiological and epidemiological considerations. *Acta. Path. Microbiol. Scand. Sect. A*, **89**, 377–387.

31. Cooperative NPC Research Group of the People's Republic of China (1979). Preliminary investigation of the epidemiology of nasopharyngeal carcinoma (NPC) in four provinces and one autonomous region in South China. In *Advances in Medical Oncology, Research and Education* (Ed J. Birch), Pergamon Press, New York, pp. 81–85.

32. Costa, J. (1981). The histopathological diagnosis of nasopharyngeal carcinoma. In *Nasopharyngeal Carcinoma*, (Eds E. Grundmann, G.R.F. Krueger, and D.V. Ablashi), Gustav Fischer Verlag, Stuttgart, pp. 7–10.

33. Creely, J.J., Jr., Lyons, G.D., Jr., and Trail, M.L. (1973). Cancer of the nasopharynx: a review of 114 cases. *Sth. Med. J.*, **66**, 405–409.

34. Cutler, S.J., and Young, J.L., Jr. (Eds), (1975). Third National Cancer Survey: incidence data. *Natl. Cancer Inst. Monogr.*, **41**, 1–454.

35. Desgranges, C., Wolf, H., de-The, G., Shanmugaratnam, K., Cammoun, N., Ellouz, R., Klein, G., Lennert, K., Munoz, N., and zur Hausen, H. (1975). Nasopharyngeal carcinoma. X. Presence of Epstein–Barr genomes in separated epithelial cells of tumors in patients from Singapore, Tunisia and Kenya. *Int. J. Cancer*, **16**, 7–15.

36. de-The, G. (1980). Role of Epstein–Barr virus in human diseases: infectious mononucleosis, Burkitt's lymphoma, and nasopharyngeal carcinoma. In *Viral Oncology* (Ed G. Klein), Raven Press, New York, pp. 769–797.

37. de-The, G., and Geser, A. (1974). Nasopharyngeal carcinoma: recent studies and outlook for a viral etiology. *Cancer Res.*, **34**, 1196–1206.

38. de-The, G., Ho, J.H.C., and Muir, C. (1976). Nasopharyngeal carcinoma. In *Viral Infections of Humans* (Ed A.S. Evans), Plenum, New York, pp. 539–563.

39. de-The, G., and Ito, Y. (Eds) (1978). *Nasopharyngeal Carcinoma: Etiology and Control*, IARC Sci. Publ. No. 20, IARC, Lyon.

40. Deutsch, M., Mercado, R., Jr., and Parsons, J.A. (1978). Cancer of the nasopharynx in children. *Cancer*, **41**, 1128–1133.

41. Dobson, W.H. (1924). Cervical lymphosarcoma. *Chin. Med. J.*, **38**, 786–787.

42. Donaldson, S.S., Castro, J.R., Wilbur, J.R., and Jesse, R.H., Jr. (1973). Rhabdomyosarcoma of head and neck in children; combination treatment by surgery, irradiation, and chemotherapy. *Cancer*, **31**, 25–35.

43. Easton, J.M., Levine, P.H., and Hyams, V.J. (1980). Nasopharyngeal carcinoma in the United States: a pathologic study of 177 U.S. and 30 foreign cases. *Arch. Otolaryngol.*, **106**, 88–91.

44. Editorial Committee (Eds) (1979). *Atlas of Cancer Mortality in the People's Republic of China.*

China Map Press, Shanghai.

45. Ellouz, R., Cammoun, M., Ben Attia, R., and Bahi, J. (1978). Nasopharyngeal carcinoma in children and adolescents in Tunisia: clinical aspects and the paraneoplastic syndrome. In *Nasopharyngeal Carcinoma: Etiology and Control* (Eds G. de-The, and Y. Ito), IARC Sci. Publ. No. 20, IARC, Lyon, pp. 115–129.

46. Enterline, P.E., and Marsh, G.M. (1982). Mortality among workers in a nickel refinery and alloy manufacturing plant in West Virginia. *JNCI*, **68**, 925–933.

47. Epstein, M.A., and Achong, B.G., (Eds) (1979). *The Epstein–Barr Virus*, Springer-Verlag, Berlin.

48. Ewing, J. (1929). Lymphoepithelioma. *Am. J. Pathol.*, **5**, 99–197.

49. Fernandez, C.H., Cangir, A., Samaan, N.A., and Rivera, R. (1976). Nasopharyngeal carcinoma in children. *Cancer*, **37**, 2787–2791.

50. Fraumeni, J.F., Jr., and Mason, T.J. (1974). Cancer mortality among Chinese Americans, 1950–69. *JNCI*, **52**, 659–665.

51. Freeman, C., Berg, J.W., and Cutler, S.J. (1972). Occurrence and prognosis of extranodal lymphomas. *Cancer*, **29**, 252–260.

52. Fu, Y.S., and Perzin, K.H. (1974). Non-epithelial tumors of the nasal cavity, paranasal sinuses, and nasopharynx: a clinicopathologic study. I. General features and vascular tumors. *Cancer*, **33**, 1275–1288.

53. Fu. Y.S., and Perzin, K.H. (1976). Non-epithelial tumors of the nasal cavity, paranasal sinuses and nasopharynx. V. Skeletal muscle tumors. *Cancer*, **37**, 364–376.

54. Fu, Y.S., and Perzin, K.H. (1976). Non-epithelial tumors of the nasal cavity, paranasal sinuses, and nasopharynx: a clinicopathologic study. VI. Fibrous tissue tumors (fibroma, fibromatosis, fibrosarcoma). *Cancer*, **37**, 2912–2928.

55. Fu, Y.S., and Perzin, K.H. (1979). Non-epithelial tumors of the nasal cacity, paranasal sinuses and nasopharynx: a clinicopathologic study. X. Malignant lymphomas. *Cancer*, **43**, 611–621.

56. Gajwani, B.W., Devereaux, J.M., and Beg, J.A. (1980). Familial clustering of nasopharyngeal carcinoma. *Cancer*, **46**, 2325–2327.

57. Gao, Y.-T. (1982). Cancer incidence in Shanghai during 1973–77. *Natl. Cancer Inst. Monogr.*, **62**, 43–46.

58. Geser, A., Charnay, N., Day, N.E., Ho, H.C., and de-The, G. (1978). Environmental factors in the etiology of nasopharyngeal carcinoma: report on a case–control study in Hong Kong. In *Nasopharyngeal Carcinoma: Etiology and Control* (Eds G. de-The, and Y. Ito), IARC Sci. Publ. No. 20. IARC, Lyon, pp. 213–229.

59. Goodman, M.L., Levine, P.H., and Miller, D. (1980). Nasopharyngeal carcinoma patients in Massachusetts. In *Third International Symposium on Prevention and Detection of Cancer* (Ed. H.G. Nieburgs), Marcel Dekker, New York, vol. 2, part II, pp. 1605–1612.

60. Greene, M.H., Fraumeni, J.F., Jr., and Hoover, R. (1977). Nasopharyngeal cancer among young people in the United States: racial variations by cell type. *JNCI*, **58**, 1267–1270.

61. Grufferman, S., Wang, H.H., DeLong, E.R., Rimm, S.Y.S., Delzell, E.S., and Falletta, J.M. (1982). Environmental factors in the etiology of rhabdomyosarcoma in childhood. *JNCI*, **68**, 107–113.

62. Haenszel, W., Kurihara, M., and Segi, M. (1972). Stomach cancer among Japanese in Hawaii. *JNCI*, **49**, 969–988.

63. Hakulinen, T., Pukkala, E., Hakama, M., Lehtonen, M., Saxen, E., and Teppo, L. (1981). Survival of cancer patients in Finland in 1953–1974. *Ann. Clin. Res.*, **13**, Suppl. 31.

64. Henderson, B.E. (1978). Nasopharyngeal cancer. In *Cancer in China* (Eds H.S. Kaplan, and P.J. Tsuchitani), A.R. Liss, New York, pp. 83–100.

65. Henderson, B.E., Louie, E., Jing, J.S.H., Buell, P., and Gardner, M.B. (1976). Risk factors associated with nasopharyngeal carcinoma. *N. Engl. J. Med.*, **295**, 1101–1106.

66. Henle, G., and Henle, W. (1976). Epstein–Barr virus-specific IgA serum antibodies as an outstanding feature of nasopharyngeal carcinoma. *Int. J. Cancer*, **17**, 1–7.

67. Henle, W., and Henle, G. (1972). Epstein–Barr virus: the cause of infectious mononucleosis-a review. In *Oncogenesis and Herpesvirus* (Eds P.M. Biggs, G. de-The, and L.N. Payne), IARC, Lyon, pp. 269–274.

68. Hirayama, T. (1978). Descriptive and analytical epidemiology of nasopharyngeal cancer. In *Nasopharyngeal Carcinoma: Etiology and Control* (Eds G. de-The, and Y. Ito), IARC Sci. Publ. No. 20, IARC, Lyon, pp. 167–189.

69. Hirayama, T. (1979). Diet and cancer. *Nutr. Cancer*, **1**, 67–81.

70. Hirayama, T., and Ito, Y. (1981). A new view of the etiology of nasopharyngeal carcinoma. *Prev. Med.*, **10**, 614–622.

71. Ho, H.C. (1975). Epidemiology of nasopharyngeal carcinoma. *J.R. Coll. Surg. Edinb.*, **20**, 223–235.

72. Ho, J.H.C., Chan, C.L., Lau, W.H., Au, G.K.H., and Loo, L.C. (1982). Cancer in Hong Kong: some epidemiologic observations. *Natl. Cancer Inst. Monogr.*, **62**, 47–55.

73. Ho, H.C., Kwan, H.C., Ng, M.H., and de-The, G. (1978). Serum IgA antibodies to Epstein–Barr virus capsid antigen preceding symptoms of nasopharyngeal carcinoma. *Lancet*, **1**, 436.

74. Ho, J.H.C. (1972). Nasopharyngeal carcinoma (NPC). In *Advances in Cancer Research* (Eds G. Klein, S. Weinhouse, and A. Haddow), Academic Press, New York, pp. 57–92.

75. Ho, J.H.C. (1978). An epidemiologic and clinical study of nasopharyngeal carcinoma. *Int. J. Radiat. Oncol. Biol. Phys.*, **4**, 183–198.

76. Huang, D.P., Gough, T.A., and Ho, J.H.C. (1978). Analysis for volatile nitrosamines in salt-preserved foodstuffs traditionally consumed by southern Chinese. In *Nasopharyngeal Carcinoma: Etiology and Control* (Eds G. de-The, and Y. Ito), IARC Sci. Publ. No. 20, IARC, Lyon, pp. 309–314.

77. Huang, D.P., Saw, D., Teoh, T.B., and Ho. J.H.C. (1978). Carcinoma of the nasal and paranasal regions in rats fed Cantonese salted marine fish. In *Nasopharyngeal Carcinoma: Etiology and Control* (Eds G. de-The, and Y. Ito), IARC Sci. Publ. No. 20, IARC, Lyon, pp. 315–328.

78. Huang, S.C. (1980). Nasopharyngeal cancer: a review of 1605 patients treated radically with Cobalt-60. *Int. J. Radiat. Oncol. Biol. Phys.*, **6**, 401–407.

79. Jenkin, R.D.T., Anderson, J.R., Jereb, B., Thompson, J.C., Pyesmany, A., Wara, W.M., and Hammon, D. (1981). Nasopharyngeal carcinoma – a retrospective review of patients less than thirty years of age: a report from Children's Cancer Study Group. *Cancer*, **47**, 360–366.

80. Joncas, J.H., Rioux, E., Wasitaux, J.P., Leyritz, M., Robillard, L., and Menezes, J. (1976). Nasopharyngeal carcinoma and Burkitt's lymphoma in a Canadian family. I: HLA typing, EBV antibodies and serum immunoglobulins. *Can. Med. Assoc. J.*, **115**, 858–860.

81. Kamaraju, L.S., Levine, P.H., Sundar, S.K., Ablashi, D.V., Faggioni, A., Armstrong, G.R., Bertram, G., and Kreuger, G.R.F. (1983). Epstein–Barr virus-related lymphocyte stimulation inhibitor: a possible prognostic tool for undifferentiated nasopharyngeal carcinoma. *JNCI*, **70**, 643–647.

82. King, H., and Haenszel, W. (1973). Cancer mortality among foreign- and native-born Chinese in the United States. *J. Chronic Dis.*, **26**, 623–646.

83. King, H., and Locke, F.B. (1980). Cancer mortality among Chinese in the United States, *JNCI*, **65**, 1141–1148.

84. Kirk, R.L., Blake, N.M., Serjeantson, S., Simons, M.J., and Chan, S.H. (1978). Genetic components in susceptibility to nasopharyngeal carcinoma. In *Nasopharyngeal Carcinoma: Etiology and Control* (Eds G. de-The, and Y. Ito), IARC Sci. Publ. No. 20, IARC, Lyon, pp. 283–297.

85. Klein, G. (1979). The relationship of the virus to nasopharyngeal carcinoma. In *The Epstein–Barr Virus* (Eds M.A. Epstein, and B.G. Achong, Springer-Verlag, Berlin, pp. 339–346.

86. Klein, G. (Ed) (1980). *Viral Oncology*, Raven Press, New York.

87. Klein, G., Giovenalla, B.C., Lindahl, T., Fialkow, P.J., Singh, S., and Stehlin, J.S. (1974). Direct evidence for the presence of Epstein–Barr virus DNA and nuclear antigen in malignant epithelial cells from patients with poorly differentiated carcinoma of the nasopharynx. *Proc. Natl. Acad. Sci.*, **71**, 4737–4741.

88. Klein, G., and Purtilo, D.T. (Eds) (1981). Symposium on Epstein–Barr virus-induced lymphoproliferative diseases in immunodeficient patients. *Cancer Res.*, **41**, 4209–4304.

89. Krueger, G.R.F., and Wustrow, J. (1981). Current histological classification of nasopharyngeal carcinoma (NPC) at Cologne University. In *Nasopharyngeal Carcinoma* (Eds E. Grundmann, G.R.F. Krueger, and D.V. Ablashi), Gustav Fischer Verlag, Stuttgart, pp. 11–15.

90. Lanier, A. (1977). Survey of cancer incidence in Alaskan natives. *Natl. Cancer Inst. Monogr.*, **47**, 87–88.

91. Lanier, A., Bender, T., Talbot, M., Wilmeth, S., Tschopp, C., Henle, W., Henle, G., Ritter, D., and Terasaki, P. (1980). Nasopharyngeal carcinoma in Alaskan Eskimos, Indians and Aleuts; a review of cases and study of Epstein–Barr virus, HLA, and environmental risk factors. *Cancer*, **46**, 2100–2107.

92. Lanier, A.P., Bender, T.R., Tschopp, C.F., and Dohan, P. (1979). Nasopharyngeal carcinoma in an Alaskan Eskimo family: report of three cases. *JNCI*, **62**, 1121–1124.

93. Lanier, A.P., Henle, W., Bender, T.R., Henle, G., and Talbot, M.L. (1980). Epstein–Barr virus-specific antibody titers in

seven Alaskan Natives before and after diagnosis of nasopharyngeal carcinoma. *Int. J. Cancer*, **26**, 133–137.

94. Levine, P.H., Connelly, R.R., and Easton, J.M. (1980). Demographic patterns for nasopharyngeal carcinoma in the United States. *Int. J. Cancer*, **26**, 741–748.

95. Levine, P.H., Connelly, R.R., and McKay, F.W. (1983). The influence of residence, race, and place of birth on the incidence and mortality in nasopharyngeal carcinoma. In *Nasopharyngeal Carcinoma: Current Concepts* (Eds U. Prasad, D.V. Ablashi, P.H. Levine, and G.R. Pearson), University of Malaya Press, Kuala Lumpur, pp. 143–156.

96. Levine, P.H., Pearson, G.R., Armstrong, M., *et al.* (1982). The reliability of IgA antibody to Epstein–Barr virus (EBV) capsid antigen as a test for the diagnosis of nasopharyngeal carcinoma (NPC). *Cancer Detection and Prevention*, **4**, 307–312.

97. Levine, P.H., Terebelo, H., Berenberg, J., Bryarly, R., Bengali, Z., and Pointek, N. (1981). A case–control study of the specificity of IgA antibodies to Epstein–Barr virus (EBV) in patients with head and neck cancer. In *Nasopharyngeal Carcinoma* (Eds E. Grundmann, G.R.F. Krueger, and D.V. Ablashi), Gustav Fischer Verlag, Stuttgart, pp. 225–230.

98. Li, F.P. (1976). Familial Burkitt's lymphoma and nasopharyngeal carcinoma. *Lancet*, **1**, 687–688.

99. Li, F.P., and Fraumeni, J.F., Jr. (1969). Rhabdomyosarcoma in children: epidemiologic study and identification of a familial cancer syndrome, *JNCI*, **43**, 1365–1373.

100. Li, F.P., and Shiang, E.L. (1980). Cancer mortality in China. *JNCI*, **65**, 217–221.

101. Lin, T.M., Chen, K.P., Lin, C.C., Hsu, M.M., Tu, S.M., Chiang, T.C., Jung, P.F., and Hirayama, T. (1973). Retrospective study of nasopharyngeal carcinoma. *JNCI*, **51**, 1403–1408.

102. Lin, T.M., Yang, C.S., Tu, S.M., Chen, C.J., Kuo, K.C., and Hirayama, T. (1979). Interactions of factors associated with cancer of the nasopharynx. *Cancer*, **44**, 1419–1423.

103. Lombardi, F., Gasparini, M., Gianni, C., DeMarie, M., Molinari, R., and Pilotti, S. (1982). Nasopharyngeal carcinoma in childhood. *Med. Pediat. Oncol.*, **10**, 243–250.

104. Madri, J.A., and Barwick, K.W. (1982). An immunohistochemical study of nasopharyngeal neoplasms using keratin antibodies: epithelial versus nonepithelial neoplasms. *Am. J. Surg. Path.*, **6**, 143–149.

105. Malik, M.O.A., Banatvala, J., Hutt, M.S.R.,

Abu-Sin, A.Y., Hidaytallah, A., and El-Hadi, A.E. (1979). Epstein–Barr virus antibodies in Sudanese patients with nasopharyngeal carcinoma: a preliminary report. *JNCI*, **62**, 221–224.

106. Mallen, R.W., and Shandro, W.G. (1974). Nasopharyngeal carcinoma in Eskimos. *Can. J. Otolaryngol.*, **3**, 175–179.

107. Mathew, G.D., Qualtiere, L.F., Neel, H.B., III, and Pearson, G.R. (1981). IgA antibody, antibody-dependent cellular cytotoxicity and prognosis in patients with nasopharyngeal carcinoma. *Int. J. Cancer*, **27**, 175–180.

108. McKeen, E.A., Bodurtha, J., Meadows, A.T., Douglass, E.C., and Mulvihill, J.J. (1978). Rhabdomyosarcoma complicating multiple neurofibromatosis. *J. Pediatr.*, **93**, 992–993.

109. Menck, H.R., and Henderson, B.E. (1979). Cancer incidence rates in the Pacific Basin. *Natl. Cancer Inst. Monogr.*, **53**, 119–124.

110. Miller, R.W. (1978). Epidemiology. In *Cancer in China* (Eds H.S. Kaplan, and P.J. Tsuchitani), A.R. Liss, New York, pp. 39–57.

111. Miller, R.W. (1981). Contrasting epidemiology of childhood osteosarcoma, Ewing's tumor, and rhabdomyosarcoma. *Natl. Cancer Inst. Monogr.*, **56**, 9–14.

112. Miller, R.W. (1978). Cancer epidemics in the People's Republic of China. *JNCI*, **60**, 1195–1203.

113. Miller, R.W., and Dalager, N.A. (1974). Fatal rhabdomyosarcoma among children in the United States, 1960–69. *Cancer*, **34**, 1897–1900.

114. Modan, B., Mart, H., Baidatz, D., Steinitz, R., and Levin, S.G. (1974). Radiation-induced head and neck tumors. *Lancet*, **1**, 277–279.

115. Mould, R.F., and Bakowski, M.T. (1976). Adenocarcinoma of nasopharynx. *Lancet*, **2**, 1134–1135.

116. Muir, C.S. (1971). Nasopharyngeal carcinoma in non-Chinese populations with special reference to Southeast Asia and Africa. *Int. J. Cancer*, **8**, 351–363.

117. Naegele, R.F., Champion, J., Murphy, S., Henle, G., and Henle, W. (1982). Nasopharyngeal carcinoma in American children: Epstein–Barr virus-specific antibody titers and prognosis. *Int. J. Cancer*, **29**, 209–212.

118. Nevo, S., Meyer, W., and Altman, M. (1971). Carcinoma of the nasopharynx in twins. *Cancer*, **28**, 807–809.

119. Nielsen, N.H., Mikkelsen, F., and Hansen, J.P.H. (1977). Nasopharyngeal cancer in Greenland: the incidence in an Arctic Eskimo

population. *Acta. Pathol. Microbiol. Scand. A*, **85**, 850–858.

120. Nikoskelainen, J., Ablashi, D.V., Isenberg, R.A., Neel, E.U., Miller, R.G., and Stevens, D.A. (1978). Cellular immunity in infectious mononucleosis. II. Specific reactivity to Epstein–Barr virus antigens and correlation with clinical and hematologic parameters. *J. Immunol.*, **121**, 1239–1244.

121. Pakikh, S.D., and El-Ghamrawi, K.A. (1978). Cancer of the nasopharynx in Kuwait. *J. Laryngol. Otol.*, **92**, 681–691.

122. Pantangco, E.E., Basa, G.F., and Canlas, M. (1967). A survey of nasopharyngeal cancers among Filipinos: a review of 203 cases. In *Cancer of the Nasopharynx* (Eds C.S. Muir, and K. Shanmugaratnam), UICC Monogr. Series 1, Munksgaard, Copenhagen, pp. 38–42.

123. Papvasiliou, C., Pavlatou, M., and Pappas, J. (1977). Nasopharyngeal cancer in patients under the age of thirty years. *Cancer*, **40**, 2312–2316.

124. Pearson, G.R. (1980). Epstein–Barr virus: immunology. In *Viral Oncology* (Ed G. Klein), Raven Press, New York, pp. 739–768.

125. Pearson, G.R., Weiland, L.H., Neel, H.B. III, Taylor, W., Earle, J., Mulroney, S.E., Goepfert, H., Lanier, A., Talvot, M.L., Pilch, B., Goodman, M., Huang, A., Levine, P.H., Hyams, V., Moran, E., Henle, G., and Henle, W. (1983). Application of Epstein–Barr virus (EBV) serology to the diagnosis of North American nasopharyngeal carcinoma. *Cancer*, **51**, 260–268.

126. Pearson, G.R., Johansson, B., and Klein, G. (1978). Antibody-dependent lymphocyte cellular cytotoxicity against EBV-associated antigens in African patients with nasopharyngeal carcinoma. *Int. J. Cancer*, **22**, 120–125.

127. Pearson, G.R., and Orr, T.W. (1976). Antibody-dependent lymphocyte cytotoxicity against cells expressing Epstein–Barr virus antigens. *JNCI*, **56**, 485–488.

128. Pearson, G.R., Redmon, L.W., and Pearson, J.W. (1973). Serochemotherapy against a Moloney virus-induced leukemia. *Cancer Res.*, **33**, 1854–1857.

129. Percy, C., Stanek, E., III, and Gloeckler, L. (1981). Accuracy of cancer death certificates and its effect on cancer mortality statistics. *Am. J. Public Health*, **71**, 242–250.

130. Pinkston, J.A., Wakabayashi, T., Yamamoto, T., Asano, M., Harada, Y., Kumagami, H., and Takeuchi, M. (1981). Cancer of the head and neck in atomic bomb survivors: Hiroshima and Nagasaki, 1957–1976. *Cancer*, **48**, 2172–2178.

131. Prathap, K., Prasad, U., and Ablashi, D.V. (1983). The pathology of nasopharyngeal carcinoma in Malaysia. In *Nasopharyngeal Carcinoma, Current Concepts* (Eds U. Prasad, D.V. Ablashi, P.H. Levine, and G.R. Pearson), University of Malaya Press, Kuala Lumpur, pp. 55–63.

132. Purtilo, D.T., Paquin, L., DeFlorio, D., Virzi, F., and Sakhuja, R. (1979). Immunodiagnosis and immunopathogenesis of the X-linked recessive lymphoproliferative syndrome. *Semin. Hematol.*, **16**, 309–343.

133. Raney, R.B., Jr., Donaldson, M.H., Sutow, W.W., Lindberg, R.D., Maurer, H.M., and Tefft, M. (1981). Special considerations related to primary site in rhabdomyosarcoma: experience of the Intergroup Rhabdomyosarcoma Study, 1972–1976. *Natl. Cancer Inst. Monogr.*, **56**, 69–74.

134. Richter, W., Gu, S.Y., Seibl, R., and Wolf, H. (1983). A new method for examination of carcinomas of the nasopharynx. In *Nasopharyngeal Carcinoma: Current Concepts* (Eds U. Prasad, D.V. Ablashi, P.H. Levine, and G.R. Pearson), University of Malaya Press, Kuala Lumpur, pp. 25–32.

135. Rothwell, R.I. (1979). Juvenile nasopharyngeal carcinoma in Sabah (Malaysia). *Clin. Oncol.*, **5**, 353–358.

136. Saad, A. (1968). Observations on nasopharyngeal carcinoma in the Sudan. In *Cancer in Africa* (Eds P. Clifford, C.A. Linsell, and G.L. Timms), East Afr. Publ. House, Nairobi, pp. 281–285.

137. Sandler, D.P., Comstock, G.W., and Matanoski, G.M. (1982). Neoplasms following childhood radium irradiation of the nasopharynx. *JNCI*, **68**, 3–8.

138. Saxen, E. (1975). Histological classification and its implications in the utility of registry data in epidemiological studies. In *Cancer Registry* (Eds E. Grundmann, and E. Pedersen), Recent Results in Cancer Research, **50**, Springer-Verlag, New York, pp. 38–46.

139. Schmauz, R., and Templeton, A.C. (1972). Nasopharyngeal carcinoma in Uganda. *Cancer*, **29**, 610–612.

140. Shanmugaratnam, K. (1978). Histological typing of nasopharyngeal carcinoma. In *Nasopharyngeal Carcinoma: Etiology and Control* (Eds G. de-The, and Y. Ito), IARC Sci. Publ. No. 20, IARC, Lyon, pp. 3–12.

141. Shanmugaratnam, K. (1982). Nasopharynx. In *Cancer Epidemiology and Prevention* (Eds D. Schottenfeld, and J.F. Fraumeni, Jr.), W.B. Saunders Co., Philadelphia, pp. 536–553.

142. Shanmugaratnam, K., Chan, S.H., de-The, G., Goh, J.E.H., Khor, T.H., Simons, M.J., and Tye, C.Y. (1979). Histopathology of nasopharyngeal carcinoma: correlations with epidemiology, survival rates and other biological characteristics. *Cancer*, **44**, 1029–1044.

143. Shanmugaratnam, K., and Muir, C.S. (1967). Nasopharyngeal carcinoma: origin and structure. In *Cancer of the Nasopharynx* (Eds C.S. Muir, and K. Shanmugaratnam), UICC Monogr. Series 1, Munksgaard, Copenhagen, pp. 153–162.

144. Shanmugaratnam, K., and Sobin, L. (1978). *Histological Typing of Upper Respiratory Tract Tumours*. International Histological Typing of Tumours No. 19, WHO, Geneva, pp. 32–33.

145. Shanmugaratnam, K., Tye, C.Y., Goh, E.H., and Chia, K.B. (1978). Etiological factors in nasopharyngeal carcinoma: a hospital-based, retrospective, case-control, questionnaire study. In *Nasopharyngeal Carcinoma: Etiology and Control* (Eds G. de-The, and Y. Ito), IARC Sci. Publ. No. 20, IARC, Lyon, pp. 199–212.

146. Shedd, D.P., von Essen, C.F., Connelly, R.R., and Eisenberg, H. (1968). Cancer of the pharynx in Connecticut, 1935–1959. *Cancer*, **21**, 706–713.

147. Shem, P., and Armstrong, R.W. (1977). Survivorship among patients with nasopharyngeal carcinoma in Hawaii. *Hawaii Med. J.*, **36**, 348–350.

148. Shope, T., DeChairo, D., and Miller, G. (1973). Malignant lymphoma in cottontop marmosets after inoculation with Epstein–Barr virus. *Proc. Natl. Acad. Sci.*, **70**, 2487–2491.

149. Shore, R.E., Albert, R.E., and Pasternack, B.S. (1976). Follow-up study of patients treated by X-ray epilation for tinea capitis. Resurvey of post-treatment illness and mortality experience. *Arch. Environ. Health*, **31**, 21–28.

150. Simons, M.J., Chan, S.G., Wee, G.B., Day, N.E., de-The, G.B., and Shanmugaratnam, K. (1975). Probable identification of an HL-A second-locus antigen associated with a high risk of nasopharyngeal carcinoma. *Lancet*, **1**, 142–143.

151. Simons, M.J., Chan, S.H., Wee, G.B., Shanmugaratnam, K., Goh, E.H., Ho, J.H.C., Chau, J.C.W., Darmalingam, S., Prasad, U., Betuel, H., Day, N.E., and de-The, G. (1978). Nasopharyngeal carcinoma and histocompatibility antigens. In *Nasopharyngeal Carcinoma: Etiology and Control* (Eds G. de-The, and Y. Ito), IARC Sci. Publ. No. 20, IARC, Lyon, pp. 271–282.

152. Simons, M.J., and Shanmugaratnam, K. (Eds) (1982). *The Biology of Nasopharyngeal Carcinoma*, UICC Tech. Report Series, Vol. 71, Report No. 16, Hans Huber, Berne.

153. Simons, M.J., Wee, G.B., Goh, E.H., Chan, S.H., Shanmugaratnam, K., Day, N.E., and de-The, G. (1976). Immunogenetic aspects of nasopharyngeal carcinoma. IV. Increased risk in Chinese of nasopharyngeal carcinoma associated with a Chinese-related HLA profile (A2, Singapore 2). *JNCI*, **57**, 977–980.

154. Snow, J.B., Jr. (1975). Carcinoma of the nasopharynx in children, *Ann. Otol. Rhino. Laryngol.*, **84**, 817–826.

155. Sugano, H., Sawki, S., Sakamoto, G., and Hirayama, T. (1978). Histopathological types of nasopharyngeal carcinoma in a low-risk area: Japan. In *Nasopharyngeal Carcinoma: Etiology and Control* (Eds G. de-The, and Y. Ito), IARC Sci. Publ. No. 20, IARC, Lyon, pp. 27–39.

156. Sundar, S.K., Levine, P.H., Ablashi, D.V., Leiseca, S.A., Armstrong, G.R., Cicmanec, J.L., Parker, G.A., and Nonoyama, M. (1981). Epstein–Barr virus-induced malignant lymphoma in a white-lipped marmoset. *Int. J. Cancer*, **27**, 107–111.

157. Sundar, S.K., Ablashi, D.V., Kamaraju, L.S., Levine, P.H., Faggioni, A., Armstrong, G.R., Pearson, G.R., Krueger, G.R.F., Hewetson, J.F., Bertram, G., Sesterhenn, K., and Menezes, J. (1982). Sera from patients with undifferentiated nasopharyngeal carcinoma contain a factor which abrogates specific Epstein–Barr virus antigen-induced lymphocyte response. *Int. J. Cancer*, **29**, 407–412.

158. Turgman, J., Modan, B., Shilon, M., Rappaport, Y., and Shanon, E. (1977). Nasopharyngeal cancer in a total population: selected clinical and epidemiological aspects. *Br. J. Cancer*, **36**, 783–786.

159. Wara, W.M., Wara, D.W., Phillips, T.L., and Ammann, A.J. (1975). Elevated IgA in carcinoma of the nasopharynx. *Cancer*, **35**, 1313–1315.

160. Waterhouse, J., Muir, C., Shanmugaratnam, K., and Powell, J. (Eds) (1982). *Cancer Incidence in Five Continents*, vol. IV, IARC Sci. Publ. No. 42, IARC, Lyon.

161. Wen, C.P. (1974). Nasopharyngeal cancer. In *China Medicine as We Saw It* (Ed J.R. Quinn), DHEW Publ. No. NIH 75–684, Washington, DC, pp. 289–344.

162. Wolf, H., zur Hausen, H., Klein, G., Becker, V., Henle, G., and Henle, W. (1975). Attempts to detect virus specific DNA se-

quences in human tumors. III. Epstein – Barr viral DNA in non-lymphoid nasopharyngeal carcinoma cells. *Med. Microbiol. Immunol.*, **161**, 15 – 21.

163. Young, J.L., Jr., Percy, C.L., and Asire, A.J. (Eds) (1981). Surveillance, Epidemiology, and End Results: incidence and mortality data, 1973 – 1977. *Natl. Cancer Inst. Mongr.*, **57**, 1 – 1082.

164. Yu, M.C., Ho, J.H.C., Ross, R.K., and Henderson, B.E. (1981). Nasopharyngeal carcinoma in Chinese – salted fish or inhaled smoke? *Prev. Med.*, **10**, 15 – 24.

165. Zeng, Y., Liu, Y., Liu, C., Chen, S., Wei, J., Zhu, J., and Zai, H. (1980). Application of an immunoenzymatic method and an immunoautoradiographic method for a mass survey of nasopharyngeal carcinoma. *Intervirology*, **13**, 162 – 168.

166. Zeng, Y., Zhang, L.G., Li, H.Y., Jan, M.G., Zhang, Q., Wu, Y.C., Wang, Y.S., and Su, G.R. (1982). Serological mass survey for early detection of nasopharyngeal carcinoma in Wuzhou City, China. *Int. J. Cancer*, **29**, 139 – 141.

167. zur Hausen, H., Schulte-Holthausen, H., Klein, G., Henle, W., Henle, G., Clifford, P., and Santesson, L. (1970). EBV-DNA in biopsies of Burkitt tumors and anaplastic carcinomas of the nasopharynx. *Nature*, **228**, 1056 – 1058.

B
STAGING

Chapter 3

Current Problems in Clinical Staging

Robert E. Wittes
*Cancer Therapy Evaluation Program,
Division of Cancer Treatment, National
Cancer Institute, Bethesda, Maryland,
USA*

A staging system is a set of rules according to which tumours of a given histological type and primary site may be assigned a category (called a stage or a stage group) having a prognosis distinct from the other categories in the classification. The *raison d'être*, therefore, of a good staging system is that its various categories say something about the patient's prognosis. The more sharply the prognosis of one stage differs from those of adjacent stages, the better.

It turns out that the established staging systems for most cancers, and for virtually all epithelial cancers, are anatomical in character; that is, the rules for assigning tumours to the various stages are related to the physical extent of the neoplasm. Since most initial therapy these days is locoregional rather than systemic, a staging system which precisely specifies anatomical detail ought to be an effective way of grouping together tumours which require similar therapeutic approaches. Hence an effective staging system ought also to facilitate communication among physicians and permit valid comparisons of therapeutic results.

This chapter will examine the characteristics of the current systems in common use for the staging of head and neck cancers. It will be seen that, despite years of careful development, these systems do not encompass the heterogeneity of clinical behaviour of which these tumours are capable.

GENERAL COMMENTS

The TNM system has gained wide acceptance as the most appropriate vehicle for head and neck cancer staging. The general assumption on which this scheme is based is that increasing size or local invasiveness of the primary tumour, and increasing extent of regional lymph nodal involvement, adversely effect prognosis. The validity of this assumption is supported by a massive amount of evidence from a large variety of primary epithelial sites, including those of the upper aerodigestive tract.

In general, *clinical* staging is defined as that which is accomplished without the aid of a major surgical procedure, prior to the first definitive therapy; it routinely includes careful physical examination with endoscopy and any necessary radiographic and laboratory studies. Clearly, then, staging is only as reliable as the expertise of the examiner and the sensitivity and specificity of the tests used in the process. Ideally one attempts to define with these manoeuvres a clinical stage which will approximate as closely as possible the true pathological stage of the tumour at that point in time. In so far as the clinical stage approaches the true pathological stage, the 'extent of disease' workup will be maximally informative about prognosis and most useful in planning treatment. As will be seen, we are still far from this goal.

There are two major versions of the TNM system currently in use; these are set forth, respectively, in the TNM booklet of the International Union Against Cancer (UICC)[1] and in the most recent edition of the *Manual for Staging of Cancer*, published by the American Joint Committee (AJC).[2]

THE PRIMARY TUMOUR

The AJC and UICC currently have very similar or identical definitions for all sites in the head and neck area.[1,2] Definitions of the various T stages are tailored flexibly to the characteristics of the individual primary sites. The T stage increases with size of tumour or with invasion into contiguous or deep structures; evidence of such invasion may be either by physical examination (presence of mass or of functional impairment, as with lingual or laryngeal motion) or by radiographic studies (mass, bone destruction).

CERVICAL NODES

The staging of neck nodes remains significantly different for the two staging systems (Table 3.1). The UICC system uses characteristics of mobility (fixed *vs.* moveable) and laterality (homolateral vs. contralateral or bilateral) as the major criteria for classification. The AJC, by contrast, has eliminated mobility altogether because of the allegedly large subjective component in its evaluation; size, multiplicity, and laterality of involved nodes all play a role in this somewhat more complex set of definitions.

TABLE 3.1   COMPARISON OF DEFINITIONS OF N CATEGORIES

	AJC	UICC
NX	Minimum requirements to assess regional nodes cannot be met	(Same)
N0	No clinically positive node	(Same)
N1	Single clinically positive homolateral node $\leqslant$3 cm in diameter	Moveable, homolateral
N2	Single clinically positive homolateral node >3 cm and $\leqslant$6 cm in diameter (N2a) *or* multiple clinically positive homolateral nodes none >6 cm (N2b)	Moveable contralateral or bilateral
N3	Clinically positive homolateral node(s), one >6 cm diameter (N3a) *or* Bilateral clinically positive nodes (N3b) *or* Contralateral clinically positive nodes only (N3c)	Fixed nodes

An examination of Table 1 shows that it is formally possible for a cancer to be classified as N1 disease in one classification and N3 in the other. *Caveat lector.*

DISTANT METASTASES

In both classifications the simple presence or absence of distant metastases determines M stage. One of the curious features of all past and present TNM systems has been the compulsive detail with which the T and N categories are defined, as contrasted with the near-total absence of information in the M category. Much of the reason for this is undoubtedly related to the incurability of most M1 disease. Both UICC and the AJC recommend that M1 disease be further subdivided according to the distant site(s) of involvement. With accumulation of more careful information on the relation of prognosis to site and/or character of distant involvement at diagnosis, it may be possible to develop meaningful subdivisions of the M1 category.

STAGE GROUPS

Since the number of combinations of the individual T, N, and M categories is unmanageable for purposes of data analysis, both systems have defined aggregates of these stages; the four stage groups that result (Table 3.2) serve to collect the various TNM stages into convenient prognostically distinct groups. These stage groups are defined similarly by the AJC and UICC; since, however, the N stages of the two systems are not the same, the actual content of the stage groupings will differ between these two TNM versions.

TABLE 3.2   DEFINITION OF STAGE GROUPS (AJC AND UICC)

Stage	T	N	M
I	1	0	0
II	2	0	0
III	3	0	0
	1,2,3	1	0
IV	4	0,1	0
	any	2,3	0
	any	any	1

PROBLEMS WITH THE STAGING PROCESS

Required Tests not Clearly Specified

Both the UICC and the AJC have defined the essential staging studies for each system (Table 3.3). In addition the AJC has suggested for each primary site additional tests which may be 'possibly useful for staging or patient management' or 'possibly useful for future staging systems or research studies'. The performance of these tests is left to the discretion of the individual physician. The AJC has specified much more precisely than the UICC the essential radiographic studies for the individual primary sites (Table 3.3). In view of the multinational character of the UICC, it is easy to understand why the definition of certain essential elements has been left rather vague; nevertheless, a staging system will be more reproducible from centre to centre in proportion as the rules for its use are made mandatory and not discretionary.

Difficulties with T Staging

Clearly the most important aspect here is a good physical examination, including the

TABLE 3.3   STAGING PROCEDURES FOR HEAD AND NECK CARCINOMAS

		AJC	UICC
A.	Essential	Complete physical examination of the head and neck including indirect laryngoscopy and nasopharyngoscopy Biopsy of primary tumour Chest roentgenogram Roentgenograms of skull (nasopharynx) Direct examination of hypopharynx	Clinical examination laryngoscopy (for larynx cancer) radiography histological verification
B.	May be useful for staging or patient management	Multichemistry screen Soft-tissue roentgenograms of neck, CT scans Barium swallow Performance status	—
C.	May be useful for future staging systems or research studies	Panendoscopy Studies of immune competence Assays of antibodies to Epstein–Barr viral capsid antigen (nasopharynx)	—

necessary endoscopies by an experienced observer, supplemented by radiography. The examiner assesses *apparent* extent of disease, which may be significantly greater than actual anatomical involvement by tumour to the extent that infection and peritumoral oedema are present. Dr Richard Jesse was fond of observing that meticulous local care frequently resulted in significant reduction in apparent tumour volume without any antineoplastic therapy.

It is also often the case that clinical staging significantly underestimates the extent of disease. Much of the problem here is the general difficulty in assessing depth of invasion; at most head and neck sites, the 'third dimension' cannot be assessed directly with any precision, but can at most be inferred from disturbances in function (tongue fixation, trismus, vocal cord paralysis). Until fairly recently radiological imaging techniques were of limited utility in assessing involvement of many difficult areas of the upper aerodigestive tract. In 114 patients with larynx cancer, for example, using the clinical examination supplemented by indirect and direct laryngoscopy, laryngeal tomography, and contrast laryngography, Pillsbury and Kirchner[3] found that 37% of glottic, 38% of supraglottic, 50% of transglottic, and 13% of subglottic tumours were staged incorrectly. The large majority of staging errors for all sites were understagings; in fact no patient in the trans- or subglottic groups was overstaged. The main cause of this 40% error rate was failure to assess correctly the spread of the cancer outside the confines of the larynx. A fair number of the understagings observed in this study might have affected choice of a surgical procedure. In addition, the choice of radiotherapy as single-modality treatment might well have been influenced by clinical understaging.

Over the past few years the potential of computed tomography (CT) has been explored with great interest in the head and neck area, as at other sites. The rapid evolution of imaging technology, specifically the great decrease in scanning times and in thickness of tomographic cuts, has increased dramatically the level of resolution and hence the clinical usefulness of the technique. The size and extent of tumour masses and the definition of extension into the orbits or the cranial vault can be done now with an accuracy that was never before possible. With specific reference to the larynx, several studies have found CT vastly superior to other imaging tools in the assessment of cartilage invasion, invasion of paralaryngeal tissues and the pre-epiglottic space, and the definition of subglottic extension. Gamsu *et al.*[4] have reported that CT changed the endoscopically defined T stage in nine out of 25 patients with cancers of the larynx and pyriform fossa. Eight of the nine had more extensive disease than was originally suspected; six of the eight had unsuspected cartilage destruction, and seven patients had unsuspected invasion into the pre-epiglottic space. Friedman, Archer, and colleagues[5,6] have found CT far superior to contrast laryngography as a staging procedure for larynx cancer; in addition to direct assessment of extralaryngeal spread, CT seemed superior in evaluating the endolaryngeal extent of disease, including subglottic extension. Now that phonation scans have been shown to be feasible,[4] CT can be used to assess functional as well as structural abnormalities.

CT is obviously not a totally satisfactory solution to the problem of clinical staging in larynx cancer. It does not provide a histological diagnosis, and therefore is an imperfect way of differentiating tumour from secondary oedema and infection. Mucosal detail may be suboptimal; this may not be a significant problem, however, since laryngoscopy will provide this information in most cases. Sagel *et al.* [7] have noted that the transition zone between the false and true cords is often poorly defined by CT; the pyriform fossa and aryepiglottic fields may also not be clearly visualized, although phonation scans may help greatly in this regard. The presence of cartilage destruction is also often difficult to call; irregular patterns of calcification and ossification with advancing age can make limited or even moderate degrees of invasion a very subtle finding. With all these limitations, however, and despite the high cost of the test, the use of CT as a staging procedure in all but the earliest stages of larynx cancer seems justifiable, especially in patients for whom conservation surgery is being considered.

At other head and neck sites, also, CT appears to have significant advantages over other imaging modalities. For the assessment of intracranial and nasopharyngeal extension of paranasal sinus tumors, CT may be superior to angiography and tomography.[8] It may also be the best technique for imaging nasopharyngeal tumours, especially small submucosal ones.[8]

Difficulties with N Staging

The importance of ascertaining the presence or absence of neck node involvement is attested by a large volume of data which relate prognosis to the extent and distribution of positive nodes.[9-11] The probability of finding nodal involvement by cancer is a function of several variables – location of the primary site,[10] size of the primary tumour[11,12] and degree of differentiation of the primary.[13]

Evaluation of the neck has always been by physical examination. Since the fingers are not terribly sensitive probes for small nodes containing tumour, or even for rather large nodes (approximately 2 cm or so) if they happen to lie under the sternocleidomastoid muscle, a substantial false-negative rate might be anticipated. Since also many of these primary tumours are sites of local infection, the presence of reactive lymphoid hyperplasia might result in a number of false-positive evaluations as well. In fact, the error rate associated with physical assessment of the neck is indeed appreciable (Table 3.4). Both false-positive and false-negative rates are substantial, though errors are somewhat less frequent when the neck is thought to be clinically positive than when it is clinically negative (Table 3.4). The reason is probably that errors in a judgement of clinical positivity become progressively less likely as the size and number of putatively involved lymph nodes increase. Along these lines, Spiro et al.[9] have found that the accuracy of assessing the necks of 70 patients undergoing bilateral neck dissections was 93%. It may also be that certain lymph node levels in the neck are easier to evaluate than others; data from a review of oral cavity and pharynx cancers[18] suggest that the accuracy of clinical staging increases pro-

TABLE 3.4   PHYSICAL ASSESSMENT OF THE NECK

Ref.	N	C(+)H(+)	C(−)H(−)	C(+)H(−)	C(−)H(+)	Overall error rate	Clin (−) error rate	Clin (+) error rate
Sako[14]	235	81	89	31	34	28%	28%	28%
Lyall[15]	35	11	6	9	9	50%	60%	45%
Southwick[16]	158	63	31	27	29	35%	48%	30%
Kremen[17]	44	9	16	5	14	43%	47%	36%
Spiro[9]	966	471	261	93	141	25%	35%	16%

C = Clinical assessment;   H = Histological assessment

$$\text{Overall error rate} = \frac{C(+)H(-) + C(-)H(+)}{N}$$

$$\text{Clin}(-)\text{ error rate} = \frac{C(-)H(+)}{C(-)H(+) + C(-)H(-)}$$

$$\text{Clin}(+)\text{ error rate} = \frac{C(+)H(-)}{C(+)H(-) + C(+)H(+)}$$

gressively from Levels I to V. These data are difficult to interpret, however, since involvement of an increasing number of levels in the neck may be correlated with a significant increase in tumour bulk.

Since the physical examination is obviously imperfect, investigators have been exploring various imaging techniques. The most promising appears to be CT, although large-scale prospective evaluations have not yet been reported. Mancuso *et al.*[19] have compared results of CT with the clinical examination in 51 larynx cancer patients; in 13 cases a pathological evaluation of the neck dissection specimen was also performed. These retrospectively derived results, admittedly with small numbers, suggest that CT can image nodes with 'suspicious' radiological characteristics that are not detected by the physical examination. In the 13 cases where pathological confirmation was available, CT was correct in 12. On the basis of this experience, Mancuso *et al.* have embarked on a prospective trial; preliminary results suggest the same level of accuracy as was found in the retrospective review. Of the combined group of 61 patients, 13 were clinically negative but positive on CT scan; histologic confirmation was available in six with no false results.[19] Thirteen were clinically positive; CT scanning was positive in five (confirmed in four) and negative in eight (confirmed in six). There were two false results here. These authors have refined their radiological criteria for node positivity and are continuing with the prospective trial. Potential problems with CT, as with all imaging modalities, involve limits of resolution; nodes less than 0.5 cm are not consistently visualized, so that the total node counts on CT are consistently less than the total counts in the neck dissection specimen.[19] Nevertheless, it seems quite likely that CT can improve the accuracy of pretreatment staging; further careful study is clearly in order.

Various radiopharmaceuticals have also received attention. The Oak Ridge Associated Universities Cooperative Group has reported a comprehensive evaluation of gallium-67 citrate imaging in head and neck tumours.[20] Fifty-six per cent of primary head and neck tumours and their metastases were successfully imaged in 65 patients. In previously untreated patients the true-positive rate was 0.63, the false-positive rate 0.53, and the accuracy rate 0.60. For neck sites of involvement less than 3 cm, the true-positive rate was only 0.48 and the accuracy rate 0.36, both significantly less than the corresponding figures for sites $\geqslant 3$ cm (0.82 and 0.80 respectively). It seems clear, therefore, that current versions of this technique are not very promising additions to the diagnostic armamentarium.

Co-57 tagged bleomycin has also been of interest. In small series[21] studies have suggested that Co-Bleo will image 50–80% of cases with malignant head and neck tumours. Variability in technique and in cases selected for inclusion, and the small number of cases studied, make firm conclusions impossible. Cummings *et al.*[22] have studied Co-Bleo in 46 patients with a variety of histologies (many unspecified) and have reported a true-positive rate of 84% with all histologies, along with a 17% false-negative and a 10% false-positive rate. Tumours less than 2 cm in diameter could not be reliably imaged; this and the excess background radioactivity seen in many studies were largely responsible for the false-negatives. Uptake in inflammatory lesions and in benign salivary tissue accounted for several of the false-positives. This technique might increase the discrimination of neck node staging if a hotter radiopharmaceutical were used, but doing so might also result in an increase in the false-positive rate.

The potential uses of lymph node scintigraphy are discussed separately in Chapter 4.

M Staging

The clinical problem of distant metastases in head and neck cancer has always taken a back seat in importance to locoregional disease. It turns out, however, that patients dying of head and neck cancer have an incidence of distant metastases approaching 40–50% at autopsy.[23,24] Many of these patients, of course, also have uncontrolled locoregional disease, which is a more frequent cause of morbidity and mortality. On the other hand, distant metastases in the *absence* of locoregional failure is of increasing concern; at the M. D. Anderson Hospital the overall rate for all head and neck sites was 7.9%.[25] Of significance, however, was the variation in frequency of distant metastasis among sites; particularly noteworthy is the propensity for oropharynx (24%), nasopharynx (25%), and hypopharynx (23%) primaries to develop distant metastases after control of the primary tumour and neck nodes.[25] Metastases appearing in this way were most likely present at the time of initial treatment. As local control rates increase, one can certainly anticipate an increase in the rate of appearance of distant metastases. The probability of distant metastasis appears to increase with both T and N stage, particularly the latter.[25,26]

Studies which have examined the frequency of detectable distant metastasis in patients with primary head and neck cancer have without exception reported a very low yield. In several series of patients heavily weighted by advanced stages of disease, liver scans showed true-positives in 0/116,[27] 4/105,[28] 0/87,[29] and 0/132.[30] The yield with bone scans seems little better; positive scans were seen in 7%,[27] 2.4%,[28] and 2%,[30] some of which were false-positives. It seems clear, therefore, that use of these tests as routine screening procedures cannot be justified by the yield. Bone scans seem reasonable for patients with symptoms or with unexplained alkaline phosphatase elevations, as are liver scans for clarification of hepatomegaly or abnormal liver function tests. Even under these circumstances, however, the yield will probably be very low unless the patients have advanced locoregional disease at the time of staging.

Neglect of Other Important Tumour-related Factors

As noted above, the degree of differentiation (grade) of the tumour has been widely acknowledged to play an important role in determining prognosis;[13] generally, the less the degree of differentiation, the more probable is the presence of nodal metastasis. From the existing data it is much less clear that tumour grade has prognostic implications *within* stage; many investigators who have examined the impact of grade have overlooked this issue entirely or have not been able to do an appropriately detailed analysis because of the relatively small size of each individual series.[13,31–33]

Vascular invasion has also been alleged to have an adverse impact on survival. Poleksic and Kalwaic,[34] for example, have correlated the presence of lymphatic or venular invasion by tumour with more advanced TNM stages and with poorer survival. As with histological grade, it is not clear whether vascular invasion is an independent prognostic factor.

Previous surveys have suggested that extracapsular spread (ECS) of tumours has an adverse effect upon prognosis.[35] A recent analysis by Johnson *et al.*[36] of patients treated with surgery with or without radiotherapy suggests also that extracapsular spread is a powerful predictor of poor prognosis. For 31 patients with positive nodes but no ECS, the survival rate of 62% did not differ much from the 70% survival seen with negative node patients. For 58 patients with positive nodes and ECS the survival rate was 37%. The presence of ECS seemed independent of the number of positive nodes or the tumour grade. Although ECS patients were more likely to have Stage IV disease, the difference between ECS and no ECS persists within Stage IV. The authors' suggestion that this question be studied prospectively in a multi-institutional setting seems well-advised.

Other histological features of the primary tumour also bear mention. In addition to grade, McGavran *et al.*[37] have noted that laryngeal tumours which have nerve sheath invasion or infiltrating margins are more likely to have nodal metastases than are tumours without nerve invasion or tumours having 'pushing' margins.

Over the past decade pathologists have attempted to formulate a comprehensive morphological description of epidermoid head and neck tumours that would be useful in estimating prognosis. The initial efforts of Jakobsson for larynx cancer have been continued by Lund and his collaborators and extended to other head and neck sites.[33,38,39] This complex classification system has eight histological criteria which relate to tumour cytology, the tumour–host relationship, and the pattern of tumour growth. Each characteristic is evaluated and assigned a numerical score, from which an overall score for the tumour is derived. For laryngeal cancer[38] Lund *et al.* have found a significant correlation between the morphological score and the presence of nodal metastases, and also between the score and the probability of death. The data suggest further that a high score correlates with increased chance of local recurrence of T2, 3, and 4 lesions. Also, a high score appears to correlate with increased risk of death *within* T stages for N0 disease. All these correlations must be regarded as preliminary and need to be confirmed with much larger numbers of cases.

Lund *et al.* have obtained similar results with carcinoma of the lip.[33] The results with tongue cancer are confusing; although score seems to be related to the frequency of nodal metastases, there is no significant correlation between score and T stage, local recurrence rates, or mortality.[39]

Others have attempted the use of this or similar classification systems with less success. In a case–control study Hordijk attempted to apply the Jakobsson and Lund scale to 31 patients with glottic cancer treated with RT and followed for at least 5 years. He found no relation of overall scores to prognosis.[40] Willen *et al.* have developed a six-parameter scale including both tumour factors (differentiation, nuclear polymorphism, and mitoses) and host factors (mode of invasion, stage of invasion, and cellular response) and attempted to correlate score with outcome in 124 patients with gingival cancer seen at the Karolinska Institute

over a 10-year period.[32] A general relation between score and the tendency to nodal metastasis was found but the correlation was rather weak; from the data presented it is not clear whether any correlation exists within stages. Helweg-Larsen *et al.* found that the Jakobsson system was not a useful predictor of clinical course in larynx cancer.[41] Crissman and colleagues have applied a modification of the Jakobsson system in floor-of-mouth cancers;[42] they also found a correlation between average score and extent of disease but also noted so much overlap between groups that the system was of no predictive value in individual cases.

Numerous practical problems exist with respect to such classification systems. Interobserver variation has been substantial[41,43] and may account for some of the variability in results obtained so far; no doubt each biopsy should be graded by several pathologists who are well schooled in the classification system being used. One also must worry about the sampling error; when there is heterogeneity from field to field, Lund *et al.*[38] have advised using the one with the highest score, but it is not at all clear that this is correct. These workers have also found that not all eight parameters can be assessed in all specimens. Nevertheless such classification schemes would seem to hold promise as predictors of outcome; clearly further advances will have to be based on very large numbers of patients, with rigorous quality control and formal statistical analysis. It might turn out, for example, that a different weighting system for the individual morphological parameters would be more powerful than the methods that have been used so far. Indeed, a formal multivariate analysis might indicate that only a few of these parameters are actually important prognostic determinants.

For glottic tumours the rather heterogeneous T2 category has been examined by Harwood, who has found that patients with impaired cord mobility have lower local control rates after RT (51.1% vs 76.7%) and lower 5-year survival rates (75.2% vs 86.8%)

than those whose cord mobility was normal.[44]

Modern techniques of cell biology have been employed only recently in the study of head and neck cancer. Cinberg *et al.*[45] have examined the cell cycle characteristics of biopsy specimens from squamous head and neck primaries; preliminary results suggest that the higher the labelling index of the tumour (i.e. the greater the number of cells in S-phase), the greater the likelihood that unrecognized nodal metastases will be present.

Neglect of Host-related Factors

Both the AJC and UICC staging systems exhort the user to note the performance status (PS) of the patient in standardized fashion; PS, however, has no effect on the staging classification itself. About the effect of PS on outcome, we shall have more to say later. In addition to PS, however, many other host-related variables have been alleged to affect prognosis. In most papers such variables are analysed in a univariate way, so that the reader cannot tell whether the particular parameter of interest is exerting an independent effect on prognosis.

Age

In a survey of 371 patients with larynx cancer treated over a 17-year period, advancing age appeared to have an adverse impact on tumour-related survival;[46] the authors state that the stage distribution did not differ significantly among the various age cohorts but provide no information concerning potential treatment-related biases as a function of age. By contrast, in a study of T3 glottic cancer, Harwood and colleagues[47] found that the 5-year control rate for men less than 60 years old was significantly worse than that for men greater than 60 (34% vs 52%). Interestingly, one large series[48] has suggested that supraglottic and glottic primaries may behave differently from each other, with supraglottic tumours showing a negative effect of age on prognosis and glottic cancers no effect. Young patients with nasopharynx cancer do better than older ones,[49,50] a relation-

ship which appears to hold within stages as well.[49]

Sex

The data here are no less confusing. A recent review of the epidemiology of oral and pharyngeal cancer in the US suggests that females with 'localized' cancers do worse than their male counterparts.[51] On the other hand Harwood's data suggest that females may have a significant advantage over men in both local control and survival from T3 glottic cancer.[47] An interim analysis of the RTOG's comparative trial of preoperative and postoperative radiotherapy[52] suggested that females were superior to males at several sites for both local control and survival at 2 years; application of Cox modelling to the data showed that for local control of supraglottic larynx disease and for survival from oropharyngeal cancer, female sex was a statistically significant prognostic factor. For nasopharynx cancer in Hong Kong, sex appears not to be a determinant of outcome, even when examined carefully within stages and within age cohorts.[49] Old data from Memorial Hospital suggest that females survive both tongue and gingival cancer better than males but more favourable site and stage may account for this.[53,54] For cancers of the palate[55] and tonsil[56] from the same institution, females also show superior survivorship but no comparative data on stage are presented. Yet another Memorial report on the radical surgical treatment of advanced mouth cancer shows no difference in outcome of the two diseases.[57]

Immune Status

Over the past 10 years much effort has been directed towards defining the relation between tests of immune function and the clinical course of patients with various malignancies. Head and neck cancer has excited particular interest because many of these patients show evidence of decreased immune competence relatively early in the course of their disease. For example, studies at Memorial Sloan–Kettering Cancer Center have shown that 8 of 24 patients with T1 or 2 N0 disease failed to react to DNCB;[58] patients with more advanced diseases had a higher percentage of anergy. Moreover, for T1 or 2 N0 patients skin test non-reactivity had an adverse effect on survival;[58] node-positive patients failed to show this relationship, but numbers were very small. In an extension of these studies, involving tests of delayed hypersensitivity to several antigens and *in vitro* response to mitogens, a correlation of immune parameters with prognosis was evident only for DNCB skin tests; depressed reactivity to DNCB was associated with an increased recurrence rate in Stages I and II, though not in III and IV.[59] *In vitro* tests failed to correlate significantly with outcome. Progressive impairment in T cell function occurred with increasing stage.

In contrast to the Memorial results Ryan *et al.*[60] found that *in vitro* studies were also predictive; responses to PNA and CON-A were greater in patients remaining tumour-free after treatment. These results held within stages as well, though the numbers of patients were small. Curiously there was no significant difference in reactivity overall across stages irrespective of outcome.

The fact that certain circulatory serum proteins can depress lymphocyte reactivity to mitogens *in vitro* led Chretien and colleagues to look for a relationship between levels of these proteins and prognosis.[61] An increase in haptoglobin and alpha$_1$ acid glycoprotein occurred in patients with head and neck cancer compared with controls; levels of these proteins were also lower in cured patients than in those with untreated disease. Among untreated cases, levels of alpha$_1$ acid glycoprotein and alpha$_1$ antitrypsin generally paralleled the anatomic extent of disease.

ATTEMPTS AT ALTERNATIVE SYSTEMS

Additions to the AJC and UICC Classifications

As previously noted, both systems have

encouraged users to enter host factors, expressed as performance status, and histological grade as formal components of the medical record. The AJC has allotted these factors the notation H and G, with numerical subscripts corresponding to the various possible categories. H and G have not, however, been incorporated into the definition of the stage groups and therefore will probably not be used widely.

STNMP

Rapidis *et al.*[62] have developed a formal modification of the TNM system for oral cancer in which site (S) and pathological characteristics (P) are appended to the traditional categories. Nine sites and seven histologies are defined. The UICC definitions of the N stages are modified to include a category for equivocal nodal involvement; also, distant metastases are classified according to whether they are absent (M0), suspected (M1), or proved (M2). Each of the 29 individual S, T, N, M, and P categories is assigned a numerical value; a patient's numerical score is the sum of the scores of the individual components. The patient's score then determines into which of four stage groupings the patient falls.

Rapidis *et al.* have classified 136 patients with oral cancer at the London Hospital according to the STNMP system and have compared its ability to discriminate prognosis with the stage groupings derived from the TNM definitions of Sakai and Masaki.[63] These latter groupings differ from the present UICC system in the definitions of T3 and T4, and also in the placing of $T_{1-3} N_2$ disease into Stage III rather than IV. The net effect of these differences is to make the Stage III of Sakai and Mosaki a more advanced stage than in the present UICC system. Rapidis *et al.* claim that discrimination of prognosis in the STNMP system is superior to TNM, particularly in its ability to define a group of patients with good prognosis.[62] The analysis used by these authors, however, does not employ survival curves and does not use survival information in a maximally informative way. They give no justification for the assignment of particular numerical weights to each staging sub-category; this seems to have been done arbitrarily. In short, the STNMP system has not been shown to be superior to the simpler TNM systems in its power to discriminate prognosis.

Feinstein's System

The most interesting modification in staging systems is one proposed by Feinstein several years ago for larynx cancer.[64] In an analysis of the clinical course of 192 patients, Feinstein found that survival probability was related most prominently to anatomic extent of disease (A), types of symptoms (S), and associated major co-morbid ailments (C). Contrary to what one might suppose, the case distribution among the various categories suggests that the S and A systems are independent of each other; in other words the anatomical extent of disease, as defined in this system, is not the sole determinant of symptoms. Within each anatomical stage, the progression from less to more severe symptomatic categories is associated with a worsening survival probability. Similarly, survival of patients in combined symptomatic–anatomical stages decreases with the presence of major co-morbid disease. Accordingly, the authors have defined a series of four S-A-C stages based on these considerations. None of the other variables considered (age, sex, smoking, anaemia, and duration of symptoms prior to diagnosis) had a significant additional effect on prognosis.

The authors show that the S-A-C system defines prognostic gradients more clearly than the TNM system in use at that time. This is true whether one looks at individual T categories or the TNM stage groups I to IV. Within each TNM-defined stage group the S-A-C stages show a clear prognostic gradient (though some of the categories have small numbers of patients); within each S-A-C stage, however, the existence of a prognostic gradient from TNM stage groups I to IV is somewhat less clear.

This staging system is, to say the least, unconventional. It de-emphasizes the importance of anatomical detail; indeed, the anatomical characteristics of the cancers are specified only as 'localized', 'intermediate', or 'distant'. Instead, it introduces elements from the history and general medical evaluation into a position of major importance. Feinstein's major conclusion from this work is that the medical history gives information about tumour biology and clinical course that is both very important and unavailable from a purely anatomical evaluation.

CONCLUSION

This chapter began by restating the goals of a good staging system: to provide (1) prognostic information; (2) guidance in the choice of therapy; and (3) a universal language to facilitate communication. The existence of heterogeneity of prognosis within the stages of the currently used systems might suggest that the systems themselves are inadequate. It is indeed unsettling if adjacent stages in a staging system exhibit significant overlap in prognosis. Even if there is not overlap, substantial heterogeneity within stages may be a nuisance; for example, the variable prognosis within Stage IV[65] or the considerable anatomical variations that occur within this stage make treatment planning based on stage alone impossible. On the other hand, since prognosis is a continuous variable, getting rid of 'all' heterogeneity would require the creation of a very large number of stage groups, such that the staging system itself would be unmanageably cumbersome. In addition, before one could begin to accomplish this, the effect on prognosis of the several variables examined in this chapter would have to be examined more carefully than has yet been done.

Since, therefore, a certain amount of heterogeneity will persist within the stages of any decent system, how is one to construct the best possible classification? The answer undoubtedly depends upon the principal uses for which the system has been constructed. If a staging classification exists mainly as anatomical shorthand to serve the needs of the surgeon and radiotherapist in treatment planning, then what is needed may simply be further attention to the kind of anatomical detail which has received so much attention already. Indeed, there is still unhappiness with aspects of both major systems, for example, regarding anatomical definition in the larynx[66,67] and the staging of small tumours of the nasopharynx.[49] If, on the other hand, accurate prognostication is to be staging's major purpose, then the spectrum of incorporated variables will have to be broadened to include at least some of those discussed above. Feinstein's study has suggested that for best possible staging the anatomical extent of a head and neck cancer is best regarded as one part of the total medical evaluation of the patient; indeed, his work has re-emphasized that what we should in fact be doing is staging *patients* with cancer rather than staging the cancers themselves.

Head and neck cancers are not unique in this respect. For years the various stages of Hodgkin's disease have been divided into A and B, according to whether the patient exhibits certain tumour-related signs[2] not having anything directly to do with the demonstrable anatomical extent of disease. The staging of soft-tissue sarcomas now recognizes explicitly the importance of grade in defining stage groupings.[2] It seems quite likely that the future staging of breast cancer will include oestrogen-receptor status[68] and the presence or absence of peritumoral lymphatic permeation[69] in the stage groupings.

The major constraint on the design of any staging system is the necessity for avoiding excessive detail such that the system becomes unusable. In recognition of the fact that even the present TNM systems are approaching the limits of complexity, both the AJC and UICC have issued pocket-sized handbooks for ready reference in examining rooms. Certainly the more complex a system is, the more frequent will be mistakes in its use. In a study assessing the accuracy with which the definitions of the 1977 AJC system were applied, Kaufman and Lore found that the stage assignments made by

the surgeon disagreed with those made by a computer from the clinical descriptions of the cancers in 44% of T stagings and 25% of N stagings; apparent errors by the clinician occurred in 35% and 20% of cases, respectively.[70] These authors have proposed that clinicians confine themselves to a description of the anatomical lesion on standardized coding forms, from which a computer could assign the stage according to any set of definitions desired.

Another possibility, far more radical than any discussed so far, would involve abandoning the current concept of stage as a discrete category. In recognition that the probability of surviving past some fixed time point is a continuous variable, one might use techniques of multivariate analysis to generate mathematical functions of the most important prognostic variables; the function would describe a relation between these variables and the probability of survival. This function could be used to calculate the expected probability of survival for a patient based on that patient's particular combination of prognostic variables. Such techniques have, of course, been used for years by many investigators, notably Gehan *et al.*[71] for identification and analysis of prognostic variables in acute leukaemia. Recently similar attempts to use mutivariate analysis to predict the probability of response to treatment have been shown to be feasible for testicular cancer[72] and these techniques are currently being employed to select patients for experimental approaches. As such, this procedure is really a means of dividing patients with Stage III testis cancer into distinct prognostic groups. In so far as staging systems are to be maximally informative about prognosis, future versions of our current systems will have to take explicit account of important non-anatomical variables that exert potent effect on prognosis.

REFERENCES

1. Harmer, M.H. (Ed.) (1978). *TNM Classification of Malignant Tumours*. UICC, Geneva, 3rd edition.
2. Beahrs, O.H., and Myers, M.H. (Eds) (1983).

Manual for Staging of Cancer. American Joint Committee on Cancer, 2nd edition, J.B. Lippincott Company, Philadelphia.

3. Pillsbury, H.R.C., and Kirchner, J.A. (1979). *Arch. Otolaryngol.*, **105**, 157.

4. Gamsu, G., Webb, W.R., Shalit, J.B., and Moss, A.A. (1981). *Am. J. Roentgenol.*, **136**, 577.

5. Friedman, W.H., Archer, C.R., Yeager, V.L., and Katsantonis, G.P. (1981). *Otolaryngol. Head Neck Surg.*, **89**, 579.

6. Archer, C.R., Sagel, S.S., Yeager, V.L., Martin, S., and Friedman, W.H. (1981). *Am. J. Roentgenol.*, **136**, 571.

7. Sagel, S.S., Aufder Heide, J.F., Armberg, D.J., Stanley, R.J., and Archer, C.R. (1981). *Laryngoscope*, **91**, 292.

8. Mancuso, A.A. (1982). Computed tomography in the diagnosis and evaluation of primary head and neck cancer. Chapter 6 in R.J. Steckel, and A.R. Kagan (Eds): *Cancer Diagnosis: New Concepts and Techniques*, Grune and Stratton, N.Y., pp. 127–160.

9. Spiro, R.H., Alfonso, A.E., Farr, H.W., and Strong, E.W. (1974). *Am. J. Surg.*, **128**, 562.

10. Lindberg, R. (1972). *Cancer*, **29**, 1446.

11. Harrold, C.C. (1971). *Am. J. Surg.*, **122**, 487.

12. Farr, H.W., and Arthur, K. (1972). *J. Laryngol. Otol.*, **86**, 243.

13. Arthur, K., and Farr, H.W. (1972). *Am. J. Surg.*, **124**, 489.

14. Sako, K., Pradier, R.N., Marchetta, F.C., and Pickren, J.W. (1964). *Surg. Gynecol. Obstet.*, **118**, 989.

15. Lyall, D., and Shetlin, C.F. (1952). *Ann. Surg.*, **135**, 489.

16. Southwick, H.W., Slaughter, D.P., and Trevino, E.T. (1960). *Arch. Surg.*, **80**, 905.

17. Kremen, A.J. (1967). In J. Conley (Ed.) *Cancer of the Head and Neck*, Butterworths, Washington, pp. 183–185.

18. Farr, H.W., Goldfarb, P.M., and Farr, C.M. (1980). *Am. J. Surg.*, **140**, 563.

19. Mancuso, A.A., Maceri, D., Rice, D., and Hanafee, W. (1980). *Am. J. Roentgenol*, **136**, 381.

20. Teates, C.D., Preston, D.F., and Boyd, C.M. (1980). *J. Nucl. Med.*, **21**, 622.

21. Woolfenden, J.M., Alberts, D.S.,Hall, J.N., and Patton, D.D. (1979). *Cancer*, **43**, 1652.

22. Cummings, C.W., Larsen, S.M., Dobie, R.A., Weymuller, E.A., Rudd, T.G., and Merello, A. (1981). *Laryngoscope*, **91**, 529.

23. Dennington, M.L., Carter, D.R., and Meyers, A.D. (1980). *Laryngoscope*, **90**, 196.

24. Gowen, G.F., and Desoto-Nagy, G. (1963). *Surg. Gynecol. Obstet.*, **116**, 603.

25. Merino, O.R., Lindberg, R.O., and Fletcher, G.H. (1977). *Cancer*, **40**, 145.

26. Probert, J.C., Thompson, R.W., and Bagshaw, M.A. (1974). *Cancer*, **33**, 127.

27. Wolfe, J.A., Rowe, L.D., and Lowry, L.D. (1979). *Ann. Otol. Rhinol. Laryngol.*, **88**, (1), 832.

28. Martin, G.F., Gullane, P.J., and Heeneman, H. (1981). *J. Otolaryngol*, **10**, 383.

29. Felix, E.L., Bagley, D.H., Sindelar, W.F., Johnson, G.S., and Ketcham, A.S. (1976). *Cancer*, **38**, 1137.

30. Belson, T.P., Lehman, R.H., Chobanian, S.L., and Malin, T.C. (1980). *Laryngoscope*, **90** (8, Pt.1), 1291.

31. Bennett, S.H., Futrell, J.W., Roth, J.A., Hoye, R.C., and Ketcham, A.S. (1971). *Cancer*, **28**, 1255.

32. Willen, R., Nathanson, A., Moberger, G., and Anneroth, G. (1975). *Acta Otolaryngol.*, **79**, 146.

33. Lund, C., Søgaard, H., Elbrønd, O., Jørgensen, K., and Anderson, A.P. (1975). *Acta Radiol. (Ther.)*, **14**, 465.

34. Poleksic, S., and Kalwaic, H.J. (1978). *Plast. Reconst. Surg.*, **61**, 234.

35. Zoller, M., Goodman, M., and Cummings, C.W. (1978). *Laryngoscope*, **88**, (1,Pt.1) 135.

36. Johnson, J.T., Barnes, E.L., Myers, E.N., Schramm, V.L., Borochovitz, D., and Sigler, B.A. (1981). *Arch. Otolaryngol.*, **107**, 725.

37. McGavran, M.H., Bauer, W.C., and Ogura, J.H. (1961). *Cancer*, **14**, 55.

38. Lund, C., Jorgensen, K., Hjelem-Hansen, M., and Anderson, A.P. (1979). *Acta Radiol. Oncol. Radiat. Phys. Biol.*, **18**, 497.

39. Lund, C., Sogaard, H., Elbrond, O., Jorgensen, K., and Anderson, A.P. (1975). *Acta. Radiol. (Ther.)*, **14**, 513.

40. Hordijk, G.J. (1980). *Arch. Otolaryngol.*, **106**, 621.

41. Helweg-Larsen, K., Graem, N., Meistrup-Larsen, K., and Meistrup-Larsen, O. (1978). *Acta Pathol. Microbiol. Scand.*, **86A**, 499.

42. Crissman, J.D., Gluckman, J., Whiteley, J., and Quenelle, D. (1980). *Head Neck Surg.*, **3**, 2.

43. Graem, N., Helweg-Larsen, K., and Keiding, N. (1980). *Acta Pathol. Microbiol. Scand.*, **88**, 307.

44. Harwood, A.R. (1980). *Cancer*, **45**, 991.

45. Cinberg, J.Z., Chang, T.H., Bases, R., and Molnar, J. (1980). *Laryngoscope*, **90**, (6,Pt.1), 920.

46. Huygen, P.L.M., Van den Broek, P., Kazem, I. (1980). *Clin. Otolaryngol.*, **5**, 129.

47. Harwood, A.R., Bryce, D.P., and Rider, W.D. (1980). *Arch. Otolaryngol.*, **106**, 697.

48. Till, J.E., Bruce, W.R., Elwan, A., Till, M. J., Niederer, J., Reid, J., Hawkins, N.V., and Rider, W.D. (1975). *Laryngoscope*, **85**, 259.

49. Choa, G. (1981). In J.Y. Suen, and E.N. Myers, *Cancer of the Head and Neck*, Churchill, Livingstone, New York, pp. 372–414.

50. Carniol, P.J., and Fried, M.P. (1982). *Ann. Otol. Rhinol. Laryngol.*, **91**, (2,Pt.1), 152.

51. Smith, E.M. (1979). *J. Nat. Cancer Inst.*, **63**, 1189.

52. Snow, J.B., Gelber, R.D., Kramer, S., Davis, L.W., Marcial, V.A., and Lowry, L.D. (1981). *Acta Otolaryngol.*, **91**, 611.

53. Frazell, E.L., and Lucas, J.C., Jr. (1962). *Cancer*, **15**, 1085.

54. Cody, B., and Catlin, D. (1969). *Cancer*, **23**, 551.

55. Ratzer, E.R., Schweitzer, R.J., and Frazell, E.L. (1970). *Am. J. Surg.*, **119**, 294.

56. Terz, J.J., and Farr, H.W. (1967). *Surg. Gynecol. Obstet.*, **125**, 581.

57. Spiro, R.H., and Frazell, E.L. (1968). *Am. J. Surg.*, **116**, 571.

58. Lundy, J., Wanebo, H., Pinsky, C., Strong, E.W., and Oettgen, H. (1974). *Am. J. Surg.*, **128**, 530.

59. Hilal, E.Y., Wanebo, H.J., Pinsky, C.M., Middleman, P., Strong, E.W., and Oettgen, H.F. (1977). *Am. J. Surg.*, **134**, 468.

60. Ryan, R.E., Jr., Neel, N.B., III, and Ritts, R.E. (1980). *Otolaryngol. Head Neck Surg.*, **88**, 58.

61. Wolf, G.T., Chretien, P.B., Elias, E.G., Makuch, R.W., Baskies, A.M., Spiegel, H.E., and Weiss, J.F. (1979). *Am. J. Surg.*, **138**, 489.

62. Rapidis, A.D., Langdon, J.D., Patel, M.E., and Harvey, P.W. (1977). *Cancer*, **39**, 204.

63. Sakai, S., and Masaki, N. (1971). *Acta Otolaryngol.*, **72**, 370.

64. Feinstein, A.R., Schimpff, C.R., Andrews, J.F., and Wells, C.K. (1977). *J. Chron. Dis.*, **30**, 277.

65. Ucmakli, A. (1980). *Otolaryngol. Clin. North Am.*, **13**, 529.

66. Anonymous editorial (1978). *Clin. Otolaryngol.*, **3**, 323.

67. Harrison, D.F. (1978). *ORL*, **41**, 241.

68. Allegra, J.C., Lippman, M.E., Simon, R., Thompson, E.B., Barlock, A., Green, L., Huff, K.K., Do, H.M.T., Aitken, S.C., and Warren, R. (1979). *Cancer Treatment Rep.*, **63**, 1271.

69. Rosen, P.P., Saigo, P.E., Braun, D.W., Jr., Weathers, E., and De Palo, A. (1981). *Ann. Surg.*, **193**, 15.

70. Kaufman, S., and Loré, J.M. (1978). *Am. J. Surg.*, **136**, 469.

71. Gehan, E.A., Smith, T.L., and Freireich, E.J. (1976). *Semin. Oncol.*, **3**, 271.

72. Bosl, G.J., Cirrincione, C., Geller, N., Vugrin, D., Whitmore, W., and Golbey, R. (1981). *Proc. Am. Soc. Clin. Oncol.*, **22**, 393 (C-239).

Chapter 4

Use of the CO2 Laser in Diagnosis and Staging

Stanley M. Shapshay
Department of Otolaryngology, Lahey Clinic Medical Center, Burlington, Massachusetts, USA

The continuous-wave carbon dioxide surgical laser has been used in surgery of the head and neck region since 1971.[1] Patients with selected benign lesions, such as recurrent respiratory papillomatosis, which affects the larynx and trachea, were treated first. It soon became apparent that the CO_2 laser was extremely useful in the diagnosis and treatment of malignant lesions involving the upper aerodigestive tract and tracheobronchial tree.[2,3] Laser delivery systems, such as handpieces, endoscopic couplers, and microscope manipulators, have extended applicability of this relatively new technology. Advances and refinements in laser technology have produced safe instrumentation that is reliable and efficient.

The emphasis of this chapter will be on the use of the CO_2 laser as a diagnostic and staging instrument for early cancer (Stages I and II) of the head and neck. A common misconception is that the CO_2 laser is used to vaporize cancer and that it provides very little pathologic material for evaluation of margins of histological tumour. In fact, the CO_2 laser is primarily used as a precision instrument when it is attached to an operating microscope and guided by a visible aiming light with a micromanipulator (Figure 4.1). Precise removal of tissue is accomplished without vaporizing or ablating disease by use of the laser as a haemostatic cutting instrument. The amount of unwanted heat coagulation around the area of tissue ablation is smallest (50–100 µm) when laser exposure time is minimized through a series of intermittent bursts of energy.

The most effective application of laser technology in the identification of cancer of the head and neck is in the evaluation of cancer of the larynx through the laryngoscope by an endoscopic technique. Its application in the diagnosis of cancer of the oral cavity and oropharynx will also be discussed.

LASER PHYSICS AND SOFT TISSUE INTERACTION

How does the laser differ from an electrocautery if both have thermal effects on tissue? Can the biopsy specimens removed with the laser be accurately examined pathologically? How does the surgeon control the depth of penetration of the laser? Does the laser spread tumour cells when it interacts with the cancer? Does the laser seal off the lym-

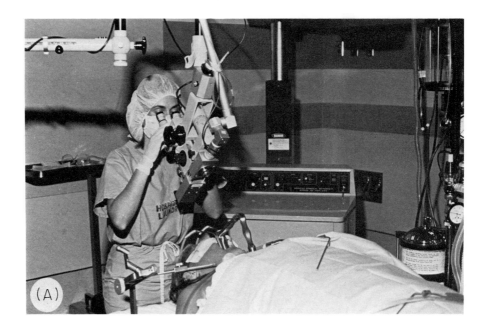

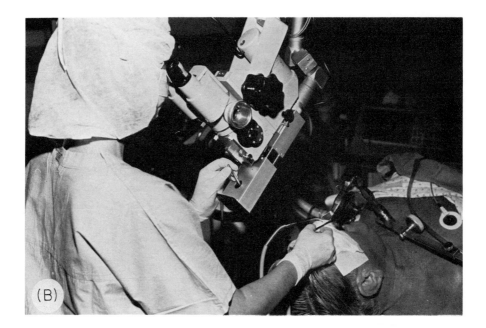

Figure 4.1 (**A**) The CO_2 laser articulating arm, attached to an operating microscope. The laser power source (40 W of CO_2) can be seen in the background.
(**B**) The surgeon's hand is on the laser micromanipulator aiming control. The beam is directed with a superimposed visible aiming light (a Hene neon red laser) through an operating laryngoscope that exposes the vocal cords. Suspension apparatus keeps the laryngoscope in place.

phatic system limiting the spread of cancer cells? To answer these questions, a basic discussion of laser physics and interaction with soft tissues is necessary.

Laser energy is non-ionizing light energy or radiation. The wavelength of the CO_2 laser, 10.6 µm, is in the infrared or invisible spectrum of electromagnetic energy. In contrast to light from an incandescent source (a light bulb), laser light has the unique properties of being coherent – all light waves are exactly in phase, collimated – the waves are parallel to each other, and monochromatic – all the waves have exactly the same wavelength (or the same colour if they are visible).

The laser light is generated by pumping an electric current through a chamber containing a mixture of CO_2 and other gases. Mirrors positioned at either end of the chamber cause the photons of light energy, all with 10.6 µm coherent waves, to reflect back and forth, amplifying the laser emission. The mirror at the output end of the tube is partially transmitting so that laser light is emitted. The laser energy is then reflected through a series of mirrors into the appropriate delivery system (for example, handpiece, microscope manipulator, or bronchoscopic coupler).

Because of the following characteristics the wavelength of the CO_2^4 laser is ideally suited for surgical removal of soft tissue:

(1) Laser light is efficiently absorbed in water. Since 70–90% of soft tissue is composed of water, flash boiling of intracellular water occurs at temperatures of about 100 °C. The steam produced is suctioned away, and carbon particles form the cell residue.

(2) The laser scattering effect from the target point is minimal, and absorption is not dependent on colour of tissue. The precision of the effect on soft tissue minimizes tissue swelling and results in unimpaired wound healing.

(3) The continuous-wave CO_2 laser does not cause a blast effect on tissue (in contrast to pulsed lasers, such as the ruby laser). Viable cancer cells are not spread.

(4) Haemostasis is achieved for small (capillary size) blood vessels. Lymphatics are sealed as well, which may be of some practical value in patients who are to undergo surgical treatment for cancer.

(5) The non-ionizing irradiation of the laser light does not cause genetic mutation.

The laser can be focused with lenses so that under the microscope the depth of laser penetration into tissue can be observed and controlled by varying the power and time exposure. The usual operating spot size of the laser beam is 0.8 mm in diameter, but this may be varied from 0.1 to 2 mm depending on the operative procedure. This no-touch surgery does not interfere with the surgeon's vision, and haemostasis further enhances visibility. Lateral destruction of tissue is limited to 50–100 µm, unlike the unpredictable thermal conductivity of the electrocautery. Postoperative pain associated with the CO_2 laser is also minimal, possibly because nerve endings are sealed and oedema of tissue is minimal. Wound healing is usually good, even in previously irradiated fields.

Other surgical lasers, such as the argon and neodymium–yttrium aluminium garnet (Nd-YAG), are currently being used for their photocoagulation effects in ophthalmology (argon) and for endoscopy (Nd-YAG) in gastroenterology, bronchology, and urology. The CO_2 instrument is currently still considered the laser of choice in head and neck surgery because of its predictable soft-tissue effects. Both argon and Nd-YAG lasers can be conducted through flexible quartz fibres that facilitate endoscopic applications. The CO_2 laser cannot at present be conducted through fibre systems.

CANCER OF THE LARYNX

The CO_2 laser becomes a unique endoscopic instrument when its micromanipulator is attached to a standard operating microscope. While illuminating the magnified operative field, laser light can be directed with pinpoint accuracy through a laryngoscope suspended in

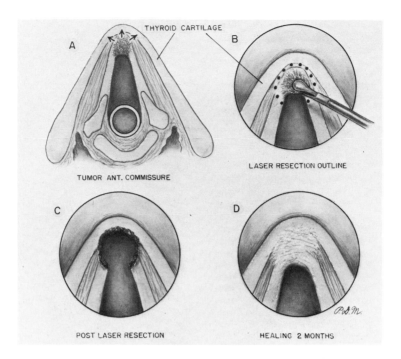

Figure 4.2 (**A**) A cancer at the anterior commissure between the vocal cords. Clinical staging is T1; however, if the cartilage is involved, the proper classification is T4.
(**B**) A microlaryngeal cup forceps applies traction on the specimen. The outline of excisional biopsy was made with the CO_2 laser on intermittent exposure.
(**C**) Area of laser excision. The specimen is submitted for pathological examination of margins. The thyroid cartilage can be seen clearly under the operating microscope. Deep biopsy specimens are obtained for control of the margin.
(**D**) Healing at 2 months after laser excision. The mild webbing at the anterior commissure can be corrected if the patient's voice is weak.

place. General anaesthesia is usually chosen for this procedure, with relaxation techniques to ensure a stationary operative field.

Correct treatment of cancer of the larynx depends on accurate biopsy sampling and precise staging according to the TNM classification.[5] Endoscopic evaluation with a large-bore fibre-optic laryngoscope allows the use of a binocular operating microscope. The small (5–6 mm), specially prepared endotracheal tube used in laser surgery can be placed posteriorly without impairing exposure of the vocal cords. Supravital staining with 2%

toluidine blue dye is commonly applied to determine areas of severe dysplasia and carcinoma *in situ*. The increased nucleic acid in these areas will stain a deep purple.

Multicentric areas of superficial cancer are easily identified with this staining technique, which helps the clinician to choose appropriate biopsy sites.[6] Areas of hyperkeratosis or white patches will not stain; areas of erythroplasia, most likely representing carcinoma *in situ*, will absorb the stain.

Incorrect staging of cancer of the larynx is common because of the shortcomings of the

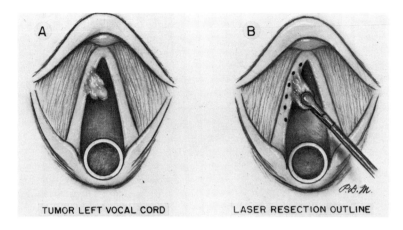

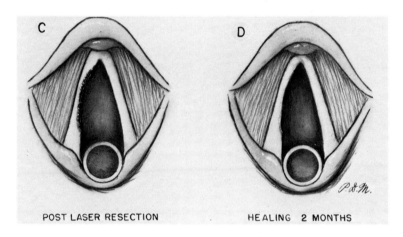

Figure 4.3   **(A)** An early invasive T1 squamous cell cancer involving the left vocal cord.
(B) A microlaryngeal cup forceps grasps the tumour and provides traction on the specimen. The outline of the CO₂ laser resection can be seen.
(C) Area of laser excision. The specimen is sent to pathology for frozen section margins. If free of tumour, no further treatment will be necessary. There is minimal functional disability postoperatively.
(D) Final healing of the left vocal cord 2 months later. The voice is usually good with only mild hoarseness, depending on the amount of vocal cord muscle resected.

TNM classification and difficulties in clinical evaluation. Fixation of the vocal cord, for instance, is easily assigned a T3 category. Impaired mobility of the vocal cord due to tumour bulk rather than to deep muscle invasion is more difficult to determine. Cancer involving the anterior commissure or the anterior junction between the vocal cords close to the thyroid cartilage would be classified as T1 cancer. Invasion of the underlying thyroid cartilage, however, is staged as T4 (Figure 4.2). Since T1 cancer is certainly treated differently from a more threatening T4 tumour, inaccurate staging leads to erroneous treatment planning. Unfortunately, because of uneven calcification of the thyroid cartilage, plain radiography and even computed tomography often miss invasion of the cartilage.

The CO_2 laser is most commonly used as a surgical, hemostatic knife for excisional biopsy of localized accessible T1 and selected T2 cancers of the vocal cord (usually for salvage after radiation failure, Figure 4.3). The laser can be used effectively to detect both invasion of vocal cord muscle and involvement of the thyroid cartilage. Pathological specimens are carefully oriented for the pathologist to evaluate tumour margins.[7] If the lesion is more invasive than was determined clinically, correct staging facilitates proper treatment planning. Since true T1 cancers that are small and localized can be excised with minimal morbidity and with retention of good function of the vocal cord, the CO_2 laser offers an alternative to radiotherapy. Control of early (carcinoma *in situ* and T1) cancer of the vocal cord by use of the CO_2 laser matches the results with radiotherapy.

The CO_2 laser can be used routinely during staging endoscopy of cancer of the larynx to shrink the tumour bulk by vaporizing the tumour after a biopsy specimen is obtained. Through microscopic control the cancer is followed to ascertain its depth of invasion into underlying structures. Accurate staging, reduction of tumour bulk for subsequent chemotherapy or radiotherapy or both, and preservation of laryngeal airway from large obstructing tumours are distinct advantages of laser application. This approach obviates the need for a tracheotomy with its potential for septic complications and possible tumour seeding.[8] Orderly treatment planning with accurate staging and maintenance of a satisfactory airway will ensure better management of the patient.

The major contraindication to endoscopic application of the CO_2 laser is inadequate exposure with a large-bore laryngoscope. Even patients with extensive bulky cancer of the larynx can benefit from reduction of tumour bulk, but these lesions are more clearly manageable by tracheotomy. Because anatomical relationships must be well known to the operating surgeon, endoscopic laser surgery requires special training and preparation.[9]

CANCER OF THE ORAL CAVITY AND OROPHARYNX

The CO_2 laser may be used effectively to diagnose early cancer of the oral cavity through excisional biopsy. It is particularly useful when combined with supravital staining (2% toluidine blue dye) for multicentric areas of dysplasia and carcinoma *in situ* often seen on the floor of the mouth in tobacco and alcohol abusers (Figure 4.4). Patchy areas of hyperkeratosis (white areas) and erythroplasia (red areas) are sometimes seen in conjunction with early invasive carcinoma. This field cancer concept is substantiated by the high incidence (10–20%) of multiple primary cancers of the head and neck.[10]

While excisional biopsy may be therapeutic if pathological margins are secure, accurate sampling is the key. Excision of specimens should be oriented carefully for the pathologist, and the histology review should include consultation with the clinician. Dialogue between clinician and pathologist is essential for proper management of the patient.

The CO_2 laser, particularly when used with the operating microscope, provides greater precision and less tissue trauma than cryosurgery or electrocautery. An adequate specimen is obtainable if the laser is used properly as a cutting instrument. A large surface area of the floor of the mouth, the tongue, and the buccal mucosa may be removed with minimal postoperative discomfort and excellent healing. Most patients are able to eat a soft, bland diet the day after the procedure and may be discharged from the hospital 24 hours after operation.

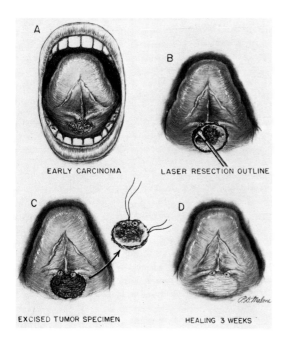

EARLY CARCINOMA   LASER RESECTION OUTLINE

EXCISED TUMOR SPECIMEN   HEALING 3 WEEKS

Figure 4.4   (**A**) Erythroplasia (carcinoma *in situ*) and keratosis in the floor of the mouth. These areas are routinely stained with 2% toluidine blue dye to identify superficial carcinoma.
(**B**) A small cup forceps applies traction on the tissue to be excised with the laser.
(**C**) Area of laser resection. The specimen is marked with long and short sutures identifying the margins for the pathologist.
(**D**) Final healing 3 weeks after laser resection. No attempt was made to identify the submaxillary ducts during surgery; rechannelling of the ducts occurs more proximally. There is minimal pain postoperatively and unimpaired tongue function.

When surface lesions are removed, secure haemostasis and minimal tissue oedema are the rule. If larger lesions (for example, of the tongue) are removed with deeper muscle margins obtained, larger blood vessels should be ligated. The CO₂ laser is haemostatic for capillary-sized blood vessels (0.5 mm).

The major contraindication for laser application is poor exposure of the operative field, which may be caused by problems with dentition or limited opening of the mouth (for example, arthritis of temporomandibular joints). More posteriorly located lesions (for example, on the base of the tongue or tonsillar pillar) are less accessible to laser application. Transoral resection of appropriate early accessible tumours of the oral cavity is associated with a low morbidity rate and is, therefore, cost-effective.[11,12]

FUTURE APPLICATIONS OF LASER TECHNOLOGY

Existing technology developed in industry as well as in military and space research has been applied to medicine. Advances and refinements in the technology of fibre-optics, computers, and lasers are being made for future application in oncology. Fibre-optic catheters capable of carrying laser light of different wavelengths can be directed through specially prepared endoscopes for use in urology, bronchology, and gastroenterology. A laserscope could also be developed for vascular application, such as removing atheromatous lesions through a percutaneous approach.

Lasers can be coupled to computers for unparalleled surgical precision, particularly for tumours of the central nervous system. Stereotaxic devices with computed tomography would map out the pathological area to be ablated, and the laser could be computed to achieve this task. The physician would be required to program its operation. Just as robotics has revolutionized the automobile industry, computerized lasers could profoundly affect certain medical disciplines.

The use of haematoporphyrin dye and laser technology is proving to be a promising diagnostic and therapeutic technique in bronchology and urology for early cancer.[13] The localization by fluorescence of systemically injected haematoporphyrin derivative in tumour tissue by laser light in the 405-mm range facilitates early detection of cancer. Tumours irradiated at the 630-μm wavelength undergo selective absorption of radiation, with destruction or regression of the tumour. Since the mortality rate for advanced cancer of the lung is at present 90%, early detection and treatment are extremely important. Spectrophotometric reading of natural tumour colour might make selective tuning of laser wavelength a future possibility.

SUMMARY

Lasers have a definite role in the diagnosis and treatment of cancer. Because of its precision and its ideal interaction with soft tissue, the CO_2 laser has been extremely useful in the diagnosis and treatment of cancer of the head and neck. Accurate diagnosis and staging of cancer are essential for proper selection of treatment. Preservation of function, excellent wound healing, and minimal destruction of surrounding tissue account for the laser's superior cost-effectiveness.

REFERENCES

1. Jako, G.J. (1972). *Laryngoscope*, **82**, 2204.
2. Strong, M.S. (1975). *Laryngoscope*, **85**, 1286.
3. Strong, M.S., Vaughan, C.W., Polanyi, T., and Wallace, R. (1974). *Ann., Otol., Rhinol., Laryngol.*, **83**, 769.
4. Mihashi, S., Jako, G.J., Incze, J., *et al.* (1976). *Ann. N.Y. Acad. Sci.*, **267**, 263.
5. American Joint Committee (1977). *American Joint Committee for Cancer Staging and End-Results Reporting*, American Joint Committee, Chicago, pp. 39–41.
6. Strong, M.S., Vaughan, C.W., and Incze, J. (1970). *Arch. Otolaryngol.*, **91**, 515.
7. Strong, M.S. (1980). *Otolaryngol. Clin. N. Am.*, **13**, 413.
8. Davis, R.K., Shapshay, S.M., Vaughan, C.W., and Strong, M.S. (1981). *Otolaryngol. Head Neck Surg.*, **89**, 209.
9. Davis, R.K., Jako, G.J., Hyams, V.J., and Shapshay, S.M. (1982). *Laryngoscope*, **92**, (Pt.1), 980.
10. Shapshay, S.M., Hong, W.K., Fried, M.P., Sismanis, A., Vaughan, C.W., and Strong, M.S. (1980). *Otolaryngol. Head Neck Surg.*, **88**, 373.
11. Strong, M.S., Vaughan, C.W., Healy, G.B., Shapshay, S.M., and Jako, G.J. (1979). *Laryngoscope*, **89**, (Pt.1), 897.
12. Strong, M.S., Vaughan, C.W., Jako, G.J., and Polanyi, T. (1979). *Otolaryngol. Clin. N. Am.*, **12**, 207.
13. Gomer, C.J., and Dougherty, T.J. (1979). *Cancer Res.*, **39**, 146.

Chapter 5

Cervical Lymphoscintigraphy

Samuel D.J. Yeh
*Memorial Sloan–Kettering Cancer Center,
1275 York Avenue, New York, NY., USA.*

Cervical lymph nodes represent not only the drainage stations of head and neck lymphatics but also the terminals for distant lymphatics elsewhere in the body. The anatomy and communications of cervical lymphatics have been well established for several centuries. Visualization of lymph nodes and lymphatics in the neck was accomplished by injecting contrast material via cannulated cervical lymphatics.[1] Large numbers of lymph nodes in the jugular, supraclavicular, spinal and retroauricular regions were clearly shown by contrast lymphangiography. Such a delicate procedure is not popular because of technical difficulties and the requirement for skilful and experienced hands. Furthermore, contrast lymphangiography carries measurable local and systemic hazards, and fatalities have been reported.[2] In contrast, radionuclide procedures are simple, non-invasive, less time-consuming, and perhaps equally effective.

Imaging lymph nodes with isotopes was introduced about 20 years ago, shortly after the demonstration of lymph node uptake of [198]Au colloid following interstitial administration.[3] Large numbers of investigations were carried out to evaluate tumour spread in the breast, pelvis, and other sites.[4-6] Scintigraphy of cervical lymph nodes was also extensively studied in Europe 10–15 years ago using [198]Au colloid.[7-9] With continuous improvement of radiopharmaceuticals and imaging equipment, many new agents with superior physical and biological properties were introduced in the last few years. The renewal of interest in imaging the lymphatic system was largely due to the extensive and fruitful work by Ege in studying internal mammary lymph nodes from patients with cancer of the breast.[10] More recently, studies have been extended to the visualization of lymph nodes directly draining prostate,[11] testes,[12] oesophagus,[13] iliopelvic area,[14] or cutaneous channels in truncal melanoma.[15] The role of cervical lymphoscintigraphy in the management of head and neck tumours, however, has not been well documented.

Head and neck cancers are relatively uncommon and represent only 5% of all malignancies. Tumour can spread very widely to the cervical lymph nodes through the rich lymphatic network in this region. The current treatment modalities require precise staging and clear knowledge of patterns of metastasis in the cervical lymph nodes. Unfortunately, many patients with advanced cancer do not have clinically detectable metastases in the cervical lymph nodes. Even for the experienced examiner, the evaluation of neck nodes by physical examination alone is plagued by many false-positives and false-negatives. Cervical lymphangiography is rarely done in the radiological laboratory because of technical difficulties, and probably has little clinical value. The isodense structures surrounding the lymph nodes would make current computed tomography less informative than CT examinations of other parts of the body.

Many tumours may show changes in proton density, T1 or T2 relaxation times on nuclear magnetic resonance imaging.[16] It is not clear whether this exciting new technology will be useful in the early detection of tumour in cervical lymph nodes. [67]Ga citrate concentrates in a large percentage of head and neck tumours, particularly those greater than 3 cm.[17] Metastases in regional lymph nodes, however, are poorly detected;[18] also, uptake of ^{67}Ga citrate is non-specific, as it is taken up in many inflammatory processes. The normal uptake in the salivary gland and increased uptake in the salivary gland following radiation[19] further increase the difficulties in interpretation. More recently, subcutaneous injections of small amounts of Ga citrate in the webs of the feet showed abnormal uptake in lymphoma-containing pelvic nodes which were cold on ^{99m}Tc colloid imaging.[20] A hot spot is certainly more easily identifiable than the defects reflecting defective phagocytic function and blockage of lymphatic channels seen in conventional lymphoscintigraphy.

Tumour localization with labelled antibodies specific for tumours has been of much recent interest.[21,22] Hoffer and Gottschalk first showed uptake of ^{131}I anti-CEA antibody in primary tonsillar carcinoma and cervical metastases.[23] Lymphangiography with radionuclide immunoglobulin or anti-CEA antibody was successful in demonstrating regional lymph node involvement in patients with lymphoma[24] and breast cancer.[25] Extensive studies are currently in progress on the localization of labelled Fab fragments or monoclonal antibodies specific to certain tumour antigens.[22] To what extent these new approaches will be useful in head and neck tumours in the future is not clear. It is apparent that we need a new and reliable modality for evaluation of the status of cervical lymph nodes and a sensitive tool for detecting early metastatic foci in the cervical lymph nodes before tumour spread is clinically apparent.

In this chapter the current status of lymphoscintigraphy in the head and neck area will be reviewed. Its potential usefulness and current difficulties will be discussed.

Lymphoscintigraphic Radiopharmaceuticals

At present it is fair to say that there is no ideal agent for lymphoscintigraphy. All of the available agents measure phagocytic activity of the lymph nodes. Labelled small colloidal particles injected subcutaneously, submucosally, intramuscularly, or interstitially inside or around tumour are transported passively through the channels to the regional lymph nodes. The trapped particles in the lymph nodes are phagocytosed by the reticuloendothelial cells. Obviously, absorption of these agents depends on the number and size of the particles, local lymphatic flow, and unknown factors which may influence the binding of these agents in the interstitial tissue. The status of lymph nodes (increase in size and number, replacement by neoplastic or inflammatory tissue, alteration in reticuloendothelial function) is reflected in the magnitude of the uptake of the trapped labelled particles.

For proper imaging of sequestered particles in the lymph nodes, a suitable radioactive tracer has to be introduced and attached to the particle uniformly and perhaps permanently. The ideal radionuclide should produce gamma emission of about 100–200 keV, optimal for currently available imaging equipment. The half-life should be sufficiently long to allow repeated examination or follow-up, yet not so long as to give an unnecessary radiation dose. The radionuclide should not contain beta emission, which would increase the dose to the patient and which does not contribute to the imaging processes. In general, small particles about 2–10 millimicrons are more efficiently taken up by the lymphatics than larger ones. The preparations must be in homogeneous colloidal dispersion with relative stability under physiological conditions. A kit preparation must be readily accessible and easy to process routinely. Certainly, every preparation must be apyrogenic and sterile, and must have been adequately tested for toxicity in animals.

Gold (^{198}Au colloid) was the first agent successfully used for lymphoscintigraphy, and a large clinical experience has been obtained. The particles are about 2–10 millimicron, the ideal size. The physical half-life of ^{198}Au is 65 hours; therefore, repeated follow-up examinations can be performed over a period of several days. The photopeak of gamma energy of 412 keV is not optimal. Because of beta emission from ^{198}Au, the radiation dose is appreciable, particularly at the site of injection. It was estimated that with a dose of 150 μCi, the average radiation dose would be 0.7 rad to the ovaries, about 30 rad to the regional lymph nodes, and 1000 rad to several millimetres around the site of injection.[26] Colloidal ^{198}Au is still used for liver imaging in some parts of the world but is no longer commercially available in the United States. According to our previous investigations in dogs, this agent is absorbed efficiently from the site of injection in the testis or subcutaneous tissue. The low rate of lymphatic transport can be easily determined by external counting. The radiation dose to the host is a relative matter; one can decrease the administered dose to decrease the radiation burden. Therefore, if there is no better substitute, ^{198}Au colloid can be still considered a possible tool for lymphoscintigraphy.

Human albumin labelled with ^{51}Cr, ^{131}I, or ^{99m}Tc can be used to measure lymph flow.[27] The molecular weight of human albumin is about 60 000. ^{51}Cr is a poor radionuclide; its half-life of 27.8 days is too long. The contribution of gamma photons at 320 keV which are useful for imaging is only 8%. Iodine (^{131}I) is available in every laboratory. The procedures for iodination of biological molecules are sim-

ple and familiar to most investigators. The half-life of 8 days and gamma energy of 345 keV are acceptable for imaging. However, the beta dose from ^{131}I represents approximately 87% of the total dose given to the patient. Although ^{123}I and ^{99m}Tc-labelled albumin can be used, the visualization of regional lymph nodes by interstitial administration of albumin is often poor.

Visualization of lymph nodes can also be achieved by interstitial administration of ^{111}In phosphate colloid.[28] The particle size is not well-defined. ^{111}In has a physical half-life of 2.81 days with gamma peaks at 173 and 247 keV. The absent beta emission during decay and relatively short physical life gives the patient a relatively low radiation dose. The 173% contribution from two ideal gamma protons is advantageous for imaging. Current interest in labelling proteins with ^{111}In chelates[29] may lead to wider use of ^{111}In labelled agents for lymphoscintigraphy. Likewise, other radionuclides such as ^{67}Ga, ^{198}Hg or ^{123}I can be used to label various colloidal particles. The recent demonstration that regional lymph nodes take up interstitially administered ^{67}Ga citrate[20] (MW 259) or labelled antibody (MW at least 150 000) challenges the conventional belief that small colloidal particles are required for lymphoscintigraphy.

^{99m}Tc has been the radionuclide of choice for routine imaging procedures in most nuclear medicine laboratories. The absence of beta emission from the decay of ^{99m}Tc and the short physical half-life of 6 hours contribute a very small radiation dose to the patient. The gamma energy of 140 keV is ideal for imaging. Our understanding of technetium chemistry has grown rapidly and has enabled us to label a great number of compounds easily. At present, one can use a number of ^{99m}Tc-labelled radiopharmaceuticals for lymphoscintigraphy. Sulphide colloid with particle size of about 100 millimicrons has been used successfully for lymph node imaging.[30] There was, however, no critical appraisal in the past comparing the efficacy of such large particles with smaller ones. We believe that conventional sulphide colloid is not efficiently trapped in lymph nodes; only rarely do we see lymph node uptake in the patient after inadvertent administration of colloid to subcutaneous sites. Nowadays, minicolloid and mini-mini-colloid preparations with smaller sizes are also available for liver or bone marrow imaging. With approval by the FDA, one could easily use these agents for lymphoscintigraphy.

In Europe and Japan,[31] [99m]Tc rhenium colloid with uniform spherical particles about 3–5 millimicrons is available for lymphoscintigraphy. The success rate was high particularly for intramucosal injections near various tumour sites.[32] Phytate labelled with ^{99m}Tc is commercially available for routine liver imaging in the United States. Ionic phytate may combine with calcium in the body to form colloidal particles which are subsequently taken up by the regional lymph nodes. Successful visualization of regional lymph nodes was demonstrated in dogs by Alavi *et al.*[33] Osborne has shown suppressed uptake of phytate by metastases in the internal mammary nodes with subsequent normal uptake of antimony colloid.[34] According to other investigators,[35,36] phytate was much inferior to antimony colloid, the agent most investigators prefer at the present time. Osborne also reported that ^{99m}Tc-labelled positively charged or neutral liposomes of average size (33 millimicrons) were well localized in the regional nodes of animals.[37] It is not clear whether such lipid spheres, with entirely different physical, chemical, and biological characteristics, present significant advantages over other colloidal particles.

At present, the best available agent is ^{99m}Tc antimony colloid. A kit with a shelf-life more than 1 year is commercially available. The labelling procedure is simple and takes about 1 hour. The material is stable and homogeneous with particles size 3–30 millimicrons, with peak at about 9 ± 2 millimicrons. Despite the final pH of 7.0, a brief period of pain is experienced by most patients. Regional lymph node uptake can be demonstrated by interstitial administration of this preparation at any site in the body. The bulk of administered material, however, remains at the site of injection. Only a small portion of the administered dose is taken up by the regional lymph nodes and reticuloendothelial cells in the liver. The labelling efficiency is high. A small amount of free pertechnetate, presumably from breakdown of labelled particles, is eventually excreted in the urine and can be imaged in the bladder area in some patients.

CLINICAL STUDIES OF CERVICAL LYMPHOSCINTIGRAPHY

Cervical lymphoscintigraphy was largely studied in Europe about 10–15 years ago using [198]Au colloid. Details and critical analysis of many of these studies are not available. Siegl *et al.* reported studies in 62 patients[7] and found 14 normal studies, 15 with increased uptake due to drainage into large lymph nodes from inflammatory foci in the ear, nose, and throat areas and poor uptake in 14 patients with malignancy and 19 patients following radical neck dissection. In 67 patients reported by Fernholz *et al.*[8] most palpable masses were cold to [198]Au, but variable patterns were seen in normal persons and normal uptakes were found in patients with small metastases. Thus they considered that this procedure had only limited clinical value. Zita showed normal scans in all 11 patients with negative lymph nodes whereas 14 abnormal studies had tumour invasion.[9] Of these, only eight had palpable masses. Schwab and Winkel[38] showed ipsilateral lymph node uptake following injection into subcutaneous tissue near the mastoid area. There was no colloid wandering into circulation, thus no accumulation in the liver. Lymph nodes along the internal jugular vein, accessory nerve, supraclavicular area and region of trapezius muscle were frequently visualized. The distribution on both sides was in general symmetrical. Even with hyaluronidase and a delay of 24 hours, about 30–50% of the injected dose was found at the site of injection. Findings in lymphoscintigraphy were identical to those seen in the contrast lymphangiogram. The specific activities in the removed lymph nodes were much higher than that in the fat and muscles.

The sites of injection varied from one laboratory to the other in these early studies. In one study,[8] submucosal injection under the tongue was found superior to other routes. More recently, [198]Au colloid and ^{67}Ga citrate were used simultaneously in a group of 46 patients with head and neck tumours.[40] Tumour uptake was demonstrated in some patients with ^{67}Ga citrate and abnormal lymphatic status was seen in others using [198]Au colloid. The procedures were complementary and provide different types of information concerning pathological processes. Hagio[41] and others studied 54 patients including 33 who had head and neck tumours. Decreased uptake was found in direct proportion to the degree of tumour invasion in regional lymph nodes. Normal patterns were seen in patients with minimal tumour metastases. About one-quarter of patients showed contralateral uptake in the lymph nodes. In this study there was no normal or nearly normal scan in patients who had a previous radical neck dissection. In the early study in Europe,[42] there was no measurable uptake in the cervical lymph nodes following radical neck dissection but some restoration was noted about 12–15 months later.

Using better radiopharmaceuticals, namely ^{99m}Tc minicolloid or antimony colloid, lymph flow was studied in some volunteers.[43] Increased flow can be demonstrated with feeding or mastication. Visualization of regional lymph nodes in a group of 45 patients showed variable distribution following submucosal injection in the oral cavity.[44] Although the average lymph nodes visualized were identical on both sides, the wide variability suggest this procedure is less reliable and clinically useful. In a small pilot series of six patients[45] with minicolloid injected immediately adjacent to the tumour in the oral cavity, no visualization of regional lymph nodes was seen in two

patients with palpable masses due to tumour involvement. Three of four patients with no clinical evidence of lymph node involvement had normal visualization of regional lymph nodes. The regional node in the fourth patient was not visualized although he had 61 negative nodes removed from surgery. Prediction of lymph node metastases was, therefore, reasonably high.

Based on the literature available, a few conclusions can be made from the previous studies on cervical lymphoscintigraphy. Regional lymph nodes can be visualized following injection of labelled particles interstitially near the mastoid or submucosally under the tongue, in the lips or buccal mucosa, or immediately adjacent to the tumor mass. In general, the distribution of lymph nodes is symmetrical on both sides in the normal individual. The number of lymph nodes visualized varies greatly, and appears much less than what is demonstrated in contrast lymphangiography or by the measurement of labelled lymph nodes removed at surgery. Although food and mastication appear to promote lymph flow following mucosal injection of antimony colloid, there is no effective method to promote greater absorption of colloidal particles from the injected sites. The value of hyaluronidase is doubtful. Prolongation of time between time of injection and imaging seems neither to alter the pattern of distribution nor to increase the number of lymph nodes visualized. Practically every investigator has found decreased uptake in lymph nodes involved by tumour, similar to contrast lymphangiography. Increased uptake was seen not only in the hyperplastic lymph nodes secondary to infection but occasionally also in nodes with tumour metastases. Lymph nodes harbouring small foci of tumour usually had a normal pattern of uptake. Crossover to the contralateral side may occur in a small but significant portion of normal individuals. Following radiation therapy or radical neck dissection, marked decrease or even absence of uptake was seen, but partial or complete restoration does take place with the passage of time. Cervical lymphoscintigraphy, therefore, does not have an established role in the management of head and neck tumours.

Forty studies were carried out in our institute using ^{99m}Tc antimony colloid in 37 patients, with bilateral subcutaneous injections of 1 mCi of radiopharmaceutical in 0.1–0.2 ml of volume to the post-auricular areas. Submucosal injections adjacent to the lesion under the tongue were done only in three patients. These 37 patients had pathological confirmation of lymphoma of the tongue in one patient, hyperplasia in another, medullary carcinoma of thyroid in three; the remaining patients had carcinoma with 17 in the tongue, four in the tonsil, four in the larynx, four in the gum, and one each in the ear, nose and parotid gland. Images were obtained 4–6 hours later. Follow-up 24 hours after injection was also done in a few patients. Scans were interpreted based on symmetry and a number of visualized lymph nodes on both sides. Surgically removed lymph nodes at various levels were available for measurement of specific activities in 16 patients. Using findings in physical examination and pathological confirmation, we had a true-positive rate of 57.5%, false-positive rate of 22.5%, false-negative rate of 12.5% and true-negative rate of 7.5%. These findings give a sensitivity of 82%, specificity of 25% and overall accuracy of 72%.

Our findings can be summarized as follows:

(1) Regional lymph nodes can be demonstrated 4–6 hours after subcutaneous or submucosal injection of a small amount of ^{99m}Tc antimony colloid. The pattern and number of visualized nodes are identical with those seen in the delayed images 24 hours later. In normal individuals the distribution appears quite symmetrical on both sides. The number of lymph nodes visualized varies greatly from patient to patient. The bulk of injected material appears to remain at the sites of injection; this interferes with proper imaging and also obscures visualization of lymph nodes near the injection sites. All patients experienced a brief period of sharp pain immediately after injection, lasting only a few seconds. No anaesthetic was necessary for this procedure. No patient refused the second study if it was indicated. There were no other adverse effects in any of our patients.

(2) Most palpable lymph nodes detectable on physical examination appeared as cold lesions in the scans. In most patients the fact that palpable masses were quite sizeable and easily detected made our examination both superfluous and less objective in interpretation. Three patients with palpable neck masses also had abnormal scans, although their lymph nodes were free from metastases on pathological examinations.

(3) Increased uptake can be found not only in patients with hyperplastic lymph nodes secondary to infection but also occasionally in patients with tumour invasion in nodes.

(4) Slight degree of asymmetry may occur in normal individuals because of abundant collateral channels in the neck area; blockage of one may lead flow to the other. Reliance on the assumption of symmetrical distribution and equal numbers of lymph nodes on both sides may be misleading.

(5) Lymph node uptake in general can be seen months or years following radical neck dissection or radiation therapy. Uptake was also seen in some patients who were supposed to have had complete removal of these nodes.

(6) Far fewer lymph nodes are visualized by lymphoscintigraphy than by contrast lymphangiography. The use of a high-sensitivity collimator, which presumably improves the detection rate of nodes with low counts, was found to be unfruitful. Many lymph nodes, normal or abnormal, with low uptake of antimony colloid are far beyond the level of our detectability with currently available equipment.

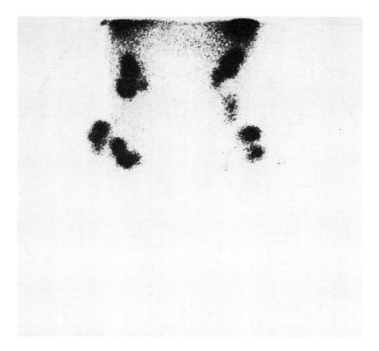

Figure 5.1

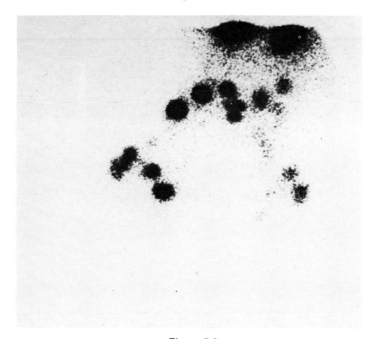

Figure 5.2

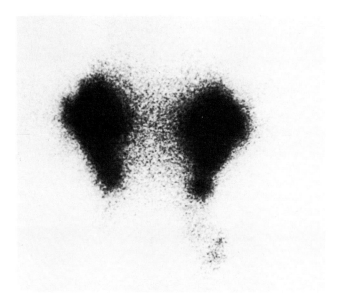

Figure 5.3

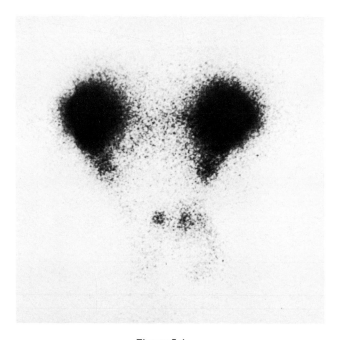

Figure 5.4

Figure 5.5

(7) Lymph nodes removed at surgery about 24 hours following injection showed much higher specific activities in the lymph nodes than the specific activities in the muscle, fat, salivary gland or tumour. Although the percentage of uptake of the dose per gram of tissue varies tremendously from patient to patient and from one lymph node to the other, submandibular and high jugular lymph nodes always had higher specific activities than nodes removed from other levels. The magnitude of the uptake may differ several hundred-fold. Only one of 16 patients studied had higher specific activities in lymph nodes containing tumor than the adjacent normal nodes. Figures 5.1 and 5.2 are examples of normal cervical lymphoscintigraphy. Figure 5.3 illustrates the lymph nodes involvement in the right side of the neck. Figure 5.4 shows lymph node uptake after bilateral radical neck dissection and radiation therapy. Figure 5.5 shows relatively abundant right

cervical nodes, although the palpable mass was cold and lymph nodes involved with tumour showed very low counts.

The advantages of cervical lymphoscintigraphy over contrast lymphangiography can be summarized as follows:

(1) Lymphoscintigraphy is a simple, non-invasive, less time-consuming procedure.
(2) There are no known adverse effects. There is no need for concern about local or systemic side-effects from contrast material or blue dye required for lymphangiography.
(3) No cannulation of small cervical lymphatic channels is required.
(4) The reproducibility is high and failure rate is nil. The sites for injections are flexible and can be tailored according to information sought.
(5) The radiopharmaceutical is more physiological than the contrast material which must be injected under pressure.
(6) Lymphoscintigraphy is a functional

measure of lymphatic patency and normality of the regional nodes. Direction and routes of regional lymphatic drainage can be easily demonstrated.

(7) The radiation dose is negligible when short-lived radionuclide such as ^{99m}Tc label is used.

(8) No anaesthetics or other preparations are required.

Pitfalls of cervical lymphoscintigraphy are many. A few examples are listed below:

(1) It provides no morphological information. It provides no clues as to tissue diagnosis. There is no specific pattern characteristic of specific diseases.

(2) There is great anatomical variability. Interpretation based on the assumption of bilateral symmetry may be misleading.

(3) Efficiency of absorption of the colloid from sites of injection is poor. The bulk of unabsorbed material not only gives a high radiation dose to the local tissue but also jeopardizes imaging procedures, and obscures visualization of neighbouring lymph nodes.

(4) Quantitation based on scan alone is difficult because of different depth levels of the lymph nodes. A large node visualized on the scan may reflect higher concentration of radionuclide in the lymph node, or a relatively large node, or a superficial location.

(5) Only two-dimensional display is possible at present. Because of low levels of uptake of the administered dose in the regional lymph nodes it is unlikely that single photon tomography would be very fruitful for cervical lymphoscintigraphy.

(6) Only a few lymph nodes can be seen in the images. It is unlikely that further improvement of imaging instrumentation will improve the detectability of lymph nodes with low levels of uptake.

(7) There are no anatomical landmarks for precise identification of various node groups, as one has with contrast lymphangiography.

(8) Specific activities in the lymph nodes, normal or abnormal, vary greatly. Hyperplastic lymph nodes may have increased uptake, and tumour-invaded lymph nodes may have either normal or increased uptake compared to neighbouring normal nodes.

(9) All of the radiopharmaceuticals available for lymphoscintigraphy at present which will show absent or decreased uptake in the involved lymph nodes are far less sensitive than the agents which produce increased uptake such as ^{67}Ga citrate or labelled antibodies.

Nevertheless, a few recommendations seem to be justified:

(1) Cervical lymphoscintigraphy is a useful technique for assessing the completeness of radical neck dissection.

(2) It can demonstrate the direction of lymphatic drainage from the tumour and possible crossover to the contralateral side.

(3) It can be used to assess response and recovery following radiation therapy.

(4) It can be used to determine development of new lymphatic channels following radical neck dissection.

(5) It is of no value in determining whether microscopic foci in the regional lymph nodes are present or not. The procedure is probably useless for detection of early metastases in the regional lymph node and is superfluous when physical examination is already positive.

(6) Unless large numbers of patients are studied, and critical evaluations of these procedures are conducted, the role of cervical lymphoscintigraphy in the management of head and neck tumour can never be established. Since this procedure is simple and free from complications, continued investigation, particularly in a

multidisciplinary setting, is certainly in order.

REFERENCES

1. Fisch, U.P., and Sigel, M.E. (1964). Cervical lymphatic system as visualized by lymphography. *Ann. Otol. Rhinol. Laryngol.*, **73**, 869.

2. Dolan, P.A. (1966). Lymphography: complication encountered in 522 examinations. *Radiology*, **86**, 876.

3. Sherman, A.I., and Ter-Pogossian M., (1953). Lymph node concentration of radioactive colloidal gold following interstititial injection. *Cancer*, **6**, 1238.

4. Hultborn, K.A., Larsson, L.G., and Rankult, J. (1955). The lymph drainage from the breast to the axillary and parasternal lymph nodes, studied with the aid of colloidal Au 198. *Acta Radiol*, **43**, 52.

5. Kazem, I., Antoniades, J., Brady, L.W., Faust, D.S., Croll, M.N., and Lightfoot, D. (1968). Clinical evaluation of lymph node scanning utilizing colloidal gold 198. *Radiology*, **90**, 905.

6. Höffer, R., and Benzer, H. (1966). Die indirekte Lymphographie der Lunge. *Radioaktive Isotope in Klinik und Forschung*, **7**, 410.

7. Siegl, H., and Washcher H. (1967). Die Szintigraphie der zervikalen Lymphbahnen. *Mschr. Ohr. Hk.*, **101**, 409.

8. Fernholz, H.J., (1967). Lymphoszintigraphie in Kopf-Hals-Bereich. *Fortschr. Röntgenstr.*, **106**, 524.

9. Zita, G. (1967). Beitrag zur zervikalen Lymphoszintigraphie. *Fortschr. Röntgenstr.*, **107**, 644.

10. Ege, G.N. (1977). Internal mammary lymphoscintigraphy in breast carcinoma: a study of 1072 patients. *Int. J. Radiat. Oncol. Biol. Phys.*, **2**, 755.

11. Whitmore, W.F., Brute, R.D., Kaplan, W.D., and Gittes, R.F. (1980). Radiocolloid scintigraphic mapping of the lymphatic drainage of the prostate. *J. Urol.*, **124**, 62.

12. Yeh, S.d.J., and Benua, R.S. (1980). Preliminary experiences with lymphoscintigraphy in patients with cancer. *Proc. Second Asia & Oceania Congr. Nucl. Med.*, p. 116.

13. Drinkwater, D.C. Jr., Wittnich, C., Bethune, D.C., and Chiu, R.C.J. (1981). Endoscopic gastrointestinal lymphoscintigraphy. *Current Surg.*, **38**, 67.

14. Ege, G.N., and Cummings, B.J. (1980). Interstitial radiocolloid iliopelvic lymphoscintigraphy: Technique, anatomy and clinical application. *Int. J. Radiat. Oncol. Biol. Phys.*, **6**, 1483.

15. Meyer, C.M., Lecklitner, M.L., Logic, J.R., Balch, C.E., Bessey, P.Q., and Tauxe, W.N. (1979). Technetium 99m sulfur colloid cutaneous lymphoscintigraphy in the management of truncal melanoma. *Radiology*, **131**, 205.

16. James, A.E. Jr., Partain, C.L., Holland, G.N., Gore, J.C., Rollo, F.D., Harms, S.E., and Price, R.R. (1981). Nuclear magnetic resonance imaging; the current state. *Am. J. Roentgenol.*, **138**, 201.

17. Teates, C.D., Preston, D.F., and Boyd, C.M. (1980). Gallium 67 citrate imaging in head and neck tumors: report of cooperative group. *J. Nucl. Med.*, **21**, 622.

18. Smith, N.J., Teates, C.D., El-Mahdi, A.M., Fitz-Hugh, G., and Constable, W. (1975). The value of gallium 67 scanning in the evaluation of head and neck malignancy. *Laryngoscope*, **85**, 778.

19. Kashima, H., McKusick, K., Malmed, L., and Wagner, H. (1974). Gallium 67 scanning in patients with head and neck cancer. *Laryngoscope*, **84**, 1078.

20. Ito, Y., Otsuko, N., Nagai, K., Murandka, A., Yonedo, M., Terashimo, H., and Yanagiomoto, S. (1982). Lymphoscintigraphy by SC injection of 67 GA citrate. *Europ. J. Nucl. Med.*, **7**, 260.

21. Mach, J.P., Buchegger, F., Forni, M., Ritschard, J., Berche, C., Lumbroso, J.D., Schreyer, M., Girardet, C., Accolla, R.S., and Carrel, S. (1981). Use of radiolabelled monoclonal anti-CEA antibodies for the detection of human carcinoma by external photoscanning and tomoscintigraphy. *Immunology Today*, **2**, 239.

22. Sfakianakis, G.N., and DeLand, F.H. (1982). Radioimmunodiagnosis and radioimmunotherapy, 1982. *J. Nucl. Med.*, **23**, 840.

23. Hoffer, P.B., and Gottschalk, A., (1974). Tumor scanning agents. *Semin. Nucl. Med.*, **4**, 305.

24. Order, S.E., Bloomer, W.D., Jones, A.G., Kaplan, W.D., Davis, M.A., Adelstein, S.J., and Hellman, S. (1975). Radionuclide immunoglobulin lymphangiography: a case report. *Cancer*, **35**, 1487.

25. DeLand, F.H., Kim, E.E., and Goldenberg, D.M. (1980). Lymphoscintigraphy with radionuclide labeled antibodies to carcinoembryonic antigen. *Cancer Res.*, **40**, 2997.

26. Winkel, K. (1972). *Lymphologie mit Radionukliden*. H. Hoffmann, Berlin.

27. Hollander, W., Reilly, P., and Durrows, B.A. (1961). Lymphatic flow in human subjects as indicated by disappearance of I-131 labeled albumin from the subcutaneous tissue. *J. Clin. Invest.*, **40**, 222.

28. Goodwin, D.A., Finston, R.A., Colombetti, L.G., Beaver, J.E., and Hupf, H. (1978). 111 In for imaging: lymph node visualization. *Radiology*, **94**, 175.

29. Khaw, B.A., Fallon, J.T., Strauss, H.W., and Haber, E. (1980). Myocardial infarct imaging of antibodies to canine cardiac myosin with indium 111 diethylenetriamine pentacetic acid. *Science*, **209**, 295.

30. Hauser, W., Atkins, H.L., and Richard, P. (1960). Lymph node scanning with 99mTc sulfur colloid. *Radiology*, **92**, 1369.

31. Nagai, K., Ito, Y., Otsuka, N., and Muranaka, A. (1982). Deposition of small 99mTc labelled colloid in bone marrow and lymph nodes. *Europ. J. Nucl. Med.*, **7**, 66.

32. Terui, S., Kato, H., Hirashima. T., Iizuka, T., and Oyamada, H. (1982). An evaluation of the mediastinal lymphoscintigram for carcinoma of the esophagus studied with 99mTc rhenium sulfur colloid. *Europ. J. Nucl. Med.*, **7**, 99.

33. Alavi, A., Staum, M.M., Shesol, B.F., and Bloch, P.H. (1978). Technetium 99m stannous phytate as an imaging agent for lymph nodes. *J. Nucl. Med.*, **19**, 422.

34. Osborne, M.P., Jeyasingh, K., Jewkes, R.F., and Burn, I. (1979). The preoperative detection of internal mammary lymph node metastases in breast cancer. *Brit. J. Surg.*, **66**, 813.

35. Ege, G.N., and Warbick, A. (1979). Lymphoscintigraphy: a comparison of 99mTc antimony sulphide colloid and 99Tc m stannous phytate. *Brit. J. Radiol.*, **52**, 124.

36. Kaplan, W.D., David, M.A., and Rose, C.M. (1979). Comparison of two technetium 99m labeled radiopharmaceuticals for lymphoscintigraphy. *J. Nucl. Med.*, **20**, 933.

37. Osborne, M.P., Richardson, V.J., Jeyasingh, K., and Ryman, B.E. (1979). Radionuclide labelled liposomes, a new lymph node imaging agent. *Int. J. Nucl. Med. Biol.*, **6**, 75.

38. Schwab, W., and Winkel, K. (1967). Der gegenwärtige Stand der Szintigraphie des zervikalen Lymphsystems. *Nucl. Med.*, **6**, 234.

39. Schwab, W., Scheer, K.E., and Winkel, K. (1964). Szintigraphie des zervikalen Lymphsystems nach radikaler Halslymphknotenausräumung. *Nucl. Med.*, **4**, 326.

40. Kessler, L., Tölle, D., and Franke, W.G. (1981). Nachweis maligner Halslymphknotenverränderungen mit Hilfe der Szintigraphie. *Laryngol. Rhinol.*, **60**, 299.

41. Hagio, R. (1963). Studies on the cervical lymph flow with radioisotope 198Au before and after the radical neck dissection. *Otologia Fukuoka*, **9**, 76.

42. Siegl, H. (1968). Szintigraphie der Kollaren Lymphbahnen nach 'neck dissection'. *Mschr. Ohr. Hk.*, **102**, 262.

43. Thommesen, P., and Jensen, F.T. (1979). Food stimulated lymph flow in the neck region. *Lymphology*, **12**, 108.

44. Thommesen, P., Buhl, J., Jansen, K., and Funch-Jensen, P. (1981). Lymphoscintigraphy in the head and neck in normals diagnostic value. *RöFo*, **134**, 80.

45. Parell, G.J., Becker, G.D., and Simpson, G.T. (1981). Prediction of lymph node metastases by lymphoscintigraphy of the neck after peri-cancer injection of a radiocolloid. Otolaryngol. *Head Neck Surg.*, **89**, 67.

46. Yeh, S.D.J., Cheung, D., Strong, E., and Benud, R.S. *Cervical Lymphoscintigraphy* (in preparation).

Chapter 6

Circulating Markers

Muhyi Al-Sarraf
Department of Oncology, Wayne State University, School of Medicine, Detroit, Michigan, USA.

INTRODUCTION

Many markers, like carcinoembryonic antigen (CEA),[1,2] α-fetoprotein (AFP),[3,4] β_2-microglobulin,[5] serum enzymes,[4] and acute phase proteins such as α_1-antitrypsin and α_1-acid glycoprotein, have been investigated as tumour markers. These substances are known to decrease with the decrease in tumour burden secondary to successful therapy.

Tumour markers have been identified and reported to be elevated in patients with head and neck cancer. Some studies have suggested correlations between the levels of circulating tumour markers, the extent of disease, and the clinical status of these patients.

Carcinoembryonic Antigens (CEA)

Plasma CEA levels have been reported to be elevated in patients with cancers of both entodermal and non-entodermal origin, as well as in patients with inflammatory and benign conditions, and in chronic cigarette smokers.

CEA levels have been investigated in patients with various stages of head and neck cancers[6-8] (Table 6.1). Silverman *et al.*[7] studied CEA in patients with epidermoid cancer of the head and neck, healthy smokers, and in non-smokers. Among 113 tumour-bearing patients, 36% had CEA levels

exceeding 5 mg/ml but only 17% exceeded 7 mg/ml. Both the incidence and level of CEA elevations correlated with the clinical stage of the cancer. The highest incidence of elevated levels occurred in patients with locally advanced cancer (Stage IV) or patients with distant involvement. Patients with elevated CEA concentrations before radical surgery had CEA elevations return to normal 1 month after operation. Of 14 patients with recurrent cancer, only four had elevated CEA levels at the time of the recurrences.

Schneider *et al.*[8] reported that 40/85 patients with head and neck cancers had levels above 5 ng/ml, but no difference was found between site or stage of the disease and the level of elevated CEA.

In 57 patients with head and neck cancer, Amiel *et al.*[9] reported 21% had elevated values of CEA (>10 ng/ml). No relationship was reported between the tumour site or stage and the incidence of elevated CEA.

Serial determinations of CEA have been used to monitor response to therapy in patients with gastrointestinal malignancies.[2] Direct correlation between CEA elevation and tumour burden has been documented.

In investigating the levels of CEA in patients with previously untreated locally advanced

TABLE 6.1   INCIDENCE OF ELEVATED CEA LEVELS IN
PATIENTS WITH HEAD AND NECK CANCERS

Authors	No. tested	Percent CEA		
		>5 ng/ml	>7 ng/ml	>10 ng/ml
Silverman et al.[7]				
Stage I	28	35	19	—
Stage II	40	20	5	—
Stage III	60	35	12	—
Stage IV	40	50	33	—
Distant	10	50	30	—
Schneider et al.[8]	85	47	—	—
Amiel et al.[9]	57	—	—	21
Al-Sarraf et al.[10,11]				
Untreated	25	32	—	—
Recurrent	17	53	—	—

TABLE 6.2   CORRELATIONS OF THE CLINICAL
RESPONSE TO THERAPY AND THE
CHANGE IN CEA VALUE

Response	Elevated CEA		Change*		
	Pre-therapy	Post-therapy	↓	=	↑
CR + PR	13/21	8/21	8	9	4
NC	5/5	5/5	—	4	1
ID	9/9	9/9	—	3	6

* 25% increase or decrease of the pre-therapy value.

epidermoid cancer of the head and neck, 20/25 (80%) and 8/25 (32%) had elevated levels above 2.5 ng/ml and 5 ng/ml respectively. In patients with recurrent disease, 14/17 (82%) and 9/17 (53%) had levels above 2.5 ng/ml and 5 ng/ml respectively.[10,11] We did not find differences in CEA values as a function of either primary site or morphology of the epidermoid cancers. CEA levels correlated with response to therapy in patients with previously untreated cancers and in patients with recurrent head and neck tumours (Table 6.2).

Glycoproteins

Many circulating glycoproteins, especially those considered as acute phase proteins (haptoglobin, α_1-antitrypsin, and α_1-acid glycoprotein) have been investigated in various cancer patients and controls. The major synthesis of these proteins is hepatic; however, production of the glycoproteins by human tumours xenotransplanted in nude mice has also been described.[12]

Significant increases in serum concentrations of α_1-acid glycoprotein, α_1-antitrypsin, and haptoglobin have been reported in advanced breast, lung, prostate, ovarian, hepatic and head and neck cancers.[13–21]

Wolf et al.[22] studied six proteins (haptoglobin, α_1-antitrypsin, α_1-acid glycoprotein, α_2-HS glycoprotein, pre-albumin, and albumin) in patients with head and neck cancers and in controls. Of the six proteins investigated, the levels of α_1-antitrypsin were significantly increased and the pre-albumin values decreased in chronic smokers as compared to non-smokers. The median levels of α_1-antitrypsin and α_1-acid glycoprotein increased progressively with increasing tumour stage and there were significant correlations between these protein values and the tumour stage. The concentrations of α_2-HS-glycoprotein, pre-albumin, and albumin were significantly lower in the head and neck cancer patients than in the normal subjects. Haptoglobin levels were significantly elevated in patients with Stage I to Stage IV tumours, but the values were similar for each stage. There were no significant differences in the serum levels of these six proteins and the tumour site. Among cured patients, the values of haptoglobin and α_1-acid glycoprotein levels were significantly lower than the levels in untreated patients, but were still higher than the levels in normal controls. Conversely, α_2-HS-glycoprotein and pre-albumin concentrations were significantly higher in cured patients than in untreated patients and did not differ from the values in normal subjects. α_1-Antitrypsin level did not differ significantly between untreated patients and normal subjects.

We have found the α_1-acid glycoprotein to be elevated in 13/25 (52%) patients with previously untreated epidermoid cancer of the head and neck and in 12/17 (70%) patients with recurrent disease.[10,11] No differences were found between the site of tumour differentiation and the incidence of elevated value of this glycoprotein. We found good correlation between the response to therapy and the incidence and level of elevations of α_1-acid glycoprotein (Table 6.3).

Patients with epidermoid cancer of the head and neck have impaired cellular immunity.[23-26] Concurrent with these demonstrations of impaired cellular immunity, sera from these patients have been shown to suppress cellular immune reactions *in vitro*.[27,28] Further analysis of the sera from these patients revealed elevation of specific glycoproteins (haptoglobin, α_1-antitrypsin, and α_1-acid glycoprotein)[13] which in other investigations suppressed *in vitro* immune reaction.[29-31] Serum levels of these glycoproteins have been correlated inversely with *in vivo* and *in vitro* parameters of cellular immunity.[20,32]

These findings suggest that serum levels of specific glycoproteins may be useful in assessing immune reactivity, tumour extent, and response to therapy.

Polyamines

The naturally occurring aliphatic polyamines – putrescine, spermidine, and spermine – are found in all types of cells. Polyamines were found to be elevated in patients with malignant diseases and may have potential value as tumour markers.[33-36] Polyamine level measurements have been made in urine specimens, CSF, plasma, and erythrocytes. Erythrocyte polyamine levels have been found to be increased in patients with advanced stages of disease and there is evidence to indicate that the levels decrease with response to treatment.[37,38]

Shideler *et al.*[39] in 1981 reported on the values of erythrocyte polyamines in patients with untreated head and neck cancers. They reported that 9/29 (31%) had elevated erythrocyte spermidine and/or spermine. Also, a positive correlation was observed between the erythrocyte spermidine levels and the stage of the tumour. In 11/12 patients the erythrocyte spermidine levels decreased after tumour therapy regardless of the pretreatment level. The erythrocyte spermine levels in these patients were more variable in their response to therapy.

Immune Complexes

Immune complexes have been found in many patients with cancers and other non-malignant diseases. Using the Raji cell test, Maxim *et al.*[40] found that immune complexes are present in over 80% of the patients with head and neck cancers as compared to less than 10% in nor-

TABLE 6.3   CORRELATIONS OF CLINICAL RESPONSE TO THERAPY AND THE CHANGE IN α_1-ACID GLYCOPROTEIN (AAG)

| Response | Elevated AAG | | Change* | | |
	Pre-therapy	Post-therapy	↓	=	↑
CR + PR	12/18	0/18	17	1	—
NC	1/3	0/3	—	3	—
ID	5/7	5/7	1	4	2

* 25% increase or decrease of the pre-therapy value.

mal control sera. These complexes persisted following treatment of these patients by surgery or radiation therapy. Others have confirmed the elevated levels of soluble immune complexes found in patients with epidermoid cancer of the head and neck.[41]

Alkaline Phosphatase

Katz *et al.*[42] reported on patients with previously untreated epidermoid cancer of the head and neck who were initially treated with chemotherapy; responses were noted more frequently in patients with elevated alkaline phosphatase levels (90%) as compared to the response rate in patients with normal alkaline phosphatase levels (50%).

Burres *et al.*[43] have recently reported on the level of alkaline phosphatase in 101 previously untreated head and neck cancer patients who were treated first by chemotherapy. The level of alkaline phosphatase was not significantly different among various tumour sites, and did not depend on tumour differentiation or response to chemotherapy. Similarly other reports[44] have not confirmed a correlation between the level of alkaline phosphatase and response to chemotherapy.

Immunoglobulins

IgA

Levels of IgA in saliva and serum are the humoral immune parameters most extensively investigated in smokers. Compared to non-smokers and patients with tumours of other histological types, serum and salivary IgA levels are elevated in chronic smokers and patients with epidermoid cancers of the head and neck.

IgA levels in salivary secretions of patients with oral cancer have been abnormal when compared to serum levels.[45,46] Serum IgA levels are increased in patients with nasopharyngeal cancer[47] and other head and neck cancers.[48,49] Brown *et al.*[45] studied the saliva and sera of patients with epidermoid cancer of the oral cavity – untreated, recurrent cancers, cured patients, and matched con-

trols. Primary oral and laryngeal cancer patients had two-fold increase of serum and salivary IgA compared to controls. Recurrent patients had even greater elevations of salivary IgA. Cured patients showed a persistent elevation of serum but a return to normal of salivary IgA.

HSVIA

Epidermoid cancer of the head and neck has been associated with herpes simplex virus (HSV) in epidemiological and serological studies.

Antibodies to a labile non-virion antigen, induced in a human tissue culture cell line by HSV, were elevated in patients with epidermoid cancer of the head and neck as compared with patients with non-epidermoid malignant lesions and normal adults.[50]

IgA antibodies to HSVIA were detected six times more frequently in the sera of smokers than in non-smoker controls.[51] Higher frequency of IgA anti-HSVIA, as well as titres of the antibody and the number of years smoking were higher in smokers who drank alcoholic beverages than in smokers who did not drink.[51]

Direct immunofluorescence studies have shown an increase in serum levels of IgA with specificity for HSV-induced antigens in chronic smokers; these levels are still higher in patients with head and neck epidermoid cancers.

Antibodies to a labelled, non-structural antigen of HSV were elevated in a large percentage of the patients with epidermoid cancers (61%) and in the heavy smokers (57%), but they were elevated in only small percentages of patients with other types of non-epidermoid cancer (11%) and non-smokers (8%).[52] Titres were higher in patients with epidermoid cancer than in smokers.

Smith *et al.* and others[52,53] correlated the extent of disease with the PHA lymphocyte response and the complement-fixing antibody titre to HSV.

EBV-Ab

Halili *et al.*[54] studied the presence of antibody

against Epstein–Barr viral capsid (EBV-VCA) in 65 patients with primary head and neck cancers. They found that 48% had detectable antibody in their sera. A rise in titre within 6 months following radiotherapy was associated with a significant incidence of recurrent disease. Elevation of antibody titres against EBV capsid (EBV-VCA) has been documented in a high percentage of patients with African Burkitt lymphoma and patients with nasopharyngeal cancer.[55,57]

Henderson *et al.*[58] have studied a small group of patients with epidermoid cancers of the hypopharynx and nasal cavity, and have shown that the antibody levels to EBV were elevated to levels similar to those of patients with nasopharyngeal cancer. They also reported elevated titres in patients with epidermoid cancers of the oropharynx and tonsils.[59]

It has also been shown that there is a relationship between antibody activity and the clinical stage of the disease or tumour burden in patients with Burkitt lymphoma and nasopharyngeal cancer.[57,60,61]

Ig Allotypes

Another group of genetic markers to which less attention has been paid in the relationship to disease association are Ig allotypes. The Gm antigens of IgG are inherited as a group with characteristic combinations for different races.

Ockhuizen *et al.*[62] recently reported on the Gm A_2m and Km allotypic markers in 40 patients with epidermoid cancers of the head and neck. Serum IgA levels, the A_2m[1] allotypic marker and antibodies against IgA1, A_2m[1] and A_2m[2] were measured quantitatively. The frequency of K_m[1] was reported to be significantly increased in patients with head and neck cancer as compared to the control population.

NASOPHARYNGEAL CANCER

EBV-Ab

The Epstein–Barr virus is a lymphocytotrophic herpes virus in man which has generally been accepted as the causative agent of infectious mononucleosis. The virus was first demonstrated in cell lines established from Burkitt's lymphoma,[63] and there is adequate documentation that EBV is associated with that disease.[64] Serological studies have shown that nasopharyngeal carcinoma (NPC) is also associated with EBV-specific IgA antibodies from different geographical locations of the world.[64–68] These patients have increased IgA antibody levels, higher than with other head and neck cancers,[56,58,69–74] which decline to low levels after treatment of the tumour.[47,65,67]

Seroepidemiological studies have shown that:

(1) significant high specific anti-EBV antibody titres are present in about 45% of Stage I NPC and in 100% of Stage IV;[56]

(2) patients with epidermoid cancers and lymphoepithelioma of the nasopharynx have elevated titres.[72,73]

The results from immunological investigations suggest that antibodies to some of the EBV-associated antigens might be of clinical importance in the diagnosis and prognosis of NPC. Levels of antibodies to the EBV-induced early antigen complex (EA) tend to increase with stage of the disease.[57,75] This is particularly true of the Ab response to the D component of this complex. Antibodies to other EBV-associated antigens also vary with stage of the disease, but these differences are not as striking as these noted with EA.[75]

Pearson *et al.*[76] reported that high Ab titres to EBV-induced early antigen complex and the presence of antibody to EBV-Ag in the IgA immunoglobulin fraction were the two most specific discriminating parameters in American patients with NPC. However, occasional patients with malignancies other than head and neck cancers or lymphoma also showed high anti-EA titres.

Glycoproteins

Baskies *et al.*[77] reported that elevated titres to EBV-associated antigens were related to tumour presence but not significantly related to clinical tumour stage. Compared with the levels in normal subjects, serum levels of acute phase proteins (haptoglobin, α_1-acid glycoprotein, and α_1-antitrypsin) were significantly increased in patients with nasopharyngeal cancer, while the values of α_2-HS-glycoprotein were significantly decreased. Serum levels of the acute phase proteins, particularly haptoglobin, were directly related to clinical NPC stage.

CONCLUSIONS

Many tumour markers have been reported in patients with head and neck cancers. The high levels and incidence of certain circulating markers in these patients are of interest. However, their usefulness as an aid in diagnosis remains doubtful since these tumours are easily accessible for direct or indirect visualization. The importance of these marker studies is derived from the need for more precise methods for the assessment of tumour extent, stage, and response to therapy. It appears that the levels of several markers may be useful in predicting the effect of therapy, but the value of such monitoring needs to be further evaluated and established.

REFERENCES

1. Kithier, K., Al-Sarraf, M., and Cejka, J. (1972). Tumor specific antigen (CEA) in tumor extracts and urine from cancer patients. In *Embryonic and Fetal Antigens in Cancer* (Eds Anderson, Coggin, Cole and Holleman), Oak Ridge National Laboratory, Oak Ridge, Tennessee, vol. 2, pp. 225–234.
2. Al-Sarraf, M., Baker, L., Talley, R.W., Kithier, K., and Vaitkevicius, V.K. (1979). The value of serial carcinoembryonic antigen (CEA) in predicting response rate and survival of patients with gastrointestinal cancer treated with chemotherapy – a Southwest Oncology Group Study. *Cancer*, **44**, 1222–1225.
3. Al-Sarraf, M., Kithier, K., Vaitkevicius, V.K., and Poulik, M.D. (1972). Alpha-fetoprotein (AFP) in human tumors. In *Embryonic and Fetal Antigens in Cancer* (Eds Anderson, Coggin, Cole and Holleman), Oak Ridge National Laboratory, Oak Ridge, Tennessee, vol. 2, pp. 309–316.
4. Al-Sarraf, M., Go, T., Kithier, K., and Vaitkevicius, V.K. (1974). Primary liver cancer: a review of the clinical features, blood groups, serum enzymes, therapy and survival, of 65 cases. *Cancer*, **33**, 547–582.
5. Kithier, K., Cejka, J., Belamaric, J., Al-Sarraf, M., Peterson, W.D., Vaitkevicius, V.K., and Poulik, M.D. (1974). β_2-Microglobulin: occurrence in fetal life and malignancy. *Clin. Chim. Acta*, **52**, 293–299.
6. Meeker, W.R., Jr., Kashmiri, R., Hunter, L., Clapp, W., and Griffin, W.O., Jr. (1973). Clinical evaluation of carcinoembryonic antigen test. *Arch. Surg.*, **107**, 266–274.
7. Silverman, N.A., Alexander, J.C., Jr., and Chretien, P.B. (1976). CEA levels in head and neck cancer. *Cancer*, **37**, 2204–2211.
8. Schneider, M., Demard, F., Chauvel, P., Gueguen, J., Vallicioni, J., Krebs, B.P., and Ramaioli, A. (1970). Carcinoembryonic antigen determinations in head and neck cancer. In *Clinical Application of Carcinoembryonic Antigen* (Eds B.P. Krebs, C.M. Lalanne, and M. Schneider), Excerpta Medica, Amsterdam–Oxford, pp. 384–387.
9. Amiel, J.L., Henry, R., Van der Brouch, C., Pico, J.L., Meriadec, B., and Froz, J.P. (1976). L'antigene embryonnaire dans le tumeurs de la tete et du cou. *Bull. Cancer (Paris)*, **63**, 519–524.
10. Al-Sarraf, M., Chu, C.Y.-T., Lai, L., Carey, M.K., and Drelichman, A. (1981). Multiple tumor markers in monitoring patients with epidermoid cancer of the head and neck. *Proc. Am. Assoc. Cancer Res.*, **22**, 285.
11. Al-Sarraf, M., Chu, C.Y.-T., Lai, L., and Carey, M.K. (1981). Tumor markers in patients with epidermoid cancer of the head and neck and the effect of therapy. *Head and Neck Surg.*, **3**, 346.
12. Yoshimura, S., Tamaoki, N., Veyama, Y., and Hata, J. (1978). Plasma protein production by human tumors xenotransplanted in nude mice. *Cancer Res.*, **38**, 3474–3478.
13. Bradley, W.P., Blasco, A.P., Weiss, J.F., Alexander, J.C., Silverman, N.A., and Chretien, P.B. (1977). Correlations among serum protein bound carbohydrates, serum glycoproteins, lymphocyte reactivity and tumor burden in cancer patients. *Cancer*, **40**, 2264–2272.
14. Cowen, D.M., Searle, F., Ward, A.M., Benson, E.A., Smiddy, F.G., Eaves, G., and Cooper, E.H. (1978). Multivariate biochemical indicators of breast cancer: An evaluation of

their potential in routine practice. *Eur. J. Cancer*, **14**, 885–893.

15. Seal, U.S., Doe, R.P., Byar, D.P., and Corle, D.K., and VA Cooperative Urological Research Group (1978). Response of serum haptoglobin to hormone treatment and the relation of pretreatment values to mortality in patients with prostatic cancer. *Cancer*, **42**, 1720–1729.

16. Newman, C.E., Ford, C.H.J., Kalsheker, N., Bradwell, A.R., and Burnett, D. (1978). Prognostic value of serum proteins in lung cancer. *Proc. Br. Assoc. Cancer Res.*, **38**, 172.

17. Chio, L.-F., and Oon, C.J. (1979). Changes in serum α_1 antitrypsin, α_1 acid glycoprotein and β_2 glycoprotein in patients with malignant hepatocellular carcinoma. *Cancer*, **43**, 596–604.

18. Mueller, W.K., Handschumacher, R., and Wade, M.E. (1971). Serum haptoglobin in patients with ovarian malignancies. *Obstet. Gynecol.*, **38**, 427–435.

19. Harris, C.C., Primack, A., and Cohen, M.H. (1974). Elevated α_1 antitrypsin serum levels in lung cancer patients. *Cancer*, **34**, 280–281.

20. Baskies, A.M., Chretien, P.B., Weiss, J.F., Makuch, R.W., Beveridge, R.A., Catalona, W.J., and Spiegel, H.E. (1980). Serum glycoproteins in cancer patients: First report of correlation with in vitro and in vivo parameters of cellular immunity. *Cancer*, **45**, 3050–3060.

21. Snyder, S., and Ashwell, G. (1971). Quantitation of specific serum glycoproteins in malignancy. *Clin. Chim. Acta*, **34**, 449–455.

22. Wolf, G.T., Chretien, P.B., Elias, E.G., Makuch, R.W., Baskies, A.M., Spiegel, H.E., and Weiss, J.F. (1979). Serum glycoproteins in head and neck squamous carcinoma. Correlations with tumor extent, clinical tumor stage and T-cell levels during chemotherapy. *Am. J. Surg.*, **138**, 489–500.

23. Eilber, F.R., Morton, D.L., and Ketcham, A.S. (1974). Immunologic abnormalities in head and neck cancer. *Am. J. Surg.*, **128**, 534–538.

24. Lundy, J., Wanebo, H., Pinsky, C., Strong, E.W., and Oettgen, H. (1974). Delayed hypersensitivity reactions in patients with squamous cell carcinoma of the head and neck. *Am. J. Surg.*, **128**, 530–533.

25 Wanebo, H.J., Jun, M.Y., Strong, E.W., and Oettgen, H.F. (1975). T-cell deficiency in patients with squamous cell cancer of the head and neck. *Am. J. Surg.*, **130**, 445–451.

26. Jenkins, V.K., Ray, P., Ellis, H.N., Griffiths, C.M., Perry, R.R., and Olson, M.H. (1976). Lymphocyte response in patients with head

and neck cancer. *Arch. Otolaryngol.*, **102**, 596–600.

27. Sample, W.F., Gertner, H.R., and Chretien, P.B. (1971). Inhibition of phytohemagglutinin-induced *in vitro* lymphocyte transformation by serum from patients with carcinoma. *J. Nat. Cancer Inst.*, **46**, 1291–1297.

28. Catalona, W.J., Sample, W.F., and Chretien, P.B. (1973). Lymphocyte reactivity in cancer patients: Correlation with tumor histology and clinical stage. *Cancer*, **31**, 65–71.

29. Arora, P., Miller, H.C., and Aronson, L.D. (1978) α_1-Antitrypsin is an effector of immunological statis. *Nature*, **274**, 589–590.

30. Israel, L., Edelstein, R., and Samak, R. (1978). *In vitro* depression of lymphocyte response to PHA by acute phase reactants. *Proc. Am. Assoc. Cancer Res.*, **19**, 10.

31. Harvey, H., Lipton, A., Sraa, D.A., Albright, C., DeLong, S., and Davidson, E.A. (1978). Inhibition of *in vitro* lymphocyte function by α_1-acid glycoprotein, tumor related glycoprotein and fibrinogen degradation products. *Proc. Am. Assoc. Cancer Res.*, **19**, 10.

32. Baskies, A.M., Chretien, P.B., Weiss, J.F., Beveridge, R.A., Makuch, R.W., Trahan, E.E., and Catalona, W.J. (1978). Serum levels of α_2 HS-glycoprotein and acute phase proteins correlate with cellular immunity in cancer patients. *Proc. Am. Assoc. Cancer Res.*, **19**, 221.

33. Russell, D.H., Levy, C.C., Schimpff, C.C., and Hawk, I.A. (1971). Urinary polyamines in cancer patients. *Cancer Res.*, **31**, 1555–1558.

34. Waalkes, T.P., Gehrke, C.W., Tormey, D.C., Zumwalt, R.W., Hueser, J.N., Kuo, K.C., Lakings, D.B., Ahmann, D.L., and Moertel, C.G. (1975). Urinary excretion of polyamines by patients with advanced malignancy. *Cancer Chemo. Rep.*, **59**, 1103–1116.

35. Lipton, A., Sheehan, L., Mortel, R., and Harvey, H.A. (1976). Urinary polyamine levels in patients with localized malignancy. *Cancer*, **38**, 1344–1347.

36. Russell, D.H. (1977). Clinical relevance of polyamines as biochemical markers of tumor kinetics. *Clin. Chem.*, **23**, 22–27.

37. Savory, J., Shipe, J.R., and Wills, M.R. (1979). Polyamines in blood cells as cancer markers. *Lancet*, **2**, 1136–1137.

38. Cooper, K.E., Shukla, J.B., and Rennert, O.M. (1978). Polyamine compartmentalization in various human disease states. *Clin. Chim. Acta*, **82**, 1–7.

39. Shideler, C.E., Johns, M.E., Cantrell, R.W., Shipe, J.R., Wills, M.R., and Savory, J. (1981). Erythrocyte polyamine determination

in patients with head and neck cancer. *Arch. Otolaryngol.*, **107**, 752–754.

40. Maxim, P.E., Veltri, R.W., Sprinkle, P.M., and Pusateri, R.J. III. (1978). Soluble immune complexes in sera from head and neck cancer patients: a preliminary report. *Otolaryngology*, **86**, 428–432.

41. Veltri, R.W., Rodman, S.M., Sprinkle, P.M., and Quick, C. (1980). Circulating soluble immune complexes and immunodepression in patients with squamous cell carcinoma of the head and neck. *Proc. Amer. Assoc. Cancer Res.*, **21**, 235.

42. Katz, A.E., Hong, W.-K., Bhutani, R., Berman, L.D., Blanchard, G.J., Koff, R.S., Shapshay, S.M., and Strong, M.S. (1980). Prognostic indicators in chemotherapy for head and neck carcinoma: alkaline phosphatase levels. *Laryngoscope*, **90**, 924–929.

43. Barres, S.A., Jacobs, J.R., Peppard, S.B., and Al-Sarraf, M. (1982). Significance of alkaline phosphatase and chemotherapy for head and neck carcinoma. *Otolaryngol. Head Neck Surg.*, **90**, 188–192.

44. Coker, D.O., Morris, D., Elias, E.G., Didolker, M.S., and Zantai, T.A. (1982). Head and neck cancer. Relationship of the pre-chemotherapy serum alkaline phosphatase levels to response rate of induction chemotherapy. *Arch. Otolaryngol.*, **108**, 28–29.

45. Brown, A.M., Lally, E.T., Frankel, A., Harwick, R., Davis, L.W., and Rominger, C.J. (1975). The association of the IgA levels of serum and whole saliva with the progression of oral cancer. *Cancer*, **35**, 1154–1162.

46. Mandel, M.A., Dvorak, K., and DeCosse, J.J. (1973). Salivary immunoglobulins in patients with oropharyngeal and bron-chopulmonary carcinoma. *Cancer*, **31**, 1408–1413.

47. Wara, W.M., Wara, D.W., Phillips, T.L., and Ammann, A.J. (1975). Elevated IgA in carcinoma of the nasopharynx. *Cancer*, **35**, 1313–1315.

48. Katz, A.E., Yoo, T.J., and Harker, L.A. (1976). Serum immunoglobulin A (IgA) levels in carcinoma of the head and neck. *Trans. Am. Acad. Ophthalmol. Otolaryngol.*, **82**, 131–137.

49. Hughes, N.R. (1971). Serum concentrations of γG, γA and γM immunoglobulins in patients with carcinoma, malanoma, and sarcoma. *J. Nat. Cancer Inst.*, **46**, 1015–1028.

50. Hollinshead, A.C., Lee, O., Chretien, P.B., Tarpley, J.L., Rawls, W.E., and Adam, E. (1973). Antibodies to Herpes virus nonvirion antigens in squamous carcinomas. *Science*, **182**, 713.

51. Smith, H.G., Horowitz, N., Silverman, N.A., Henson, D.E., and Chretien, P.B. (1976). Humoral immunity to herpes simplex viral-induced antigens in smokers. *Cancer*, **38**, 1155–1162.

52. Smith, H.G., Chretien, P.B., Henson, D.E., Silverman, N.A., and Alexander, J.C. (1976). Viral-specific humoral immunity to Herpes-induced antigens in patients with squamous carcinoma of the head and neck. *Am. J. Surg.*, **132**, 541–548.

53. Silverman, N.A., Alexander, J.C., Jr., Hollinshead, A.C., and Chretien, P.B. (1976). Correlation of tumor burden with *in vitro* lymphocyte reactivity and anti-bodies to Herpes virus tumor-associated antigens in head and neck squamous carcinoma. *Cancer*, **37**, 135–140.

54. Halili, M.R., Spigland, I., Foster, N., and Ghossein, N.A.A. (1978). Epstein–Barr virus (EBV) antibody in patients treated by radical radiotherapy for head and neck cancer. *J. Surg. Oncol.*, **10**, 457–463.

55. DeSchryver, A., Friberg, S., Jr., Klein, G., Henle, G., Henle, W., DeThé, G., Clifford, P., and Ho, H.C. (1969). Epstein–Barr virus (EBV) associated antibody patterns in carcinoma of the post-nasal space. *Clin. Exp. Immunol.*, **5**, 443–459.

56. Henle, W., Henle, G., Ho, H.C., Burtu, P., Cachin, Y., Clifford, P., Schryver, A., DeThé, G., Diehl, V., and Klein, G. (1970). Antibodies to Epstein–Barr virus in nasopharyngeal carcinoma, other head and neck neoplasms and control groups. *J. Nat. Cancer Inst.*, **44**, 225–231.

57. Henle, W., Ho, H.-C., Henle, G., and Kwan, H.C. (1973). Antibodies to Epstein–Barr virus related antigens in nasopharyngeal carcinoma. Comparison of active cases with long term survivors. *J. Nat. Cancer Inst.*, **51**, 361–369.

58. Henderson, B.E., Louie, E., Bogdanoff, E., Henle, W., Alena, B., and Henle, G. (1974). Antibodies to Herpes group viruses in patients with nasopharyngeal and other head and neck cancers. *Cancer Res.*, **34**, 1207–1210.

59. Henderson, B.E., Louie, E., Jing, J.S.-H., Buell, P., and Gardner, M.B. (1976). Risk factors associated with nasopharyngeal carcinoma. *New Engl. J. Med.*, **295**, 1101–1106.

60. DeSchryver, A., Klein, G., Henle, G., Henle, W., Cameron, H.M., Santesson, L., and Clifford, P. (1972). EB-virus associated serology in malignant disease: Antibody levels to viral capsid antigens (VCA), membrane antigens (MA) and early antigens (EA) in patients with

various neoplastic conditions. *Int. J. Cancer*, **9**, 353–364.

61. Klein, G. (1975). The Epstein–Barr virus and neoplasia. *New Engl. J. Med.*, **293**, 1353–1357.

62. Ockhuizen, T., Pandey, J.P., Veltri, R.W., Arlen, M., and Fudenberg, H.H. (1982). Immunoglobulin allotypes in patients with squamous cell carcinoma of the head and neck. *Cancer*, **49**, 2021–2024.

63. Epstein, M.A., Achong, B.G., and Barr, Y.M. (1964). Virus particles in cultured lymphoblasts from Burkitt's lymphoma. *Lancet*, **1**, 702–703.

64. Henle, G., Henle, W., Klein, G., Gunven, P., Clifford, P., Morrow, R.H., and Ziegler, J.L. (1971). Antibodies to early Epstein–Barr virus induced antigens in Burkitt's lymphoma. *J. Nat. Cancer Inst.*, **46**, 861–871.

65. Henle, G., and Henle, W. (1976). Epstein–Barr virus-specific IgA serum antibodies as an outstanding feature of nasopharyngeal carcinoma. *Int. J. Cancer*, **17**, 1–7.

66. Henderson, B.E., Louie, E.W., Jing, J.S., and Alena, B. (1977). Epstein–Barr virus and nasopharyngeal carcinoma: is there an etiologic relationship? *J. Nat. Cancer Inst.*, **59**, 1393–1395.

67. Henle, W., Ho. H.-C., Henle, G., Chau, J.C.W., and Kwan, H.C. (1977). Nasopharyngeal carcinoma: significance of changes in Epstein–Barr virus-related antibody patterns following therapy. *Int. J. Cancer*, **20**, 663–672.

68. Klein, G. (1973). The Epstein–Barr virus. In *The Herpes Viruses* (Ed. A. Kaplan), Academic Press, New York, pp. 521–555.

69. Vonka, V., Šibl, O., Suchánková, A., Simonová, I., and Závadová, H. (1977). Epstein–Barr virus antibodies in tonsillar carcinoma patients. *Int. J. Cancer*, **19**, 456–459.

70. Lin, T.M., Yang, C.S., Chiou, J.F., Tu, S.M., Lin, C.C., Liu, C.H., Chen, K.P., Ho, Y., Kawamura, A., and Hirayama, T. (1973).

Seroepidemiological studies on carcinoma of the nasal pharynx. *Cancer Res.*, **33**, 2603–2608.

71. Lin, T.M., Yang, C.S., Tu, S.M., Chen, C.H., Kuo, K.C., and Hirayama, T. (1979). Interaction of factors associated with cancer of the nasopharynx. *Cancer*, **44**, 1419–1423.

72. Miller, D., Goldman, J., and Goodman, M. (1971). Etiologic study of nasopharyngeal cancer. *Arch. Otolaryngol.*, **94**, 104–108.

73. Sako, K., Minowada, J., and Marchetta, F.C. (1975). Epstein–Barr virus antibodies in patients with carcinoma of the nasopharynx and carcinoma of other sites in the head and neck. *Am. J. Surg.*, **130**, 437–439.

74. Kottaridis, S.D., Dafnou, M., Besbeas, S., and Garas, J. (1977). Antibodies to Epstein–Barr virus in nasopharyngeal carcinoma and other neoplastic conditions. *J. Nat. Cancer Inst.*, **59**, 89–91.

75. DeThé, G., Ho, J.H.-C., Ablashi, D.V., Day, N.E., Macario, A.J.L., Martin-Berthelou, M.C., Pearson, G., and Sohier, R. (1975). Nasopharyngeal carcinoma. 9. Antibodies to EBNA and correlation with response to other EBV antigens in Chinese patients. *Int. J. Cancer*, **16**, 713–721.

76. Pearson, G.R., Coates, H.L., Neel, H.B., III, Levine, P., Ablashi, D., and Easton, J. (1978). Clinical evaluation of EBV serology in American patients with nasopharyngeal carcinoma. In *Nasopharyngeal Carcinoma: Etiology and Control* (Eds G. DeThé, and Y. Ito), IARC Scientific Publication No. 20, Lyon.

77. Baskies, A.M., Chretien, P.B., Yang, C.-S., Wolf, G.T., Makush, R.W., Tu, S.-M., Hsu, M.-M., Lynn, T.-C., Yang, H.-M., Weiss, J.F., and Spiegel, H.E. (1979). Serum glycoproteins and immunoglobulins in nasopharyngeal carcinoma. Correlations with Epstein–Barr virus associated antibodies and clinical tumor stage. *Am. J. Surg.*, **138**, 478–488.

Chapter 7

Malignancy-associated Hypercalcaemia: Mechanisms and Management

Andrew F. Stewart
Departments of Medicine, West Haven VA Medical Center, West Haven, CT, USA, and Yale University School of Medicine, New Haven, CT, USA.

INTRODUCTION

Malignancy-associated hypercalcaemia (MAHC) is the most common variety of hypercalcaemia encountered among hospitalized patients. Squamous carcinomas, including those of head and neck origin, result in hypercalcaemia with a frequency second only to breast carcinoma.[1-4] Of 50 consecutive patients with MAHC studied at our own institution, 18 (36%) had squamous carcinomas, and six (12%) had a head and neck malignancy.[4] Among patients with head and neck cancer followed longitudinally through the course of their disease, the incidence of hypercalcaemia has been reported by Ariyan *et al.*[5] to be as high as 20%. Thus, any physician caring for patients with malignancies involving the upper airways will encounter a substantial number of patients with hypercalcaemia.

Hypercalcaemia may lead to depression, lethargy, constipation, muscular weakness, polyuria, dehydration, renal failure, abdominal pain, cardiac conduction disturbances, coma, and ultimately death. Because of these complications, rapid and accurate diagnosis and treatment of MAHC are important. This review will focus on (1) the mechanisms responsible for causing hypercalcaemia in patients with cancer; (2) methods now available for diagnosing malignancy-associated hypercalcaemia, and for distinguishing this syndrome from primary hyperparathyroidism, with which it is often confused; and (3) management of hypercalcaemia in the patient with cancer.

MECHANISMS OF HYPERCALCAEMIA

Hypercalcaemia among patients with cancer may be broadly divided into two mechanistic categories. Patients with breast cancer and multiple myeloma develop hypercalcaemia as a result of direct skeletal invasion by malignant cells (local osteolytic hypercalcaemia), a phenomenon which was recognized as early as 1936.[6] Skeletal involvement by tumour, as assessed by bone scan or skeletal radiographs, is extensive.

Other patients, typically those with squamous, renal, bladder, and ovarian carcinomas, develop hypercalcaemia in the absence of skeletal metastases, or in the presence of limited numbers of skeletal metastases.[1,3,4,7-9] These patients are viewed as having hormonally mediated or humorally mediated hypercalcaemia. The term 'humoral hypercalcaemia of malignancy' is widely used to describe this syndrome. (Older terms such as 'ectopic hyperparathyroidism' or 'pseudohyperparathyroidism', as will be described below, are misnomers.) In these patients, hypercalcaemia results from secretion by tumour remote from bone of a circulating calcaemic factor (or factors) which stimulates bone resorption.

Historically, the presence of bone metastases has been viewed as excluding the presence of a humoral mechanism. Clearly, however, both humoral and local mechanisms may be operative in some patients. For example, a carcinoma of the larynx may secrete a systemic, bone-resorbing factor which leads to activation of osteoclastic bone resorption throughout the skeleton. Should this tumour have metastases in the clavicle and the base of the skull, local secretion of the same bone-resorbing factor would lead to a local component of bone resorption as well. Thus, the presence of a small number of skeletal metastases does not preclude the presence of humorally mediated bone resorption. To illustrate this point we have shown in iliac crest biopsies that striking bone resorption occurs in portions of the skeleton uninvolved by skeletal metastases[10] in hypercalcaemic patients with squamous carcinomas metastatic to bone. Thus, systemic, humoral mechanisms as well

as local ones, may both be operative in some patients.

Local Osteolytic Hypercalcaemia (LOH)

The precise mechanisms whereby malignant cells within bone lead to bone resorption remain unclear. It is known that breast cancer cells within bone may synthesize and secrete prostaglandins, and that prostaglandins may activate osteoclasts.[11] However, direct resorption of devitalized (i.e. osteoclast-free) bone by breast cancer cells has also been demonstrated.[12] The relative importance of these mechanisms in breast cancer-induced local osteolysis is unknown.

Both malignant plasma cells from patients with multiple myeloma and activated lymphocytes from normal individuals are capable of secreting osteoclast-activating factor (OAF) and prostaglandins.[13,14] Both of these substances are capable of stimulating osteoclasts to resorb bone. OAF is a protein with a molecular weight of approximately 30 000 daltons. This lymphokine is felt to play a role in the bone destruction and hypercalcaemia seen with myeloma, and perhaps with lymphoma and leukaemia as well. It is not postulated to play a role in any type of humoral hypercalcaemia. The precise fashion in which malignant plasma cells, normal lymphocytes, macrophages, and osteoclasts interact to lead to bone resorption is unclear.

Humoral Hypercalcaemia of Malignancy (HHM)

In 1941 Albright described a patient with a renal carcinoma and hypercalcaemia in the presence of a single skeletal metastasis.[15] He reasoned that if the hypercalcaemia were due to skeletal invasion by tumour, the patient ought to have been hyperphosphataemic as well as hypercalcaemic, as a consequence of delivery of both calcium and phosphorus from bone into the extracellular fluid. The observation that the patient had only a single skeletal metastasis suggested to him that a humoral or 'ectopic hormonal' mechanism was operative.

The presence of hypophosphataemia suggested that the hormone might be parathyroid hormone. In 1956 two groups demonstrated that surgical excision of tumours remote from bone could reverse hypercalcaemia,[16,17] confirming Albright's humoral hypothesis. It is now widely accepted that in some instances MAHC is due to secretion of an ectopic hormone (or hormones). Substances which have been causally implicated in HHM are discussed individually below.

Vitamin D-like Sterols

Gordan in 1966 described the presence of four phytosterols (plant-derived vitamin D-like compounds) in the plasma of hypercalcaemic women with breast cancer.[18] Haddad subsequently demonstrated that these same four phytosterols were present in similar concentrations in the plasma of normal women, lactating women, and women with breast cancer without hypercalcaemia.[19] Further, he demonstrated that the concentrations of these compounds in the plasma of hypercalcaemic patients with breast cancer were inadequate to cause bone resorption. Thus, these specific four phytosterols appear to have been excluded as possible agents of HHM. However, the rapid evolution of the field of vitamin D metabolism, and the continuing discovery of additional vitamin D metabolites, leaves open the possibility that an as yet unidentified vitamin D-like sterol could account for some instances of HHM. Yet it seems unlikely that such a factor could be present in many patients, in that no other example of a non-protein ectopic hormone has been described, and none of the known vitamin D metabolites display the metabolic effects typically encountered in patients with HHM (see below).

Prostaglandins

Klein and Raisz demonstrated in 1970 that prostaglandins, particularly PGE_2, are potent activators *in vitro* of osteoclastic bone resorption.[20] Since that time at least one animal model of prostaglandin-mediated HHM has been described.[21] That prostaglandins may be responsible for some instances of HHM seems likely, since some hypercalcaemic patients have been described in whom plasma immuno-reactive PGE_2 or urine PGE-M (a metabolite of PGE_2) are elevated, and who responded with a fall in both plasma prostaglandin levels or urine PGE-M levels and a fall in serum calcium to the administration of prostaglandin synthetase inhibitors such as aspirin or indomethacin.[22,23] The initial enthusiasm for the prostaglandin–HHM link has begun to wane, however, as a larger experience with prostaglandin synthetase inhibitors and iPGE measurements accumulates.[24-26] Plasma or tumour iPGE content has been shown to differ little between patients with and without hypercalcaemia, and only a small minority of patients appear to respond to prostaglandin synthetase inhibitors.[24-26] Further, it is now clear that a response to prostaglandin synthetase inhibitors does not necessarily indicate a systemic role for prostaglandins in HHM, as prostaglandins appear to have an important role within bone, modulating osteoclastic and osteoblastic function. In summary, prostaglandin secretion by tumours may account for a minority of instances of HHM. Patients who fit into the prostaglandin-mediated HHM category have typically been patients with renal carcinoma.

Parathyroid Hormone

Following Albright's initial postulate that parathyroid hormone may be secreted ectopically, and may account for some instances of HHM, the concept of 'ectopic hyperparathyroidism' or 'pseudohyperparathyroidism' gained increasing acceptance: patients with both primary hyperparathyroidism and HHM are hypercalcaemic, both groups are usually hypophosphataemic and are phosphaturic, and both syndromes are humorally mediated. With the advent of parathyroid immunoassays in the 1960s and 1970s a number of investigators demonstrated the presence of PTH-like immunoreactivity in plasma[27] or tumour extracts[28] from some patients with HHM. More recently, urinary cyclic AMP and nephrogenous cyclic AMP excretion have been shown to be elevated in both syndromes.[4,29-31]

Despite these similarities it is now quite clear that HHM is rarely if ever due to ectopic secretion of parathyroid hormone. The evidence that PTH is not the mediator of HHM has recently been outlined in detail,[32] and can be summarized as follows:

(1) Fractional excretion of calcium is far higher in HHM than in HPT, indicating an absence of PTH effect on the distal nephron.[4,23]

(2) Plasma 1,25-dihydroxyvitamin D levels are reduced in HHM, but are elevated in HPT.[4] 1,25-Dihydroxyvitamin D is synthesized in the proximal renal tubule in the presence of PTH. The reduced levels of plasma 1,25-dihydroxyvitamin D encountered in the plasma of patients with HHM indicates an absence of PTH interaction with the proximal tubular PTH – receptor – enzyme complex responsible for 1,25-dihydroxyvitamin D synthesis.

(3) Immunoreactive PTH concentrations are lower in the plasma or serum of patients with HHM than in those with HPT for any given serum calcium value.[4,8,27,33] In fact, in the vast majority of PTH immunoassays in which plasma from patients with HHM has been run, values are normal, low, or undetectable in contrast to the elevated values encountered among the majority of patients with HPT. (In the instances in which iPTH values have been reported to be 'normal' in HHM, the 'iPTH' measured may reflect the accumulation of inactive PTH fragments in plasma due to delayed renal clearance of these fragments, a non-suppressible component of normal parathyroid hormone secretion, or non-specific binding in a particular assay).

(4) Bone histology differs markedly in patients with HHM as compared to those with HPT.[10] In the former, marked increases in osteoclast numbers are encountered, with mean numbers of osteoclasts which are far higher than those usually seen in HPT. However, unlike the findings in HPT where osteoblastic activity is increased, osteoblastic activity is markedly reduced in patients with HHM. This striking 'uncoupling' of osteoclasts from osteoblasts has not been encountered in other metabolic bone diseases and suggests that osteoclasts are being stimulated by a factor other than PTH.

Other Factors

If HHM is due to secretion of vitamin D-like sterols, prostaglandins, and PTH in only the exceptional instance, then in the vast majority of individuals HHM must be due to an as yet unidentified substance (or substances). As noted above, we have shown that the majority of patients with HHM display elevated NcAMP excretion, an observation which suggests that the factor responsible for HHM stimulates the PTH-sensitive proximal tubular adenylate cyclase and binds to the proximal tubular PTH receptor. We have also shown that the plasma of some patients with HHM contains a factor which stimulates the distal tubular PTH receptor responsible for activity in a cytochemical bioassay for parathyroid hormone. These observations suggested to us that the factor responsible for HHM could be measured in extracts of tumours from patients with HHM using either a PTH-sensitive adenylate cyclase assay, or the cytochemical bioassay for PTH. These predictions proved to be correct when tumour extracts from patients with HHM were assayed – the extracts contain activity in both the adenylate cyclase assay and the cytochemical bioassay. That the activity is not due to PTH is apparent from the observation that the activity cannot be destroyed by PTH antisera, and appears to have a molecular weight far larger than that of PTH or its precursors.[35] Thus, we believe that the factor responsible for HHM is a protein or glycoprotein larger than and unrelated to PTH, which appears to share some, but not all, receptor sites with PTH. Further purification and characterization of this substance is under way.

DIAGNOSIS OF MALIGNANCY-ASSOCIATED HYPERCALCAEMIA

Upon discovery that a patient with cancer is hypercalcaemic, one should accept a diagnosis of MAHC only after careful exclusion of the many other disease processes which may produce hypercalcaemia. This is of critical importance because:

(1) several conditions other than malignancy which cause hypercalcaemia are also common and can be expected to occur frequently in a group of patients with cancer;

(2) attributing hypercalcaemia to malignancy usually implies the presence of a large tumour burden and a limited prognosis;[1,36,37] and

(3) in most instances, hypercalcaemia due to causes other than malignancy is readily treatable, whereas that due to malignancy is often difficult to treat.

A list of drugs, conditions, or diseases which may induce hypercalcaemia is shown in Table 7.1. In addition to being capable of producing hypercalcaemia on their own, these entities may worsen or enhance malignancy-associated hypercalcaemia. For example, the use of thiazide diuretics in a patient with MAHC would be expected to produce an additional elevation in serum calcium by interfering with renal calcium excretion. Hyperalimentation solutions containing calcium will worsen hypercalcaemia. Most oral nutritional supplements contain calcium in considerable amounts. Large amounts of calcium administered orally (more than 2 – 3 grams of

TABLE 7.1   CAUSES OF HYPERCALCAEMIA

1. Malignancy
2. Primary hyperparathyroidism
3. Excessive oral calcium administration, with or without alkali
4. Hyperthyroidism
5. Immobilization in young adults or children and in Paget's disease
6. Medications
    Vitamin D intoxication
    Vitamin A intoxication
    Thiazide diuretics
    Lithium carbonate
    Oestrogen/Tamoxifen use in breast cancer with skeletal metastases
7. Granulomatous disease – sarcoidosis, berylliosis, tuberculosis, coccidioidomycosis, histoplasmosis
8. Addisonian crisis
9. Watery diarrhoea hypokalaemic alkalosis (WDHA) syndrome, (VIP-oma)
10. Hyperproteinaemia
11. Phaeochromocytoma
12. Familial hypocalciuric hypercalcaemia[59]

elemental calcium per day) will lead to hypercalciuria and will worsen hypercalcaemia.[38] Hyperalimentation solutions and oral nutritional supplements should therefore be prepared without the addition of calcium when used in patients with MAHC. Most of the entities in Table 7.1 can be readily excluded by history or simple laboratory tests.

With great regularity the differential diagnosis is rapidly whittled down to the consideration of MAHC versus primary hyperparathyroidism (HPT). With the advent of the measurements of vitamin D metabolites, this differential diagnosis has become straightforward. It should also be borne in mind that primary hyperparathyroidism may coexist with a cancer in the same patient.[39] In fact some authors have reported that the incidence of HPT is higher among patients with cancer than in the general population.[40]

History

The duration of a patient's hypercalcaemia is an important differential point in distinguishing MAHC from HPT. With only rare exceptions, MAHC is characterized by a rapidly progressive vicious spiral of hypercalcaemia leading to polyuria and dehydration, which in turn lowers the glomerular filtration rate, limiting the patient's ability to clear calcium. Hypercalcaemia thus tends to worsen rapidly over a period of days to weeks. In contrast, hypercalcaemia in HPT is a chronic phenomenon. The discovery of an elevated serum calcium 6–12 months in the past, for example, excludes a diagnosis of MAHC and typifies HPT. Similarly, a history of nephrolithiasis suggests the presence of chronic hypercalciuria and would favour a diagnosis of HPT.

Physical Examination

Particular emphasis should be placed on the examination of the head and neck, lymph nodes, spleen, liver, breasts, ovaries, and female genital tract, as tumours of these organs are particularly apt to produce hypercalcaemia.[1–9] The examiner should be aware that tumours which are responsible for hypercalcaemia are large tumours, and will be obvious on careful examination.[1,36,37] Small 'occult' tumours do not cause hypercalcaemia.

Laboratory Studies

Simple laboratory tests should include a complete blood count (leukaemia), a serum and protein urine protein electrophoresis (multiple myeloma), and a urinalysis (renal and bladder carcinoma). Calcium, phosphorus, and creatinine in the blood and in a fasting spot urine should be measured to permit calculation and derivation of the renal phosphorus threshold (TmP/GFR) and fasting calcium excretion (FCaE). The TmP (calculated by plotting the fractional phosphorus excretion against the serum phosphorus on a simple and widely available nomogram[41]) can be calculated within hours of admission to the hospital, and rapidly provides a clue as to whether the hypercalcaemia is due to HPT or HHM (which are associated with reduced TmP/GFR values) or to LOH which is associated with normal or elevated TmP values.[4] Similarly, FCaE is rapidly calculated

(fasting urine calcium concentration ÷ urine creatinine concentration × serum creatinine), and provides an early means of distinguishing LOH and HHM, which are usually associated with marked elevation in calcium excretion, from HPT, which is regularly associated with only mild hypercalciuria in the fasting state.[4,23] Care should be taken to collect samples for FCaE and TmP/GFR while fasting and prior to the use of saline infusion or diuretics, as these manoeuvres alter the TmP/GFR and FCaE.

Plasma concentrations of 1,25-dihydroxyvitamin D $(1,25(OH)_2D)$ are elevated in the plasma of patients with HPT, reflecting the effects of elevated circulating parathyroid hormone concentration on the renal enzyme which synthesizes this vitamin D metabolite.[4,42] The elevation of $1,25(OH)_2D$ in HPT is responsible for the intestinal hyperabsorption of calcium characteristic of HPT.[42] In contrast, malignancy-associated hypercalcaemia, both humoral and local osteolytic, is associated with low–normal to frankly reduced plasma $1,25(OH)_2D$ values, reflecting a reduction in circulating PTH levels.[4] This reduction in plasma $1,25(OH)_2D$ concentration in turn results in the reduction in intestinal calcium absorption characteristic of MAHC.[43] Plasma $1,25(OH)_2D$ measurements are widely available commercially, and provide a simple and accurate means of distinguishing HPT and MAHC.[4]

The problems associated with PTH immunoassays have been alluded to earlier. While immunoreactive PTH (iPTH) values are elevated in the majority of patients with HPT, it is not correct to assume that iPTH will be reduced in patients with hypercalcaemia resulting from causes other than HPT. For a given degree of hypercalcaemia, however, iPTH values are far higher in patients with HPT than in those with MAHC.[33] For example, a patient with a serum calcium of 13.0 mg/dl due to HPT will typically have an iPTH value approximately twice the upper normal limits for a given iPTH assay. In contrast, a patient with MAHC and the same serum calcium will typically have a normal to undetectable iPTH value, depending on the assay employed.[4,8,27,33,44] Dehydrated or azotaemic patients with MAHC may display elevated iPTH values, reflecting impaired renal clearance of biologically inactive carboxyterminal PTH fragments.

Total urinary cyclic AMP (UcAMP) measurements reflect the excretion of cyclic AMP derived from two sources. Approximately 50% of UcAMP is derived from filtration of plasma cyclic AMP at the glomerulus. This component of UcAMP is non-specific. The remaining half of UcAMP is produced in the proximal tubule by the interaction of either PTH or the substance responsible for HHM, with a PTH receptor – adenylate cyclase complex in proximal tubular cells. This 'nephrogenous cyclic AMP' (NcAMP) specifically reflects circulating levels of PTH or of the factor responsible for HHM.[4,45,46] NcAMP measurement requires measurements of both plasma and urine cAMP and must be expressed in appropriate units (nmol/100 ml GFR).[46] In general, NcAMP measurements are available only in research laboratories because of the difficulties in measuring plasma cAMP. Fortunately, however, total urinary cyclic AMP excretion roughly parallels NcAMP excretion so that patients with HPT and HHM have elevated UcAMP excretion, whereas those with LOH display reduced UcAMP excretion.[46] UcAMP measurements are relatively easy to perform and are available through commercial laboratories. Care must be taken to express UcAMP excretion as nmol per 100 ml of GFR.

BONE RADIOGRAPHS AND SCANS

Typical radiological signs of hyperparathyroidism include a 'salt and pepper' appearance of the calvarium, bone cysts, subperiosteal resorption of the phalanges, and resorption of the tufts of the distal phalanges. These findings are present only in rare patients with severe long-standing hyperparathyroidism. Thus, in the majority of individuals with HPT skeletal radiographs are normal. Skeletal X-rays may reveal the presence of skeletal metastases in either HHM or LOH. No studies comparing the radiological appearance of skeletal radiographs in HHM and HPT for features of metabolic bone disease have been reported.

Bone scanning is a useful adjunct to the evaluation of suspected MAHC. If the bone scan shows extensive metastatic disease throughout the skeleton, hypercalcaemia of the local osteolytic variety is likely. A negative bone scan is compatible with HHM and with multiple myeloma. The discovery of a small number of areas of uptake is consistent with HHM, as noted earlier.

In summary, when confronted with a patient with newly discovered hypercalcaemia, one should perform a routine history and physical examination with particular emphasis on the areas described above. Fasting samples should be obtained for serum calcium, phosphorus, creatinine, $1,25(OH)_2D$ and immunoreactive parathyroid hormone. A fasting spot urine for calcium, phosphorus, creatinine, and cyclic AMP should be obtained; values should be calculated for FCaE, TmP/GFR; and urinary cyclic AMP expressed as nmol/100 ml GFR. The results of these studies readily categorize a patient as having HHM, LOH, or HPT, as shown in Table 7.2. If the patient is in good health these samples may be obtained as an outpatient, obviating the need for an extensive and fruitless tumour search in patients who eventually prove to have HPT. Bone scans in patients with suspected MAHC provide information as to the mechanism of hypercalcaemia (LOH vs HHM) and therefore suggest specific tissue diagnosis in individuals with MAHC. The demonstration of extensive skeletal metastases would favour a diagnosis of breast carcinoma, whereas the presence of few or no metastases suggests a humoral syndrome produced by a renal, squamous, bladder or ovarian tumour.

TABLE 7.2 BIOCHEMICAL DIFFERENTIAL DIAGNOSIS OF PRIMARY HYPERPARATHYROIDISM (HPT), LOCAL OSTEOLYTIC HYPERCALCAEMIA (LOH), AND HUMORAL HYPERCALCAEMIA OF MALIGNANCY (HHM)

	Serum calcium	TmP/GFR	Fasting calcium excretion	1,25-dihydroxy vitamin D	Nephrogenous cyclic AMP	Immunoreactive PTH
HPT	↑	↓	↔ ↑	↑	↑	↑
LOH	↑	↔	↑↑	↔ ↓	↓	↔ ↓
HHM	↑	↓↓	↑↑	↔ ↓	↑	↔ ↓

TABLE 7.3 PRINCIPLES OF THERAPY

1. Reduce tumour burden
2. Enhance renal calcium clearance
    Saline infusion
    Furosemide
    Dialysis
3. Inhibit bone resorption
    Mobilization
    Phosphorus
    Prostaglandin synthetase inhibitors
    Glucocorticoids
    Calcitonin
    Mithramycin
    Diphosphonates

THERAPY OF MALIGNANCY-ASSOCIATED HYPERCALCAEMIA

An enlightened therapeutic approach to MAHC requires (1) attempts at eliminating or reducing tumour bulk, (2) increasing renal calcium excretion, and (3) reducing skeletal calcium losses. These therapeutic modalities are summarized in Table 7.3.

REDUCING TUMOUR BURDEN

Over the long term the only successful means of reversing MAHC is through elimination or reduction of tumour burden. The other available therapeutic modalities listed in Table 7.3 result in toxicity or loss of response over a period of days to weeks. They should thus be viewed as temporizing therapies to be used over the short term while awaiting tumour responses consequent to radiation, surgery, or chemotherapy. A corollary of this principle is that, because other means of therapy will fail or lead to toxicity over the short term, a strategy designed to deal with tumour therapy should be formulated and initiated in patients with hypercalcaemia as soon as possible. Delays in anti-tumour therapy lead to the unhappy prospect of administering radiation or chemotherapy to a patient with mithramycin-induced thrombocytopenia, or of operating on a patient with severe hypercalcaemia who has failed calcitonin and/or steroids and who is no longer a candidate for mithramycin.

ENHANCING RENAL CALCIUM CLEARANCE

Hypercalcaemia interferes with urinary concentrating mechanism and leads to polyuria and dehydration. Dehydration, with its resultant fall in glomerular filtration rate, leads to reduced renal clearance of calcium from plasma and therefore worsening hypercalcaemia. Thus an attempt should be made to return the GFR to normal. Sodium chloride, in addition to its effects on glomerular filtration, interferes with calcium reabsorption in the proximal nephron. Saline infusion thus increases both the filtered load of calcium at the level of the glomerulus and the fractional excretion of calcium at the level of the proximal nephron.[47] Saline should be administered at 200–300 cc per hour, with close monitoring of the patient for signs of overhydration or continued dehydration.

Furosemide inhibits calcium reabsorption in the thick ascending limb of Henle's loop, and leads to a further increase in fractional calcium excretion.[47] Care should be taken to ensure that the patient is adequately hydrated before furosemide is administered. If given to a dehydrated patient it will further reduce the glomerular filtration rate leading to decreased renal calcium excretion. Furosemide is given in doses of 20–40 mg orally or intravenously one to four times a day, with careful evaluation for signs of volume depletion or electrolyte disturbance.

Dialysis against a low calcium bath is an effective means of lowering serum calcium in patients with MAHC.[1] Indeed, in the patient with MAHC and renal failure, the items other than dialysis listed in Table 7.3 are contraindicated or ineffective. While dialysis would be overzealous in many patients with MAHC, in the occasional patient with acute reversible renal failure who has a favourable prognosis from the underlying malignancy, dialysis can be life-saving.

INHIBITION OF BONE RESORPTION

Immobilization leads to osteoclastic activation and inhibition of osteoblastic bone formation.[48] This combination of events can lead to hypercalciuria and hypercalcaemia in situations where bone turnover is increased (Paget's disease, adolescence), and would be predicted to worsen skeletal calcium losses in MAHC. Patients with MAHC who are bedridden as a consequence of pain, inanition, or sedative/analgesic use should be ambulated to the extent that this is reasonable and possible.

Phosphorus therapy is effective in reducing serum calcium. Increases in serum phosphorus concentration inhibit osteoclastic bone resorption, stimulate osteoblasts to form new bone, and, through an increase in the calcium × phosphorus ion product, lead to calcium phosphate salt deposition in bone and possibly other sites.[49] Which of these is most important in leading to a reduction in serum calcium remains open to question. Many, and perhaps most, patients with MAHC become hypophosphataemic in the course of their disease as a result of anorexia, tumour-induced phosphaturia, saline and furosemide therapy, hypercalcaemia and other factors. This hypophosphataemia can be expected to worsen or accelerate osteoclastic bone resorption. For these reasons, oral phosphorus in a dose of 500–1500 mg of elemental phosphorus per day is appropriate in patients with serum phosphorus values below the normal range. Guidelines for interconverting millimolar and milligram concentrations of phosphorus are available.[50] Serum calcium, phosphorus, and creatinine should be closely followed during phosphorus administration because of the possibility of renal dysfunction. Phosphorus should be discontinued at the earliest sign of a fall in glomerular filtration rate. Intravenous phosphorus therapy is particularly hazardous and should be used only in the exceptional patient with marked hypophosphataemia who cannot tolerate oral phosphorus and in whom other means of reducing serum calcium have failed or are contraindicated. The amount of phosphorus infused should not exceed 500–1000 mg per 24 hours, and serum calcium, phosphorus, and creatinine concentrations should be followed meticulously.

Prostaglandin synthetase inhibitors such as aspirin and indomethacin appear to be effective in reversing hypercalcaemia in only a minority of patients.[24–26] Their use should be reserved for the occasional patient with mild hypercalcaemia in whom other means of therapy have failed or are contraindicated, and in whom control of serum calcium is not urgent. Aspirin has been used in a dose of 1.8–4.8 grams per day, and indomethacin in a dose of 50 mg three times a day.[23]

Glucocorticoids, in doses of 40–60 mg of prednisone or equivalent, are particularly effective in reversing the hypercalcaemia associated with multiple myeloma and breast cancer.[51] Glucocorticoids probably act through several mechanisms including (1) tumour lysis, (2) inhibition of prostaglandin synthesis, and (3) inhibition of OAF synthesis. The effectiveness of glucocorticoids in reversing humoral hypercalcaemia such as that associated with squamous carcinomas remains to be studied carefully. In so far as HHM appears to be caused by a substance similar in some respects to PTH, and in view of the fact that glucocorticoids do not alter the serum calcium appreciably in HPT, one might predict that glucocorticoids would be ineffective in HHM. In practice the availability of other agents, as well as the drawbacks associated with glucocorticoid use (osteopenia, immunosuppression, long response time) allow little role for these agents in managing HHM.

Calcitonin produces a rapid fall in serum calcium in the range of 2 or 3 mg/dl. Unfortunately, the effects of calcitonin, even when given continually in high dose, are transient, lasting only a matter of days.[52,53] Thus the limited fall in serum calcium, the high cost of the drug, the ephemeral nature of the response, and the unpredictability of response do not recommend calcitonin as a front-line drug in managing MAHC. The dose suggested by the manufacturer is 4 MRC units/kg given subcutaneously or intramuscularly every 12 hours. Recently, the suggestion has been made that a combination of glucocorticoids together with calcitonin may result in more substantial falls in serum calcium.[53] Whether the 'escape' from calcitonin can be prevented by glucocorticoid use remains to be determined.

Mithramycin continues to be the agent of choice for the management of severe hypercalcaemia.[54] It reliably induces return to normal serum calcium values over a period of 48–72 hours. Mithramycin appears to interfere with osteoclastic bone resorption, although the precise mechanism through which this occurs is uncertain. It is given in a dose of 25 μg/kg in 50 cc of 5% dextrose intravenously over 2–4 hours and may be repeated at intervals exceeding 72 hours. The drug is toxic to the kidneys and the liver, interferes with both thrombopoiesis and platelet aggregation, and should be used with caution and in reduced dose in patients with renal disease, liver disease, or bone marrow suppression. Mithramycin toxicity of the above types is common when large antitumour doses (eg 250 μg/kg over several days) are used.[55] No toxicity from a single 25 μg/kg dose of mithramycin has been reported in patients free of liver, renal, or haematopoietic disorders. However, its continued use over a period of weeks is likely to lead to one or more of the above toxicities.

The diphosphonates are a class of compounds which inhibit osteoclast activity and, to a varying degree, bone mineralization. These drugs have been used with dramatic success in reversing MAHC in clinical trials in the United States and Europe.[56–58] Although none of these drugs is available for use in the United States at present, it seems likely that one or more diphosphonate derivatives will become the keystone of MAHC management in years to come.

In most instances, combinations of the agents listed in Table 7.3 will be utilized in most patients. For example, a bedridden patient with severe hypercalcaemia, hypophosphataemia, and dehydration, resulting from a carcinoma of the larynx will benefit from a combination of saline, lasix, oral phosphorus replacement, ambulation, and mithramycin. A patient with multiple myeloma and mild hypercalcaemia may simply require oral hydration, ambulation, and moderate doses of glucocorticoids. In each case ultimate control of hypercalcaemia will only be established through successful antitumour therapy.

ACKNOWLEDGEMENT

This work was supported by the Veteran's Administration, West Haven, CT, USA, by National Institutes of Health Grant RR 125 and AM 30102, and by the General Clinical Research Center of the Yale–New Haven Hospital.

REFERENCES

1. Rodman, J.S., Sherwood, L.M. (1978). In *Metabolic Bone Disease*, vol. 2 (Eds L.V. Avioli, and S.M. Krane), Academic Press, New York, p.247.
2. Myers, W.P.L. (1960). *A.M.A. Arch. Surg.*, **80**, 308.
3. Omenn, G.S., Roth, S.I., and Baker, W.H. (1969). *Cancer*, **24**, 10034.
4. Stewart, A.F., Horst, R., Deftos, L.J., Cadman, E.C., Lang, R., and Broadus, A.E. (1980). *New Engl. J. Med.*, **303**, 1377.
5. Aryian, S., Farber, L.R., Hamilton, B.P., and Papac, R.J. (1974). *Cancer*, **33**, 159.
6. Gutman, A.B., Tyson, T.L., and Gutman, E.B. (1936). *Arch. Intern. Med.*, **57**, 379.
7. Lafferty, F.W. (1966). *Medicine (Baltimore)*, **45**, 247.
8. Powell, D., Singer, F.R., Murray, T.M., Minkin, C., and Potts, J.T. (1973). *New Engl. J. Med.*, **289**, 176.
9. Skrabanek, P., McPartlin, J., and Powell, D.M. (1980). *Medicine (Baltimore)*, **50**, 262.
10. Stewart, A.F., Vignery, A., Silverglate, A., Ravin, N.D., LiVolsi, V., Broadus, A.E., and Baron, R. (1982). *J. Clin. Endocrinol. Metab.*, **55**, 219.
11. Bockman, R.S. (1980). *Clin. Endocrinol. Metab.*, **9**, 317.
12. Eilon, G., and Mundy, G.R. (1978). *Nature*, **276**, 726.
13. Yoneda, T., and Mundy, G.R. (1979). *J. Exp. Med.*, **149**, 279.
14. Mundy, G.R., Raisz, L.G., Cooper, R.A., Schecter, G.P., and Salmon, S.E. (1974). *New Engl. J. Med.*, **291**, 1041.
15. Albright, F. (1941). *New Engl. J. Med.*, **225**, 789.
16. Plimpton, C.H., and Gellhorn, A. (1956). *Am. J. Med.*, **21**, 750.
17. Connor, T.B., Thomas, W.C., and Howard, J.E. (1956). *J. Clin. Invest.*, **35**, 697.
18. Gordan, G.S., Fitzpatrick, M.E., and Lubich, W.P. (1967). *Trans. Assoc. Am. Phys.*, **80**, 183.
19. Haddad, J.G., Couranz, S.J., and Avioli, L.V. (1970). *J. Clin. Endocrinol. Metab.*, **30**, 174.
20. Klein, D.C., and Raisz, L.G. (1970). *Endocrinology*, **86**, 1436.
21. Tashjian, A.H. (1978). *Cancer Res.*, **38**, 4138.
22. Robertson, R.P., Baylink, D.J., Marini, J.J., and Adkison, H.W. (1975). *J. Clin. Endocrinol. Metab.*, **41**, 164.
23. Seyberth, H.W., Segre, G.V., Morgan, J.L., Sweetman, B.J., Potts, J.T., and Oates, J.A. (1975). *New Engl. J. Med.*, **293**, 1278.
24. Tashjian, A.H. (1975). *New Engl. J. Med.*, **293**, 1317.
25. Metz, S.A., McRae, J.R., and Robertson, R.P. (1981). *Metabolism*, **30**, 299.
26. Brenner, D.E., Harvey, H.A., Lipton, A., and Demers, L. (1982). *Cancer*, **44**, 556.
27. Benson, R.C., Riggs, B.L., Pickard, B.M., and Arnaud, C.D. (1974). *Am. J. Med.*, **56**, 821.
28. Mavligit, G.M., Cohen, J.L., and Sherwood, L.M. (1971). *New Engl. J. Med.*, **285**, 154.
29. Shaw, J.W., Oldham, S.B., Rosoff, L., Bethune, J.E., and Fichman, M.P. (1977). *J. Clin. Invest.*, **59**, 14.
30. Rude, R.K., Sharp, C.F., Fredericks, R.S., Oldham, S.B., Elbaum, N., Link, J., Irwin, L., and Singer, F.R. (1981). *J. Clin. Endcrinol. Metab.*, **52**, 765.
31. Kukreja, S.C., Shemerdiak, W.P., Lad, T.E., and Johnson, P.A. (1980). *J. Clin. Endocrinol. Metab.*, **51**, 167.
32. Stewart, A.F. (1982). *Mineral Electrolyte Metab.*, **8**, 215.
33. Riggs, B.L., Arnaud, C.D., Reynolds, J.C., and Smith, L.H. (1971). *J. Clin. Invest.*, **50**, 207A.
34. Goltzman, D., Stewart, A.F., and Broadus, A.E. (1981). *J. Clin. Endcrinol. Metab.*, **53**, 889.
35. Stewart, A.F., Insogna, K.L., Goltzman, D., Jones, R., and Broadus, A.E. (1982). *Clin. Res.*, **30**, 405A.
36. Angel, M., Stewart, A.F., Pensak, M.L., Pillsbury, H.R.C., and Sasaki, C.T. (1982). *Head Neck Surg.*, (In press).
37. Stewart, A.F., Romero, R., Schwartz, P.E., Kohorn, E.I., and Broadus, A.E. (1982). *Cancer*, **49**, 2389.
38. Adams, N.D., Gray, R.W., and Lemann, J. (1979). *J. Clin. Endocrinol. Metab.*, **48**, 1008.
39. Vichayanrat, A., Avramides, A., Gardner, B., Wallach, S., and Carter, A.C. (1976). *Am. J. Med.*, **61**, 136.
40. Farr, H.W., Fahey, T.J., Nash, A.G., and Farr, C.M. (1973). *Am. J. Surg.*, **126**, 539.
41. Walton, R.J., and Bijvoet, O.L.M. (1975). *Lancet*, **2**, 309.
42. Broadus, A.E., Horst, R.L., Lang, R., Littledike, E.T., and Rasmussen, R.H. (1980). *New Engl. J. Med.*, **302**, 421.
43. Coombes, R.C., Ward, M.K., Greenberg, P.B., Hillyard, C.J., Tulloch, B.R., Morrison, R., and Joplin, G.F. (1976). *Cancer*, **38**, 2111.
44. Raisz, L.G., Yajnik, C.H., Bockman, R.S., and Bower, B.F. (1979). *Ann. Intern. Med.*, **91**, 739.

45. Broadus, A.E., and Rasmussen, H.R. (1981). *Am. J. Med.*, **70**, 475.
46. Broadus, A.E. (1981). *Rec. Prog. Horm. Res.*, **37**, 667.
47. Suki, W.N., Yium, J.J., Von Minden, M., Saller-Hebert, C., Eknoyan, G., and Martinez-Maldonado, M. (1970). *New Engl. J. Med.*, **283**, 836.
48. Minaire, P., Meunier, P., Edouard, C., Bernard, J., Courpron, P., and Bourret, J. (1974). *Calcif. Tiss. Res.*, **17**, 57.
49. Breuer, R.I., and LeBauer, J. (1967). *J. Clin. Endocrinol. Metab.*, **27**, 695.
50. Lentz, R.D., Brown, D.M., and Kjellstrand, C.M. (1978). *Ann. Intern. Med.*, **89**, 441.
51. Watson, L., Moxham, J., and Fraser, P. (1980). *Lancet*, **1**, 1320.
52. Hosking, D.J. (1980). *Met. Bone Dis. Rel. Res.*, **2**, 207.
53. Binstock, M.L., and Mundy, G.R. (1980). *Ann. Intern. Med.*, **93**, 269.
54. Perlia, C.P., Gubisch, N.J., Wolter, J., Edelberg, D., Dederick, M.M., and Taylor, S.G. (1970). *Cancer*, **25**, 389.
55. Kennedy, B.J. (1970). *Am. J. Med.*, **49**, 494.
56. Jung, A. (1982). *Am. J. Med.*, **72**, 221.
57. Jacobs, T.P., Siris, E.S., Bilezikian, J.P., Baquiran, D.E., Shane, E., and Canfield, R.E. (1981). *Ann. Intern. Med.*, **94**, 312.
58. Douglas, E.L., Russell, R.G.G., Preston, C.J., Prenton, M.A., Duckworth, T., Kanis, J.A., Preston, F.E., and Woodhead, J.S. (1980). *Lancet*, **1**, 1043.
59. Marx, S.J. (1980). *New Engl. J. Med.*, **303**, 810.

C
TREATMENT AND PREVENTION

Chapter 8

Overview of Conventional Surgery and Radiotherapy

James E. Marks*
Stanley E. Thawley†
and
Joseph H. Ogura†
* Division of Radiation Oncology,
Mallinckrodt Institute of Radiology
† Department of Otolaryngology,
Washington University School of
Medicine, St Louis, Missouri, USA

BACKGROUND

Surgery and radiotherapy, alone or in combination, are the methods used to treat the majority of patients with head and neck cancer. These methods of treatment are available to most patients and are capable of eradicating the primary tumour and its lymphatic metastases in 50–75% of all who enter the clinic.[26,28–32,36,46] Local–regional treatment failures after conventional surgery and/or irradiation range from 25% to 50% and distant metastases from 10% to 25%.[26,28–32,36,46] Salvage of initial local–regional failures by additional surgery and/or irradiation ranges from 0% to 80% and is largely dependent on the stage and site of the original tumour. It is clear from these statistics that the majority of patients with head and neck cancer would benefit most from improved local–regional control. Some would benefit from early detection of local–regional recurrence and others from effective systemic treatment for distant metastases.

BIOLOGICAL BEHAVIOUR

Head and neck cancers are a complex set of diseases whose biological behaviour depends on their pathology, size, and site of origin. Patterns of *local invasion* depend upon the anatomical barriers present at each anatomical site, as well as the pathology of the primary tumour. Cancers of the larynx are impeded by the laryngeal skeleton, membranes and ligaments,[19] while cancers of the tongue spread easily along muscular bundles. Perineural invasion is extremely common for adenoid

TABLE 8.1 PERCENTAGES OF CERVICAL LYMPH
NODE METASTASES BY SITE FOR
SQUAMOUS CELL CARCINOMAS OF
THE HEAD AND NECK[22] (*n* = 2044)

Site	Unilateral	Bilateral	Total
Lateral			
Floor of mouth	26	4	31
Oral tongue	29	5	35
Anterior faucial pillar Retromolar trigone	40	5	45
Tonsillar fossa	64	11	76
Hypopharynx	65	11	76
Midline			
Soft palate	28	16	44
Oropharyngeal wall	42	17	59
Supraglottic larynx	39	16	55
Base of tongue	49	29	78
Nasopharynx	39	49	87

cystic carcinomas and less common for squamous carcinomas. *Lymphatic metastases* are a function of pathology and tumour location. Verrucous and adenoid cystic carcinomas seldom metastasize to lymph nodes, although lymphoepitheliomas commonly do so. Tonsillar, nasopharyngeal, base of tongue, and hypopharyngeal carcinomas metastasize to lymph nodes more often than do cancers of a number of other sites; and bilateral or contralateral lymph node metastases are more common for midline tumours than for those that arise more laterally (Table 8.1).[22] *Distant metastases* are pathology- and site-dependent. Adenoid cystic carcinomas metastasize haematogenously to distant sites more commonly than squamous carcinomas. The incidence of distant metastases is less than 10% for squamous carcinomas of the vocal cord, faucial arch, oral cavity, and paranasal sinuses; 15% for cancers of the supraglottis and oropharynx; and approximately 25% for cancers of the hypopharynx and nasopharynx (Table 8.2)[33] Distant metastases seldom occur in the absence of lymphatic metastases and are more common for large than small tumours. Certain subgroups of patients have a particularly high incidence of distant metastases; 35% of large pyriform sinus cancers[30] and 50% of nasopharyngeal cancers metastastic to

both necks[6] develop distant metastases. It is important to understand that head and neck cancers differ in their behaviour depending on their pathology, size, and site of origin if we are to improve treatment strategies and define those questions that need asking.

HOST CHARACTERISTICS

The management of head and neck cancers by surgery and irradiation is influenced greatly by the condition of the host as well as

TABLE 8.2 PERCENTAGES OF DISTANT
METASTASES BY SITE FOR
SQUAMOUS CELL CARCINOMAS
OF THE HEAD AND NECK[33]
(*n* = 5019)

Site	Incidence
Vocal cord	3
Faucial arch	7
Oral cavity	7
Paranasal sinus and nasal cavity	9
Supraglottic larynx	15
Oropharynx proper*	15
Hypopharynx	24
Nasopharynx†	28
Total	11

* Tonsillar fossa, base of tongue, pharyngeal wall.
† Includes lymphoepitheliomas.

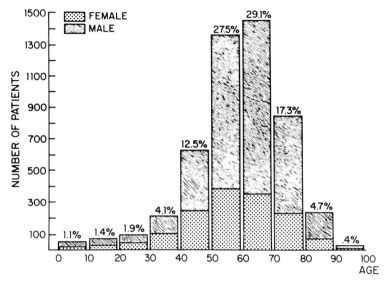

Figure 8.1   Frequency histogram demonstrating the age distribution of males and females with head and neck cancer (Mallinckrodt Institute of Radiology, 1965–80).

biological, anatomical, and functional considerations. Patients with head and neck cancer are chronologically and physiologically an aged group whose sex is predominantly male (Figure 8.1). They are heavy smokers and drinkers and present with varying degrees of nutritional deprivation. Because of their age and smoking, they are frequently afflicted by cardiac and chronic pulmonary obstructive disease. All of these factors significantly influence selection of treatment, surgical operability, tolerance of irradiation, post-surgical complications, and ultimately survival. Patients who are too weak and nutritionally deprived to withstand aggressive surgery and irradiation are treated with palliative intent. Patients with advanced cardiac and pulmonary disease are often declared medically unfit for operation and referred for irradiation. Those who are weak and nutritionally deprived tolerate irradiation poorly and frequently require nasogastric intubation to prevent dehydration and further loss of weight. Patients with nutritional deprivation or hepatic or renal disease heal poorly and suffer a high rate of post-surgical complications. These numerous conditions of the host greatly influence treatment selection, tolerance, and

complications. Moreover, the status of the host influences life expectancy and must be considered along with the stage and biology of the cancer in any study of prognostic factors.

ANATOMY AND FUNCTION

Head and neck cancers arise in a variety of sites whose anatomy and function differ greatly, and which act simultaneously and separately to perform a variety of functions that are essential to the well-being of the patient. Concentrated in the head and neck region are the major senses of sight, hearing, smell, and taste; this region of the body is also responsible for breathing, eating, and speech. Extirpative surgery can result in considerable cosmetic deformity and functional loss, while high-dose irradiation may cause significant fibrosis, ablation of functioning tissues, and late radiation sequelae. Any surgeon or radiotherapist who must explain the functional losses that result from surgery and irradiation realizes the impact of these losses upon the patient. Consequently, radical surgery and radical irradiation should be used only when absolutely necessary, and avoided whenever possible.

As we have improved our knowledge of the processes of local invasion and lymphatic metastases as a function of pathology and site of origin, we have seen an evolution in patient selection, treatment methodology, and end results. We now understand that certain lesions are biologically less aggressive than others and require less aggressive treatment. We recognize that surgery can be performed and irradiation delivered in ways that preserve anatomy and function without compromising tumour control; and it seems there have been measureable improvements in local – regional control[26] as well as significant advances in preservation of anatomy and function.[39] Individualization of treatment techniques to spare anatomy and function is nowhere more important than in the head and neck region.

CONSERVATION SURGERY

Appropriate surgical therapy of head and neck tumours requires an understanding of the general biological behaviour of the primary neoplasm. Location is the main factor influencing behaviour and mode of spread and therefore determines the surgical procedure to be employed. Accurate tumour localization, improved technical ability, and early diagnosis have resulted in the increasing use of conservation types of head and neck tumour surgery. Conservation surgical techniques combined with radiation therapy have resulted in preserving functions of the head and neck area while not sacrificing tumour cure rate. The ability to

preserve the appearance and function of such areas as the lips, mouth, and larynx is extremely important to patients who are afflicted with head and neck tumours.

Since it is beyond the scope of this report to discuss conservation surgery, reconstructive techniques, and complications for all sites in the head and neck, we will limit our discussion to carcinomas of the lips, tongue, and supraglottis.

Lip

The lip is very prominent and easily visible; relatively minor changes in appearance may produce pronounced overall cosmetic changes to the facial area. Partial loss of function of the lip area may result in speech problems, eating difficulties, and drooling. Smaller lesions of the lip may be resected and the defects closed primarily without significant loss of function or cosmesis. Larger defects require reconstruction with some type of local or distant tissue. Reconstruction techniques have utilized: (1) remaining adjacent lip, (2) advancement of cheek tissue, (3) a cross-lip flap, or (4) a distant flap. A defect of up to 80% of the lip may be repaired by the advancement of an orbicularis oris myocutaneous flap[17] (Figure 8.2). This flap preserves the neurovascular supply from the labial branches of the facial artery and nerve, and the functional and cosmetic results of this reconstruction are much better than with the use of a dynamic flap. Defects greater than 80% of the lip may be successfully reconstructed using a cheek advancement flap.

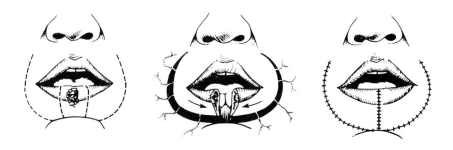

Figure 8.2   Lip repair with orbicularis myocutaneous flap.

This is also a myocutaneous flap and maintains a neurovascular supply to the orbicularis oris and the buccinator components of the flap. The results of this reconstruction are very acceptable for function and cosmesis. The cross-lip and distant flaps have largely been supplanted by the myocutaneous flaps since this type of reconstruction maintains function of the flap itself. Because of their good blood supply they are able to withstand postoperative radiation therapy with virtually no complications. Cure rates for $T_1 - T_2$ lip lesions are in the 80–90% range. Cancer control in patients with cervical metastases is about 50%.[2]

Tongue

Tongue lesions are generally divided into those tumours anterior to the circumvallate papillae and those lesions posterior to the papillae (the base of tongue). In general, those lesions in the anterior tongue are more easily treated and cure rates and functional results are generally higher than for those lesions involving the base. In considering surgical therapy of tongue lesions, small tumours of less than 2 cm in diameter may be treated locally with a partial glossectomy. Traditionally, adequate margins have been considered to comprise a 1 cm margin of tissue which is grossly normal to vision and palpation. However, tumours in the tongue are notoriously more extensive than clinically apparent, and wider margins of 2–3 cm may be necessary to improve local control rates. Adequacy of the margins may be determined by frozen sections. Lesions of the lateral aspect of the tongue are more easily encompassed by a surgical resection, and reconstruction is facilitated by the location. Lesions crossing the midline require more extensive resection, and reconstruction is more difficult. Lesions which extend beyond the tongue generally require a composite resection including portions of the tongue, mandible, and neck. Usually in these extensive procedures the mandibular branch of the seventh nerve, the lingual nerve, hypoglossal nerve, and spinal accessory nerve may be preserved. Most patients having composite resections are able to swallow and speak acceptably and do not require any type of prosthesis in the intraoral area.

Many of the intraoral defects may be closed with the use of a myocutaneous flap. Postoperative radiation therapy may be combined with this procedure and is usually started approximately 3 weeks after the initial surgery. The myocutaneous flap withstands radiation therapy very well. Advanced tumours crossing the midline or involving the middle third of the tongue may require total glossectomy in order to encompass these lesions. These tumours are usually greater than 3 cm in diameter and preoperatively patients have difficulty with swallowing and speech because of tongue fixation. In the past these patients were frequently treated with total glossectomy accompanied by a total laryngectomy. With a total glossectomy and preservation of the larynx most patients had significant problems with aspiration, necessitating a completion laryngectomy at a later date. Recently the use of the pectoralis major myocutaneous flap for reconstruction for soft tissue bulk in the inferior oral cavity has allowed some patients to have total glossectomy with preservation of the larynx. This has been a major advance in the reconstruction of this area as it allows total glossectomy and preservation of laryngeal function. Smaller lesions of the anterior tongue have cure rates of 60–75%. With larger lesions and cervical metastases the cure rate decreases to 30–40%.[58]

Tumours of the base of the tongue are frequently associated with early cervical metastases.[22] For smaller lesions, radiation therapy with surgical salvage of failures is usually optimal. For larger lesions, combined radiation therapy and surgery is usually recommended. Access to the base of the tongue may be accomplished either through a cervical approach or intraorally by splitting the mandible and the tongue anteriorly. In our experience the approach is usually cervical. This may or may not be combined with mandible resection or mandibulotomy. Extensive tumours in the base of the tongue area generally require total glossectomy and reconstruction with a myocutaneous flap. This may or may not be combined with a total laryngectomy depending on extent of disease and the patient's general health. Tumours that are more inferior and extend into the supraglottic area may be approached by an extended supraglottic laryngectomy. If at least one-half of the base of the tongue is able to be preserved, frequently swallowing and phonation will be adequate. Cure rates for base of tongue lesions are low (10–30%).

Over the past 25 years many larynx-sparing procedures have been developed. Conservation laryngeal surgery for properly selected tumours allows preservation of function without increasing the incidence of local recurrence.[39] Treatment philosophies vary. At some centres, radiation therapy is used almost exclusively for primary therapy and surgery is reserved for radiation failures.[14] We have tended to use more surgical therapy and combinations of surgery and radiation in a planned treatment protocol rather than using surgery strictly for radiation failures.[26,39]

Supraglottis

Certain supraglottic carcinomas are amenable to conservation surgery. Histological observation supports the concept of a barrier at the level of the anterior commissure and ventricle which prevents the downward extension of cancer of the epiglottis and false vocal cords.[19] The supraglottic portion of the larynx develops from the buccal–pharyngeal anlage whereas the glottic and subglottic portions develop from the tracheal–bronchial anlage. As a result these two portions of the larynx have separate lymphatic systems. The supraglottic region drains superiorly through the thyrohyoid membrane, while the glottic and subglottic regions drain inferiorly. The principles of supraglottic laryngectomy involve removal of the supraglottic area in continuity with the pre-epiglottic space and the lymphatic channels which drain through the thyrohyoid membrane. This membrane, with its associated lymphatic channels, serves as the point of attachment of the neck dissection. Therefore, supraglottic laryngectomy with neck dissection adheres to the concept of en-bloc resection of the primary tumour with its associated lymphatic drainage channels and lymph nodes.[39] Supraglottic carcinoma does not usually invade the thyroid cartilage, but instead spreads in the mucosa superiorly and frequently invades the pre-epiglottic space and the epiglottic cartilage. Since most of the hyoid bone is removed in a supraglottic resection, the pre-epiglottic space which may be occupied with cancer is just as well encompassed by a supraglottic resection as by a total laryngectomy. Supraglottic carcinoma that extends below the anterior commissure frequently invades the thyroid cartilage and is not amenable to conservation surgery. The supraglottic area is reconstructed by attaching perichondrial laryngeal flaps to the base of tongue area. Even without an epiglottis and false vocal cords, these patients do not aspirate and their phonation is quite good. Patients who have isolated pyriform lesions or involvement of pyriform sinus from extension of a supraglottic tumour may be candidates for a partial laryngopharyngectomy. This resection usually includes the supraglottic area, the aryepiglottic fold, the arytenoid, and the involved areas of the pyriform fossa.[39] The technique is similar to a supraglottic laryngectomy but the arytenoid is removed and the ipsilateral vocal cord is then fixed in the midline to prevent aspiration. With properly applied conservation surgery, patients should have acceptable phonation; they should be able to swallow without aspiration, and they should have an adequate airway and not require a permanent tracheostomy. Survival rates for patients with supraglottic cancers are in range of 80% for T_1, 75% for T_2, 60–70% for T_3, and 60% for T_4 lesions.[39]

IRRADIATION TECHNIQUES

Like the surgeon, the radiotherapist must have an intimate knowledge of patterns of local invasion and lymphatic spread for each cancer of the head and neck. This knowledge will enable him to design irradiation techniques that will ablate the cancer while preserving the functioning tissues within the radiation field.

The optimal field perimeter is that which encompasses the primary tumour and its local and regional extensions, and prevents regrowth of the tumour at the margins of the irradiated volume. The optimal dose distribu-

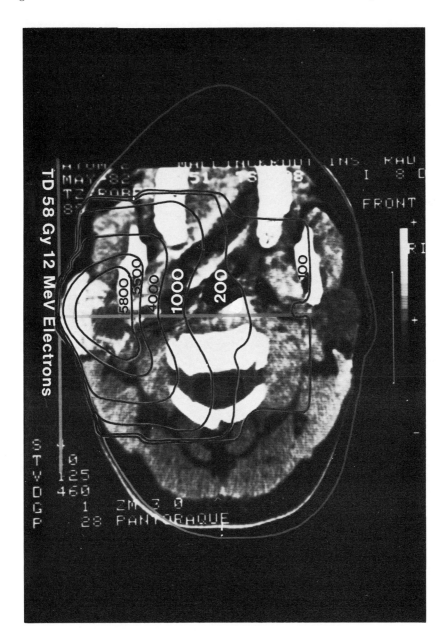

Figure 8.3   Dose distribution of unilateral electron-beam irradiation demonstrating reduction in dose to the spinal cord and parotid opposite the side of the lesion. Ipsilateral parotid is opacified with pantopaque used for sialogram.

tion is that which prevents regrowth of the tumour and spares normal anatomy and function without damaging normal structures in the irradiated volume. Radiotherapy is a complex art that requires careful follow-up of the irradiated patient and revision when rates of tumour regrowth are too great or radiation complications become excessive.

Electron-beam irradiation is a valuable modality as well. Electrons penetrate tissue to a depth which depends on their energy; then dose to the tissue falls precipitously in a short distance. This peculiarity in dose distribution is advantageous because it spares sensitive midline and contralateral structures in the head and neck. For instance, we commonly use electrons to irradiate lymph nodes in the posterior cervical triangle to spare the underlying spinal cord. Electrons are also used to irradiate patients with parotid and skin cancers and small lateralized tumours of the oral cavity and oropharynx that have low rates of contralateral neck metastases (Table 8.1);[22] electron beam irradiation confines the dose to the side of the tumour and spares the opposite parotid (Figure 8.3). The importance of preserving parotid function is illustrated nicely by a chronological study of body weight as a function of number of parotids irradiated (Figure 8.4). Body weight is not altered for patients whose parotids have not received irradiation; it declines slightly and temporarily for those who have had one parotid irradiated; and it declines and does not return to normal in those who have had both parotids irradiated.[42] Therefore, preservation of one functioning parotid allows patients with head and neck cancer to maintain a near-normal state of nutrition.

High-energy X-rays (greater than 10 MeV) are also valuable. Because they are more penetrating than lower-energy X-rays and gamma-rays from ^{60}Co, they enable the radiotherapist to concentrate dose centrally with relative sparing of more superficial structures, such as temporomandibular joints, muscles of mastication, and mandible (Figure 8.5). This peculiarity in dose distribution is useful in the irradiation of midline cancers of the nasopharynx and palate. The use of high-energy X-rays reduces the dose to the temporomandibular joints and muscles of

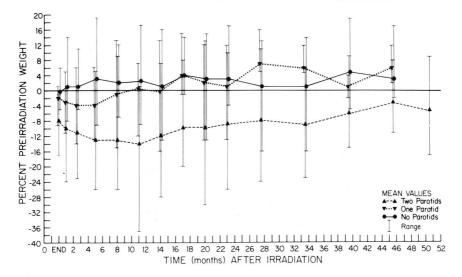

BODY WEIGHT vs. NUMBER OF PAROTIDS IRRADIATED

MEAN VALUES
▲--▲ Two Parotids
▼···▼ One Parotid
●—● No Parotids
| Range

Figure 8.4   Body weight of head and neck cancer patients after irradiation of none, one, or two parotids.

mastication sufficiently to decrease the late effects of irradiation on these structures. Preliminary analysis shows that incisor and gum separations are greater for patients irradiated by high-energy X-rays than those irradiated by ^{60}Co.[25] It also seems that the mouth is more moist after high-energy X-rays than after ^{60}Co; this impression has been difficult to quantify, as salivary flow is immeasurable in most patients whose salivary

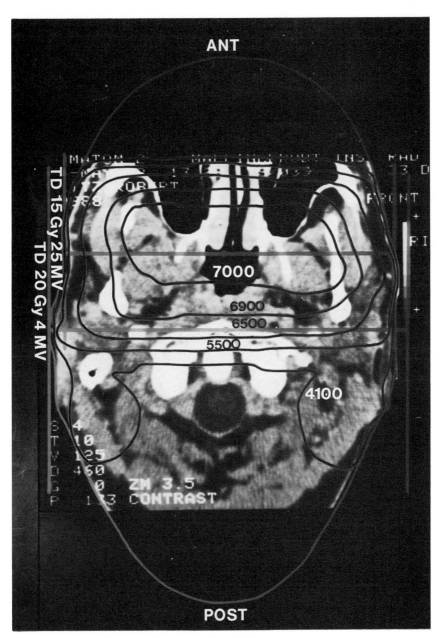

Figure 8.5   Dose distribution of combined 4 MeV and 25 MeV X-rays used to irradiate midline tumours with relative sparing of superficial tissues.

glands have received doses of 4000 rad or greater.[27] Recent measurements of oral moisture using Schirmer paper have established higher levels of oral moisture in patients who have received 50 Gy than patients who received 60 – 70 Gy.[8]

Sophisticated linear accelerators, simulators, treatment aids, and computerized methods of reconstructing dose distribution have definitely advanced the state of radiotherapy for head and neck cancer. Equally important are the training and technical expertise of the radiotherapist. Head and neck cancers are more likely to receive effective treatment in institutions that have sophisticated technology and well-trained personnel.

POST-SURGICAL COMPLICATIONS

Many factors are involved in dertermining the risk of developing some type of postoperative surgical complication: (1) age of patient, (2) nutritional status, (3) anaesthesia risks, (4) cardiac – pulmonary status, (5) area of resection, (6) type of reconstruction, (7) function of reconstructed area, (8) history of smoking – alcoholic intake, (9) hypertension, (10) renal status, and (11) diabetes mellitus.

When one considers the age group and the medical history of most of these patients, it is apparent that most head and neck tumour patients began their therapy with some type of medical problem. This may or may not be responsive to preoperative medical treatment and many times the tumour surgeon is operating on patients who are not good operative risks. This, combined with preoperative or postoperative radiation therapy, leads to a significant number of postoperative complications. The psychological problems of many of these patients are great. The diagnosis of cancer commonly produces a significant reaction in the patient and in the family. The long postoperative course and associated radiation therapy course is depressing to patient and family.

In *lip* resections for carcinoma, the complications primarily are cosmetic and functional. The cosmetic ones usually result from an extensive resection with narrowing of the mouth inlet; many of these may be avoided by proper planning at the initial resection with the use of myocutaneous flaps for reconstruction. Functional problems lead to difficulty in speech, mastication, and drooling. Again, with proper surgical planning, most of these complications can be avoided and a functional mouth inlet should be the end result.

Resections of the oral area commonly lead to dysphagia, inability to swallow properly, and speech difficulties. Resections of the tongue commonly result in shortening of the tongue with decreased mobility. The resultant speech is usually intelligible, but certainly different from preoperative speech. If mobility is significantly restricted, then difficulty in swallowing may result. If the resection extends to the palate, then velopharyngeal incompetence, poor speech, and reflux of oral contents into the nasal cavity commonly occur. This problem can be corrected by a prosthesis worn in the roof of the mouth and extending back into the palate area. Fistulas may arise in the oral area following large resections. These may be secondary to tightness of closure or to poor healing due to poor general health and/or associated radiation therapy. With good surgical planning, fistulas seldom occur. Tight closures can almost always be eliminated by the use of local or distant flaps, especially the myocutaneous flap. If wound breakdown occurs, exposure of the mandible may result in osteomyelitis with sequestration of the bone. This occurs more commonly in patients who have had radiation implants in the oral area. Again, anticipation of this problem during the resection will usually allow prevention by use of good vascular flaps to cover the anticipated problem area.

The problems associated with resection of the larynx or pharynx generally are related to poor medical condition of the patient, or to incorrect surgical planning and technique. If large resections of the pharynx are performed without proper technique for reconstruction, then tight closures ensue with stenosis, dysphagia, and inability to swallow. In laryngeal resections, improper reconstruction results either in stenosis of the supraglottic or glottic area producing an inadequate airway or, in some cases, too large a glottic airway with improper closure and significant postoperative aspiration. Partial laryngeal resections commonly produce voice changes. The voice is usually intelligible but hoarse. Those who have had supraglottic laryngectomies commonly have the best voice because the true vocal cords are still intact.

Commonly, patients with head and neck tumours have tracheostomies either temporarily or permanently. Tracheitis and crustiness of the tracheal area commonly occurs. This can usually be treated with local measures. The problem with tracheal stenosis is becoming less because of proper tracheostomy techniques as well as the use of low-pressure cuffs on tracheostomy tubes. Avoidance of low tracheostomies decreases the chance of innominate artery rupture.

The major complications in the neck include

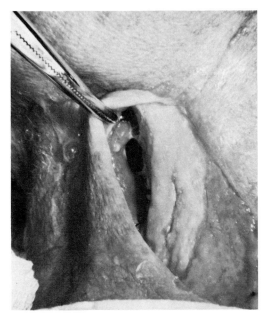

Figure 8.6   Pharyngeal–cutaneous fistula. White area is an epithelialized dermal graft protecting the carotid artery.

fistula, carotid artery exposure and blow-out, and infection with loss of skin flaps. Most fistulas occurring in the pharyngeal area will close with local care. Some fistulas will require local flap closure. With the development and more aggressive use of flaps for primary closure, the rate of fistula formation has decreased. If a fistula develops and saliva is draining directly over the exposed carotid artery, then the chances for a carotid blow-out increase. At the time of the initial surgery, most surgeons place a dermal graft over the carotid so that it may epithelialize and protect the blood vessel if a fistula develops (Figure 8.6).

Infection and loss of skin flaps can usually be kept to a minimum by ensuring that the flap has a good vascular supply and by avoidance of fistulas. If skin loss does occur, skin grafts or flap coverage may be necessary.

Patients who have had preoperative radiation therapy are certainly more prone to develop postoperative complications than those who have not received any radiation. The difference in complication rate between patients receiving preoperative and postoperative radiation therapy depends on the series.[24,38,53] This is a difficult area to study because of the multiple factors involved with the patient's medical condition, as well as the surgery and reconstruction performed and the size, type, and location of the tumour. Generally, most studies have shown that patients receiving postoperative radiation tolerate surgery as well as, or better than, patients receiving preoperative treatment (Table 8.3).[53] On the basis of our clinical experience we feel that patients receiving postoperative radiation therapy generally have fewer complications. Again, this is difficult to quantify because surgical techniques, especially the use of myocutaneous flaps, have improved with time and this may also be influencing the decrease in postoperative complications.

RADIATION COMPLICATIONS

Ionizing radiation affects any functioning or

TABLE 8.3   COMPLICATIONS OF
SUPRAGLOTTIC LARYNGECTOMY
AFTER PRE- AND POSTOPERATIVE
IRRADIATION[53]

Complications	Preoperative	Postoperative
Infarction	1 (1.4%)	2 (11.8%)
Skin slough	2 (2.8%)	0 (9%)
Fistula	4 (5.6%)	0 (9%)
Carotid rupture	0 (0%)	9 (0%)
Insufficiency	5 (6.9%)	3 (17.6%)
Death	2 (2.8%)	1 (5.9%)
Chondritis	2 (2.8%)	0 (0%)
Hospital time	25 days	21 days

non-functioning tissue within the radiation field. The resulting biological effect is determined by the total dose of irradiation, the size of each increment, and the total time. Tissues that are reproducing rapidly are acutely affected by irradiation and those that divide slowly or not at all manifest the effects of irradiation later. These principles that govern the biological effect of irradiation on normal tissue are readily demonstrated in the head and neck region.

Irradiation of oral, pharyngeal, and endolaryngeal *mucosa* gradually produces an acute mucositis that only resolves after cessation of treatment. The rapidly dividing stem cells that remain in small islands of residual mucosa and at the periphery of the radiation field grow to re-epithelialize the irradiated area. Irradiation of *vasculoconnective tissues* causes microscopic deposition of collagen and narrowing and obliteration of small vessels; these changes undoubtedly explain the mucosal atrophy, telangiectasia, alveolar bone exposure, and subcutaneous induration that we later see. Irradiation of *muscles* of mastication and temporomandibular *joints* likewise causes fibrosis of the muscles and joint capsule; this fibrosis causes variable degrees of trismus and limits the patient's ability to chew. Irradiation of mandible, maxilla, and temporal *bone* destroys osteocytes, marrow, and small vessels; the remaining bone is, for all intents and purposes, inert and would easily become infected and necrotic were it not for

the protection of surrounding mucosal, submucosal, and subcutaneous soft tissues. Irradiation of major *salivary glands* preferentially damages serous acini causing a diffuse deposition of collagen in the gland; the patient complains of a dry mouth and difficulty clearing thick mucous saliva. The saliva loses its buffering capacity due to a reduction in bicarbonate and becomes more acidic; bacterial flora change and the *teeth* are more susceptible to decay. Excessive irradiation of the *central nervous system* may cause demyelination and necrosis of white matter after a delay of 1 – 3 years. The resulting neurological sequelae of cerebral radionecrosis and radiation myelopathy are truly calamitous for the patient.

The acute effects of irradiation are managed easily by adequate hydration and caloric intake, but the late effects of irradiation are not so easily managed and are best avoided by delivering no more than the maximum dose in small increments over a long period of time. The tolerance of normal tissues in the head and neck region ranges from 50 Gy in 5 weeks for the central nervous system to nearly 70 Gy in 7 weeks for bone. Late radiation sequelae are avoided by protecting more sensitive tissues, such as spinal cord, once they have received their maximum tolerated dose. It is clear that large daily increments of irradiation over short periods of time and excessive total doses of irradiation are associated with a greater incidence of late radiation damage than are conventional fractionation schemata. Consider the experience of Fletcher *et al.*[11] for cancers of the vocal cord (Table 8.4). By

TABLE 8.4   LARYNGEAL OEDEMA AND
NECROSIS ACCORDING TO
RADIATION DOSE, TIME AND
FRACTIONATION[11]

Dose in Gray	Duration in weeks	Fraction size in Gray	Oedema or necrosis
50	4	2.5 ⎫	6/68 (9%)
60	5	2.4 ⎭	
60	5½	2.14 ⎫	3/330 (1%)
70	6½	2.12 ⎭	

reducing fraction size and increasing the total dose to maintain the same approximate biologically equivalent nominal standard dose (NSD),[9] Fletcher was able to reduce significantly the incidence of laryngeal necrosis.

RADIATION RESPONSE

Response of tumours to irradiation is a function of their pathology, size, and morphology. Undifferentiated tumours are more responsive than differentiated ones; small lesions are more easily controlled by irradiation than large ones; and exophytic lesions are more responsive to irradiation than endophytic, ulcerating ones. The experienced clinician can usually select those lesions that will respond to irradiation and thereby predict radiocurability. Understanding the selection process for any particular treatment is important in interpreting the results of treatment. Interpret cautiously claims of treatment superiority in those publications that report only part of a patient population and conveniently avoid discussion of patient selection.

Those lesions that disappear by the end of full-course irradiation are less likely to recur than those that remain (Table 8.5).[23] This dictum was contested by one publication,[52] but was subsequently confirmed when the same data were reviewed again along with the records of additional patients from the same institution.[3] Others have also correlated radioresponsiveness with radiocurability.[23,48]

Continuous irradiation to doses of 60–70 Gy utilizing *conventional fractionation* of 2 Gy per day has been compared to *split-course* and *unconventional fractionation* schemes using NSD equivalents[9] of continuous irradiation. Though unproven by clinical trial, the existing evidence indicates that continuous irradiation yields greater tumour control than either split-course or unconventional fractionation schema using larger fractions and smaller total doses.[7,40] Apparently split-course irradiation, i.e., a continuous course with a rest midway, reduces the biological effect of the irradiation on the tumour.[40] It also seems that unconventional fractionation schemata or NSD equivalents of continuous irradiation are not biologically equivalent in their effect on the tumour.[7]

Clinical dose–response correlations are available for a variety of head and neck tumours and normal tissues (Figure 8.7), but are less than ideal for a number of reasons. Most patients in the megavoltage era have been treated within a narrow dose range between 50 and 70 Gy; consequently, little is known about the effects of irradiation for doses above or below that narrow range. Another problem is the small number of patients at each dose level, making it statistically impossible to separate the radiation effects at one dose level from those at another. Also, there are significant discrepancies in dose–response information from different institutions for similar-stage tumours in the same site; one suspects that tumour size, pathological differentiation, and tumour morphology are not comparable. All of these factors, of course, are important

TABLE 8.5   RECURRENCE OF HEAD AND NECK CANCER IN RELATION TO TUMOUR REGRESSION AT THE END OF RADIATION[23]

Tumor size at end of radiation	No recurrence within 2 years		Recurrence within 2 years
Disappears ($n = 26$)	18 (69%)	$P = 0.009$	8 (31%)
Decreased, no change or no information ($n = 84$)	34 (40%)		49 (58%)

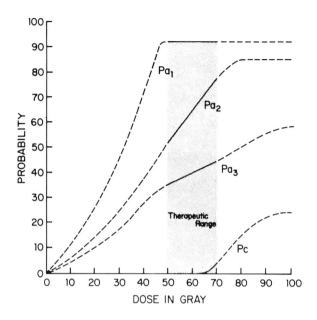

Figure 8.7 Graph of the probability of ablation for a small tumour (Pa₁), for an intermediate tumour (Pa₂), for a large tumour (Pa₃), and the probability of complication (Pc) for normal tissues of the head and neck as a function of dose. Note the usual therapeutic range of dose between 50 and 70 Gy.

determinants of response to irradiation and influence greatly any dose–response analysis.

Review of available dose–response information shows minimal or no variation in tumour control between 50 and 70 Gy for very small and very large tumours;[26] there seems to be a modest improvement in tumour control within the therapeutic range for intermediate size tumours (Figure 8.7).[45] It is likely that a dose–response could be appreciated at doses lower than 50 Gy for small tumours and at doses greater than 70 Gy for larger tumours (Figure 8.7). The incidence of normal tissue complications begins to rise between 65 and 70 Gy and should influence choice of dose for a particular tumour. The decision to prescribe a dose in the upper part of the therapeutic range, and thereby risk radiation damage to normal tissues, should be reserved for those tumours which show significant improvement in tumour control within the therapeutic range.

A common mistake is to prescribe high doses and risk radiation complications when there is little hope that the higher dose will improve the overall rate of tumour control. Dose is best prescribed by a radiotherapist who understands in depth the clinical dose–response relationships for tumours and normal tissues of the head and neck.

ENDPOINTS

Treatment success for cancers of the head and neck is better measured by endpoints other than patient survival. Patient survival is an accurate method of measuring success of treatment when death is invariably due to the cancer, as is the case with glioblastoma multiforme. Patients with head and neck cancer, however, die from causes other than the cancer in significant proportions that vary for each individual site (Table 8.6). Deaths

TABLE 8.6   PERCENTAGES OF PATIENTS WHO
DIE OF CAUSES OTHER THAN
CANCER BY HEAD AND NECK SITE

Site	Percentage
Vocal cord[37]	88
Supraglottic larynx[28]	61
Oral tongue[31]	52
Floor of mouth[32]	54
Base of tongue[43]	45
Tonsil[41]	50
Pyriform sinus[30]	38
Pharyngeal wall[29]	35
Transglottic larynx[36]	35
Nasopharynx[5]	21
Unknown primary[46]	21

due to intercurrent disease, complications of treatment, second primary cancers, and unknown reasons are not uncommon, and, on the average, occur as often as deaths due to tumour. It therefore seems to us that more direct measurements of treatment success are preferable to the traditional reporting of survival. Specifically, we would like to know how often our treatment eradicates the primary tumour and regional lymphatic metastases without regrowth for a period of follow-up adequate to detect the majority of recurrences. This endpoint, known as tumour (T) and nodal (N) control, is a direct measure of our ability to successfully treat head and neck cancers by surgery and irradiation. It is also important to record the preservation of specific anatomy and function that is associated with specific sites in the head and neck. For example, we always report how often larynx and voice are preserved for cancers of the larynx. The abilities of laryngectomy and subtotal supraglottic laryngectomy to control the tumour may be comparable, but the conservation procedure is superior because it more often spares voice.

Measurements of treatment benefit, such as tumour control and anatomical function, should be accompanied by measurements of treatment risk. One particular treatment may control the tumour as well as another, but be rejected because of excessive morbidity or mortality. The ideal treatment by surgery and irradiation is that which achieves T + N control and preserves anatomy and function with the least risk and cost to the patient.

MANAGEMENT BY SITE

The designation 'head and neck cancer' is a deceptively simple label for a variety of cancers in a number of individual sites. There is no consensus on the best approach to the treatment of each particular site; rather, treatment varies according to the bias and experience of each individual practitioner, group, or institution. There have been few well-conducted clinical trials that compare conventional methods of surgery and irradiation for individual sites and it is often impossible to compare retrospective reviews with one another for a number of reasons: (1) selected groups of patients are reported, instead of whole populations; (2) patterns of selection are not addressed; and (3) analysis of end-results are often not comparable. In the reporting of end-results, we think it is important to define treatment goals and patient selection and to report entire populations of patients treated in a particular institution. We also think it is important to analyse tumour control, preservation of anatomy and function, and risk of treatment. Analysis of risk and benefit can then be used to search for improved or optimum treatment strategies.

The limited scope of this chapter precludes an in-depth summary of management for all tumours of the head and neck. We will therefore focus our attention on three tumours whose management differs because of different anatomical location, patterns of local and lymphatic spread, and biological behaviour. The first, carcinoma of the nasopharynx, is a tumour for which there is no selection of treatment. The second, carcinoma of the oral tongue, is a tumour for which there is selection of progressively more aggressive treatments as a function of increasing tumour stage. The third, carcinoma of the supraglottic larynx, is a tumour for which there is controversy about the best primary method of treatment, surgery, or irradiation. The contrast that exists in the management of these three tumours points out the necessity to study separately each head and neck site. The issues of management for one head and neck cancer are not the same for others and investigators should avoid the pitfall of 'conglomerate study' of a variety of sites.

NASOPHARYNX

Goals

The goal in the management of this tumour is a high rate of tumour and nodal control without an excessive incidence of late radiation complications.

Selection

All patients are irradiated.

Radiation Alone

Nasopharyngeal cancer is a difficult tumour to irradiate because of its close proximity to the central nervous system and the fact that the tumour requires more radiation dose than the brain and spinal cord will tolerate. Accurate definition of tumour extent is essential before the radiotherapist can design a field perimeter that encompasses the tumour and excludes the central nervous system. Polytomography and, more recently, computed tomography have proven invaluable in the staging of nasopharyngeal cancer. In our institution the percentage of $T_3 - T_3$ nasopharyngeal cancers has increased from approximately 50% before 1969 to 80% now;[26] we attribute this change to the advent of polytomography in 1969 which accurately demonstrates base of skull destruction (T_4) and tumour beyond the confines of the nasopharynx (T_3). Despite the diagnosis of more advanced tumours in recent years we have seen an improvement in T and N control from 50% to 70%, which we have attributed to staff sub-specialization and greater technical expertise.[26] Review of portal films has shown fewer inadequate portals and less shielding of

the nasopharynx in recent years.[26] Technical accuracy correlated with improved tumour control, and we concluded that repetitive daily delivery of dose was critical for the successful eradication of nasopharyngeal cancer. Some have supplemented the external irradiation with intracavitary irradiation but the benefit of this supplemental dose is unproven.[55]

Issues

The central issue for a tumour that is treated by radiation alone is the optimum dose of irradiation that will produce maximum tumour control without excessive complications. Late radiation complications of varying degrees of severity occur frequently (Table 8.7)[26] and might be reduced were it possible to reduce dose without compromising tumour control. Three keys to the reduction of dose to normal tissues are: (1) dose optimization or concentration of dose in the region of tumour with relative sparing of normal tissues, (2) selection of patients who require lower doses, and (3) understanding the relationship between dose, complications, and tumour control. We routinely reduce dose to normal tissues by using high-energy X-rays to concentrate dose centrally in the region of the tumour with relative sparing of superficially located normal tissues (Figure 8.5). Patients with undifferentiated carcinomas, lymphoepitheliomas, and small tumours probably require lower doses to control their tumours than those with well-differentiated or larger tumours.[15,34] Since complications are dose-dependent and begin to occur in the upper part of the therapeutic range of dose, dose-response analysis for the tumour becomes critical. Study of our patients with nasopharyngeal carcinoma failed to show improvement in tumour control within the therapeutic range for either $T_1 - T_2$ or $T_3 - T_4$ tumours[26] (Figure 8.8). Consequently, we prescribe no more than 6500 rad in $6\frac{1}{2}$ weeks for lymphoepitheliomas and small tumours; we do, however, continue to prescribe 7000 rad in 7 weeks for large tumours in the belief that the late effects of

TABLE 8.7   LATE RADIATION COMPLICATIONS FOR
NASOPHARYNGEAL CARCINOMA,
MALLINCKRODT INSTITUTE OF RADIOLOGY[26],
1950−78 (*n* = 118)

	No.	(%)
Severe		
Unable to eat/aspiration	4*	(3)
Pharyngeal stricture	2*	(2)
Suspected radiation myelopathy	2	(2)
Ankylosis of TM joints	1	(1)
Osteonecrosis of mandible (fracture)	1	(1)
Mastoiditis	1	(1)
Growth retardation	1	(1)
Total†	10	(8)
Mild		
Neck fribrosis	19	(16)
Trismus	14	(12)
Dental caries	11	(9)
Serous otitis	8	(7)
Perforated eardrum	6	(5)
Bone sequestrum	7	(6)
Bone exposure	2	(2)
Cellulitis of cheek	2	(2)
Furunculosis	1	(1)
Laryngitis	2	(2)
Cranial nerve palsies	4	(3)
Swelling of tongue	1	(1)
Hypothyroidism	3	(3)
Total	44	(37)

* Five fatalities due to complications.
† Patients may have had more than one complication.

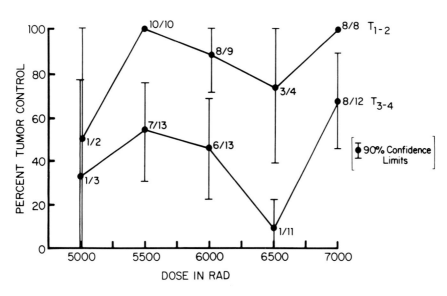

Figure 8.8   Dose−response analysis for T_1-T_2 and T_3-T_4 nasopharyngeal carcinomas. (Reproduced by permission of *Cancer.*)

radiation are acceptable given any chance for improvement in tumour control.

Distant metastases develop in a high proportion of patients with undifferentiated nasopharyngeal cancers and those with bilateral neck metastases.[6] The usefulness of chemotherapy for these particular patients needs to be tested, since many of the patients are young and suitable candidates for aggressive treatment.

ORAL TONGUE

Goals

The goal in the management of these tumours is uncomplicated ablation of the primary tumour and neck nodes with preservation of mandible and tongue for mastication and speech.

Selection

In our institution, small surface lesions have been treated by local excision (LE), $T_1 - T_2$, N_0 lesions have been treated by radiation alone (RA) and larger lesions and those with palpable lymph nodes have been treated by preoperative radiation and surgery (R + S).[31]

Surgery Alone

There is a small subset of patients with surface lesions who are suitable for local excision. These tumours exhibit only superficial invasion of underlying muscle, have a low rate of lymph node metastases (10%) and are salvageable by additional treatment.[31] The patients survive long periods and develop a high rate of second primary cancers.[31] Because of a significant rate of complications, we avoid interstitial implant for these lesions unless the margins of excision contain tumour. We also avoid external elective irradiation because of the low rate of sub-clinical lymphatic metastases and because we wish to preserve parotid function. Careful follow-up is essential.

Surgical excision of $T_1 - T_2 N_0$ lesions (invading tongue) without adjunctive irradiation

TABLE 8.8 PERCENTAGES OF PRIMARY AND NECK FAILURES AFTER LOCAL EXCISION OF CANCERS OF THE ORAL TONGUE[49] ($n = 185$)

Tongue recurrence	21
Neck recurrence ($N_0 \rightarrow N_+$)	
$T_1 N_0$	29
$T_2 N_0$	43
$T_3 N_0$	77

TABLE 8.9 PERCENTAGES OF ELECTIVE NECK IRRADIATION (ENI) FOR CANCERS OF THE ORAL TONGUE AND FLOOR OF MOUTH

Dose in Gray	Neck recurrence ($N_0 \rightarrow N_+$)	
	ENI	No ENI
40^{16}	5	37
$45 - 50^{35}$	0	35
60^1	0	17

is best avoided because of a significant rate of tumour regrowth in the tongue and necks[49,57] (Table 8.8) and because elective irradiation of N_0 necks effectively eradicates subclinical lymphatic metastases[1,16,35] (Table 8.9).

Radiation Alone

External irradiation and interstitial implant are considered optimum treatment in many institutions for $T_1 - T_2$, N_0 lesions of the oral tongue because there is a high rate of tumour control with preservation of mandible and tongue. Study of our own patients treated by RA showed ultimate T + N control of 88% for $T_1 N_0$ lesions and 53% for $T_2 N_0$ lesions.[31] Because of poor tumour control and a high rate (25%) of late radiation complications (Figure 8.9) we no longer treat the $T_2 N_0$ lesions by RA.[31] These lesions are simply excised and the tongue and neck are irradiated postoperatively by electron beam to spare the opposite parotid. If the margins of excision contain tumour, interstitial implant of the tongue is done. As long as the tip of the tongue is preserved, speech is quite good.

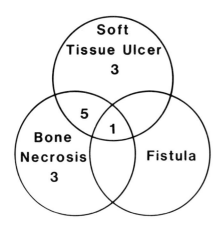

Figure 8.9   Venn diagram of late radiation complications after external and interstitial irradiation for carcinoma of the oral tongue (1962–76).

Surgery and Irradiation

For larger tumours of the oral tongue and those with palpable lymph nodes (T_3–T_4, N +) combined surgery and irradiation are indicated because tumour control by either method alone is poor. After combined R + S our tumour control for these lesions was 57% and no patient who recurred in the tongue and/or neck was successfully retreated.[31] The mandible was preserved in roughly half of these patients by pull-through glossectomy or mandibulotomy plus partial glossectomy and in-continuity neck dissection.[31] Patients with advanced tongue cancer are a very poor risk group as one-third die of causes other than cancer within 2 years after treatment.

Issues

Can the incidence of late radiation complications associated with external irradiation and implant be reduced by combinations of conservative surgery and irradiation without compromising tumour control? Is elective irradiation of the ipsilateral neck sufficient for lesions of the lateral border of the tongue? How often can mandible be preserved for advanced lesions? Can tumour control of advanced lesions be improved by more radical

treatment or is the host simply too weak to withstand the treatment? There needs to be better definition of patient selection for particular methods of treatment and continued search for improved treatment strategies.

SUPRAGLOTTIC LARYNX

Goals

The goal in the management of carcinoma of the supraglottic larynx is control of the primary tumour and lymph nodes with preservation of voice whenever possible.

Selection

The treatment of choice is surgery in some institutions and radiotherapy in others. Most of our patients, for instance, are treated by adjunctive irradiation and conservation surgery to preserve voice. Only a few do not undergo this operation because of poor medical condition or discovery that the tumour is transglottic. Patients are probably unselected in those institutions that favour radiation alone, with surgery reserved for salvage of radiation failures.

Radiation Alone

Full-course irradiation controls the primary tumour and lymph nodes and preserves voice in three-quarters of those with T_1–T_2 and 40% of those with T_3–T_4 carcinomas of the supraglottis[4,10,12,13,56] (Table 8.10). Radiation failures can be salvaged by laryngectomy and/or neck dissection in roughly one-half of the small lesions and one-quarter of the larger ones.

TABLE 8.10   TUMOR CONTROL AND VOICE PRESERVATION BY STAGE AND TYPE OF TREATMENT FOR CARCINOMA OF THE SUPRAGLOTTIC LARYNX

T + N Control and voice preservation	RA[4,10,12,13,56]	R + S[28]
T_1–T_2	230/312 (74%)	62/84 (74%)
T_3–T_4	156/391 (40%)	51/76 (67%)

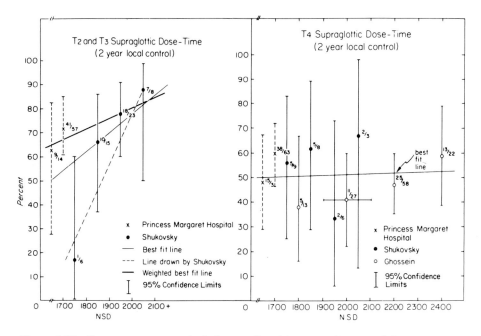

Figure 8.10   Dose–response analysis for small and large carcinomas of the supraglottic larynx. (Reproduced from Harwood *et al.* (in press), *International Journal of Radiation Oncology, Biology and Physics.*)

Dose–response curves for early cancer of the supraglottis show a moderate improvement in tumour control within the range of doses commonly used, but the curve is not as steep as many believe.[45] Harwood *et al.* have nicely demonstrated how small numbers of patients at each dose level can be statistically misleading giving the impression that the curve is steep when, in fact, it is not[14] (Figure 8.10). There is moderate improvement in tumour control with increasing doses of irradiation for $T_2 - T_3$ supraglottic cancers but little improvement for T_4 lesions (Figure 8.10). The dose–response information available indicates there is some value to increasing dose for small, but not for large, carcinomas of the supraglottis. The radiotherapist must remember that laryngeal oedema and cartilage necrosis are more common in the upper parts of the therapeutic dose range.

Surgery and Radiation

Conservation surgery with adjunctive irradiation controls the primary tumour and lymph nodes in three-quarters of those with $T_1 - T_2$ and two-thirds of those with $T_3 - T_4$ cancers of the supraglottic larynx[28] (Table 8.10). Voice is preserved in 70% of all patients who enter the clinic.[28] Major complications occur in 16% and the operative mortality is 4%.[28] The cost of surgical treatment is three to four times greater than the cost of irradiation. The value of elective irradiation of the necks and adjunctive irradiation in general is not as well established for carcinomas of the supraglottis as it is for other sites; nevertheless, it is used rather routinely and has proven somewhat effective in one clinical trial.[47]

Issues

The major controversy in the management of carcinoma of the supraglottis surrounds the choice of the primary method of treatment; will surgery or irradiation give the best results? Radiation therapy successfully controls as many $T_1 - T_2$ cancers of the supraglottis as conservation surgery and saves the voice with less risk and cost than surgery (Table 8.10). Conservation surgery, on the other hand, more often controls tumour and saves voice for larger $T_3 - T_4$ cancers of the supraglottis (Table 8.10).

Radiation success depends on tumour size and is greater for small than for large tumours. If large tumours are irradiated and subsequently fail, they are salvaged by total laryngectomy with loss of voice. Alternatively, many large cancers of the supraglottis can be managed by conservation surgery because they remain compartmentalized and amenable to subtotal supraglottic laryngectomy.[19,39,44] As a result, tumour control and voice preservation are greater for conservation surgery than full-course irradiation in the treatment of advanced cancers of the supraglottis (Table 8.10). Probably the best approach is to irradiate the small lesions for cure and to perform conservation surgery for the larger lesions.

CLINICAL TRIALS

Clinical trials that have tested the value of conventional surgery and irradiation for head and neck cancer will be summarized in chronological order.

Strong, E.W. (1969)[50]

This important trial from Memorial Sloan–Kettering demonstrated the value of low-dose preoperative irradiation (20 Gy in 1 week) in reducing neck recurrence for a variety of tumours that required radical neck dissection as part of their treatment. The addition of radiation to the neck dissection was particularly valuable for patients with advanced nodal disease involving multiple levels in the neck.

Ketcham, A.S. et al. (1969)[18]

This trial tested the value of a single dose of 10 Gy the day before surgery for head and neck cancers. This dose of preoperative irradiation caused a significant number of post-surgical complications but failed to improve tumour control. The data were relatively inconclusive because of inability to accession adequate numbers of patients into the sites under study.

Lawrence, W.L. et al. (1974)[21]

This prospective trial tested the value of 14 Gy in two treatments 24–48 hours before surgery for 143 patients with cancers of the oral cavity, oropharynx, and larynx. The SA (74) and R + S (69) groups had comparable rates of recurrence (35% vs 22%), distant metastases (16% vs 18%), surgical complications (20% vs 24%), and 3-year survival (48% vs 61%). No risk or benefit could be demonstrated for this schedule of pre-operative irradiation.

Vanderbrouck, C. et al. (1977)[54]

This trial from the Gustave Roussy Institute compared high-dose pre- and postoperative irradiation (55 Gy in $5\frac{1}{2}$–6 weeks) for carcinomas of the hypopharynx. A control group treated by SA was not included and only 49 of 177 patients seen in the institution over 2 years were considered eligible for randomization. The trial was terminated prematurely because of a prohibitive rate of fatal complications in

TABLE 8.11   COMPARISON OF COMPLICATIONS AND SURVIVAL AFTER PRE- AND POSTOPERATIVE IRRADIATION FOR CANCERS OF THE HYPOPHARYNX[54]

	Preoperative[25]	Postoperative[24]
Carotid artery haemorrhage	38%	0%
Breakdown of cutaneous sutures	44%	13%
Pharyngocutaneous fistulae	38%	45%
Mean hospital stay	98 days	23 days
Five-year survival	36%*	56%

* Postoperative deaths due to complications excluded.

the pre-operatively irradiated group. Rates of carotid artery haemorrhage, breakdown of cutaneous suture lines, and deaths due to these complications were significantly higher in the preoperative than the postoperative group (Table 8.11). Pharyngocutaneous fistulae were comparable for the two groups, but the average time required to heal the fistulae was 98 hospital days for the preoperative group and only 23 days for the posteropative group. Administration of high doses of irradiation before surgery significantly delayed healing in these patients. Survival of patients who received irradiation postoperatively was significantly greater than survival of those who received it preoperatively (Table 8.10).

Strong, M.S. et al. (1978)[51]

This trial failed to demonstrate any value for low-dose preperative irradiation (20 Gy in 1 week) in addition to surgery for cancers of the oropharynx and hypopharynx. Tumour control, complications, and 3-year survival were comparable for the SA and R + S groups.

Snow, J.B. et al. (1981)[47]

This trial, conducted by the Radiation Therapy Oncology Group, compared pre- and postoperative irradiation plus surgery for cancers of the oral cavity, oropharynx, supraglottic larynx, hypopharynx, and maxillary sinus; in addition, patients with cancers of the oral cavity and oropharynx were randomized to a third arm, radiation alone. Aside from a suggested improvement in local-regional control for the postoperatively irradiated patients with cancers of the supraglottis, there were no significant differences in local – regional control or survival for any of the treatment methods used for any particular site. Surgical complications for the pre- and postoperatively irradiated groups were comparable for the oral cavity patients (42% vs 44%), 2.5 times greater for the preoperatively irradiated patients with cancers of oropharynx (27% vs 10%), 1.4 times greater for the preoperatively irradiated patients with cancers of the supraglottic larynx

(45% vs 33%), and 1.5 times greater for the postoperatively irradiated patients with cancers of the hypopharynx (39% vs 58%). The last finding differs from the results of the Gustave Roussy trial and is unexplained by differences in preoperative dose, as doses for both studies were roughly comparable (50 Gy in the RTOG study and 55 Gy in the Gustave Roussy study).

The major problems with the clinical trials conducted thus far have been their limited scope and failure to access adequate numbers of patients with cancers of particular sites and stages. Trials have been terminated prematurely and conclusions drawn from 'conglomerate analysis' of a number of sites. Another problem in recent trials has been the lack of a control group of patients treated by surgery alone. It is not enough to assume that the addition of irradiation will improve upon the results of surgery alone; it needs to be proven. Out of four trials[18,21,50,51] that have compared SA and R + S, only the Memorial trial[50] has shown an advantage to the addition of preoperative irradiation. To address the timing of adjunctive irradiation, i.e., pre- or postoperative, is important; but we think it even more important to first confirm the value of adjunctive irradiation for given stages and sites of disease.

ULTIMATE POTENTIAL

We doubt that the maximum potential of conventional surgery and radiotherapy has been realized for head and neck cancer. It may have been reached in a few major institutions, but probably not in many smaller ones. Consider the findings of the Patterns of Care Study which was funded by the National Cancer Institute to characterize the quality of radiotherapy in the United States.[20] The investigators studied a variety of institutions, large and small, public and private, associated and not associated with educational programmes. The workup and outcome of treatment for a variety of neoplasms, including

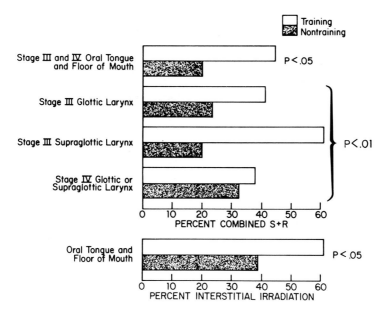

Figure 8.11   Histogram of type of treatment used in training and non-training institutions for cancers of the oral cavity and larynx.

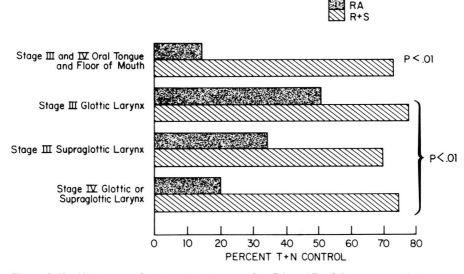

Figure 8.12   Histogram of treatment outcome after RA and R + S for cancers of the oral cavity and larynx.

head and neck cancer, were studied. Compliance with existing standards of workup and better treatment results were more often achieved in major teaching institutions than smaller, non-teaching institutions.[20] Combined use of surgery and external and interstitial irradiation in the treatment of head and neck cancer was more often practised in major institutions (Figure 8.11) and was thought to account for the better outcome of treatment in these institutions[20] (Figure 8.12).

Conventional surgery and radiotherapy

may have maximized tumour control in major institutions, but even these institutions can make progress in the preservation of anatomy and function. Efforts to improve the quality of physician education and training must continue so that smaller hopsitals will eventually become staffed by physicians better qualified to treat head and neck cancer. In the meantime, centralized referral of patients to major centres is probably the most practical way of guaranteeing quality care for the patient with head and neck cancer. We think periodic re-evaluation of paterns of care and treatment outcome for patients with head and neck cancer is desirable. Hopefully, this re-evaluation will ultimately demonstrate that the potential of conventional surgery and radiotherapy is being achieved for this group of diseases.

REFERENCES

1. Bagshaw, M.A., and Thompson, R.W. (1971). Elective irradiation of the neck in patients with primary carcinoma of the head and neck. *JAMA*, **217**, 456–458.
2. Baily, B.J. (1977). Management of carcinoma of the lip. *Laryngoscope*, **87**, 250–260.
3. Barkley, H.T., and Fletcher, G.H. (1977). The significance of residual disease after external irradiation of squamous cell carcinoma of the oropharynx. *Radiology*, **124**, 493–495.
4. Bataini, J.P., Ennuyer, A., Poncet, P., and Ghossein, N.A. (1974). Treatment of supraglottic cancer by radical high dose radiotherapy. *Cancer*, **33**, 1253–1262.
5. Bedwinek, J.M. (1982). Unpublished data, Mallinckrodt Institute of Radiology.
6. Bedwinek, J.M., Perez, C.A., and Keys, D.J. (1980). Analysis of failures after definitive irradiation for carcinoma of the nasopharynx. *Cancer*, **45**, 2725–2729.
7. Cox, J.D., Byhardt, R.W., Komaki, R., and Greenberg, M. (1980). Reduced fractionation and the potential of hypoxic cell sensitizers in irradiation of malignant epithelial tumors. *Int. J. Radiat. Oncol. Biol. Phys.*, **6**, 37–40.
8. Davis, C., Marks, J.E., and Purdy, J.A. (1982). Quantifying oral moisture levels after parotid irradiation. Unpublished data, Mallinckrodt Institute of Radiology.
9. Ellis, F. (1968). The relationship of biological effects to dose-time-fractionation factors in radiotherapy. In M. Ebert, and A. Howard (Eds), *Current Topics in Radiation Research*, vol. 4, Amsterdam, North Holland, pp.357–397.
10. Fletcher, G.H., Jesse, R.H., Lindberg, R.D., and Koons, C.R. (1970). The place of radiotherapy in the management of squamous cell carcinoma of the supraglottic larynx. *Am. J. Roentgenol. Radium Ther. Nucl. Med.*, **108**, 19–26.
11. Fletcher, G.H., Lindberg, R.D., Manberger, A., and Horiot, J.C. (1975). Reasons for irradiation failure in squamous carcinoma of the laynx. *Laryngoscope*, **85**, 987–1003.
12. Fu, K.K., Eisenberg, L., Dedo, H.H., and Phillips, T.L. (1977). Results of integrated management of supraglottic carcinoma. *Cancer*, **40**, 2874–2881.
13. Ghossein, N.A., Bataini, J.P., Ennuyer, A., Stacey, P., and Krishnaswamy, V. (1974). Local control and site of failure in radically irradiated supraglottic cancer. *Radiology*, **112**, 187–192.
14. Harwood, A.R., Beale, F.A., Cummings, B.J., Keane, T.J., Payne, D.G., Rider, W.D., Rawlinson, E., and Elhakim, T. (1983). Supraglottic laryngeal carcinoma: An analysis of dose-time volume factors in 410 patients. *Int. J. Radiat. Oncol. Biol. Phys.*, **9**, 311–319.
15. Hoppe, R.T., Williams, J., Warnke, R., Goffinet, D.R., and Bagshaw, M.A. (1978). Carcinoma of the nasopharynx: the significance of histology. *Int. J. Radiat. Oncol. Biol. Phys.*, **4**, 199–205.
16. Horiuchi, J., and Adachi, T. (1971). Some considerations on radiation therapy of tongue cancer. *Cancer*, **28**, 335–339.
17. Jacoby, M.E., Clement, R.L., and Orcult, T.W. (1977). Myocutaneous flaps in lip reconstruction: applications of the Karapandzic principle. *Plast. Reconstr. Surg.*, **59**, 680–688.
18. Ketcham, A.S., Hoye, R.C., Chretien, P.B., and Brace, K.C. (1969). Irradiation twenty-four hours properatively. *Am. J. Surg.*, **118**, 691–697.
19. Kirchner, J.A., and Sorn, M.L. (1971). Clinical and histological observations on supraglottic cancer. *Ann. Otol. Rhinol. Layngol.*, **70**, 638–645.
20. Kramer, S. (1981). An overview of process and outcome data in the Patterns of Care Study. *Int. J. Radiat. Oncol. Biol. Phys.*, **7**, 795–800.
21. Lawrence, W.L., Terz, J.J., Rogers, C., King, R.E., Wolf, J.S., and King, E.R. (1974). Preoperative irradiation for head and neck cancer: a prospective study. *Cancer*, **33**, 318–323.

22. Lindberg, R. (1972). Distribution of cervical lymph node metastases from squamous cell carcinoma of the upper respiratory and digestive tracts. *Cancer*, **29**, 1446–1449.

23. Mäntylä, M., Kertekangas, A.E., Valevaava, R.A., and Nordman, E.M. (1979). Tumor regression during radiation treatment as a guide to prognosis. *Br. J. Radiol.*, **52**, 972–977.

24. Marcial, V.A., Gelber, R., Kramer, S., Snow, J.B., Davis, L.W., and Vallecillo, L.A. (1982). Does preoperative irradiation increase the rate of surgical complications in carcinoma of the head and neck? A Radiation Therapy Oncology Group report. *Cancer*, **49**, 1297–1301.

25. Marks, J.E., Baglan, R., and Purdy, J.A. (1982). Study of temporomandibular joints and muscles of mastication. Unpublished results, Mallinckrodt Institute of Radiology.

26. Marks, J.E., Bedwinek, J.M., Lee, F., Purdy, J.A., and Perez, C.A. (1982). Dose–response analysis for nasopharyngeal carcinoma: an historical perspective (in press). *Cancer*, **50**, 1042–1050.

27. Marks, J.E., Davis, C.C., Gottsman, V.L., Purdy, J.A., and Lee, F. (1981). The effects of radiation on parotid salivary function. *Int. J. Radiat. Oncol. Biol. Phys.*, **7**, 1013–1019.

28. Marks, J.E., Freeman, R.B., Lee, F., and Ogura, J.H. (1979). Carcinoma of the supraglottic larynx. *Am. J. Roentgenol. Radium Ther. Nucl. Med.*, **132**, 255–260.

29. Marks, J.E., Freeman, R.B., Lee, F., and Ogura, J.H. (1978). Pharyngeal wall cancer: an analysis of treatment results, complications and failures. *Int. J. Radiat. Oncol. Biol. Phys.*, **4**, 587–593.

30. Marks, J.E., Kurnik, B., Powers, W.E., and Ogura, J.H. (1978). Carcinoma of the pyriform sinus: an analysis of treatment results and patterns of failure. *Cancer*, **41**, 1008–1015.

31. Marks, J.E., Lee, F., Freeman, R.B., Zivnuska, F.R., and Ogura, J.H., (1981). Carcinoma of the oral tongue: a study of patient selection and treatment results. *Laryngoscope*, **91**, 1548–1559.

32. Marks, J.E., Lee, F., Smith, P.G., and Ogura, J.H. (1983). Floor of mouth cancer: patient selection and treatment results. *Laryngoscope*, **93**, 475–480.

33. Merino, O.R., Lindberg, R.D., and Fletcher, G.H. (1977). An analysis of distant metastases from squamous cell carcinoma of the upper respiratory and digestive tracts. *Cancer*, **40**, 145–151.

34. Mesic, J.B., Fletcher, G.H., and Goepfert, H.

(1981). Megavoltage irradiation of epithelial tumors of the nasopharynx. *Int. J. Radiat. Oncol. Biol. Phys.*, **7**, 447–453.

35. Million, R.R. (1974). Elective neck irradiation for T_XN_0 squamous carcinoma of the oral tongue and floor of mouth. *Cancer*, **34**, 149–155.

36. Mittal, B., Marks, J.E., and Ogura, J.H. (1984). Transglottic carcinoma. *Cancer*, **53**, 151–161.

37. Mittal, B., Rao, D.V., Marks, J.E., and Perez, C.A. (1982). Role of radiation in the management of early vocal cord carcinoma. Submitted to *Ann. Otol. Rhinol. Laryngol.*

38. Mantravadi, R.V.P., Skolnik, E.M., and Applebaum, E.L. (1981). Complications of postoperative and preoperative radiation therapy in head and neck cancer. *Arch. Otol.*, **107**, 690–693.

39. Ogura, J.H., and Thawley, S.E. (1977). Conservation laryngeal surgery and radical neck dissection. In *Otolaryngology*, vol. 5, Harper and Row, chapter 36.

40. Parsons, J.T., Bova, F.J., and Million, R.R. (1980). A re-evaluation of split-coarse technique for squamous cell carcinoma of the head and neck. *Int. J. Radiat. Oncol. Biol. Phys.*, **6**, 1645–1652.

41. Perez, C.A. (1982). Unpublished data, Mallinckrodt Institute of Radiology.

42. Rao, D.V., and Marks, J.E. (1982). Body weight in relation to parotid irradiation. Unpublished data, Mallinckrodt Institute of Radiology.

43. Rollo, J., Rozenbom, C.V., Thawley, S.E., Korba, A., Ogura, J.H., Perez, C.A., Powers, W.E., and Bauer, W.C. (1981). Squamous carcinoma of the base of the tongue: a clinical pathologic study of 81 cases. *Cancer*, **47**, 333–340.

44. Shah, J.P., and Tollefsen, H.R., (1974). Epidermoid carcinoma of the supraglottic larynx. *Am. J. Surg.*, **128**, 494–499.

45. Shukovsky, L.J., (1979). Dose, time, volume relationships in squamous cell carcinoma of the supraglottic larynx. *Am. J. Roentgenol. Radium Ther. Nucl. Med.*, **108**, 27–29.

46. Silverman, C.L., Marks, J.E., Lee, F., and Ogura, J.H. (1983). Treatment of epidermoid and less differentiated carcinoma from occult primaries presenting in cervical lymph nodes. *Laryngoscope*, **93**, 645–648.

47. Snow, J.B., Gelber, R.de., Kramer, S., Davis, L.W., Marcial, V.A., and Lowry, L.D. (1981). Comparison of preoperative and postoperative radiation therapy for patients with carcinoma of the head and neck. *Acta.*

Otolaryngol., **91**, 611–626.

48. Sobel, S., Rubin, P., Keller, B., and Poulter, C. (1976). Tumor persistence as a predictor of outcome after radiation therapy of head and neck cancers. *Int. J. Radiat. Oncol. Biol. Phys.*, **1**, 873–880.

49. Spiro, R.A., and Strong, E.W. (1971). Epidermoid carcinoma of the mobile tongue: treatment by partial glossectomy alone. *Am. J. Surg.*, **122**, 707–710.

50. Strong, E.W. (1969). Preoperative radiation and radical neck dissection. *Surg. Clin. N. Am.*, **49**, 271–276.

51. Strong, M.S., Vaughan, C.W., Kayne, H.L., Aral, I.M., Ucmakli, A., Feldman, M., and Healy, B.G. (1978). A randomized trial of preoperative radiotherapy in cancer of the oropharynx and hypopharynx. *Am. J. Surg.*, **136**, 494–500.

52. Suit, H., Lindberg, R., and Fletcher, G.H. (1965). Prognostic significance of tumor regression at completion of radiation therapy. *Radiology*, **89**, 1100–1103.

53. Thawley, S.E. (1981). Complications of combined radiation therapy and surgery for carcinoma of the larynx and inferior hypopharynx. *Laryngoscope*, **91**, 677–700.

54. Vanderbrouck, C., Sancho, H., LeFur, R., Richard, J.M., and Cachin, Y. (1977). Results of a randomized clinical trial of preoperative irradiation versus postoperative in treatment of tumors of the hypopharynx. *Cancer*, **39**, 1445–1449.

55. Wang, C.C., Busse, J., and Gitterman, M.S. (1975). A simple afterloading applicator for intracavitary irradiation of carcinoma of the nasopharynx. *Radiology*, **115**, 737–739.

56. Wang, C.C. (1973). Megavoltage radiation therapy for supraglottic carcinoma. *Radiology*, **109**, 183–186.

57. Whitehurst, J.O., and Droulias, C.A. (1977). Surgical treatment of squamous carcinoma of the oral tongue. *Arch. Otolaryngol.*, **103**, 212–215.

58. Yarrington, C.T. (1980). A protocol for combined treatment of cancer of the oral cavity and tongue. *Laryngoscope*, **90**, 2004–2020.

Chapter 9

Brachytherapy

Bhadrasain Vikram
*Memorial Sloan – Kettering Cancer Center,
Department of Radiation Therapy, 1275
York Avenue, New York, NY, USA*

INTRODUCTION

Radium was discovered by Marie and Pierre Curie in 1898. Soon thereafter early applications of radium for the treatment of cancer, along with many other diseases, were undertaken in different parts of the world. By 1904 surface and intracavitary applications of radium were being employed in Paris by Danlos. Abbe in New York used celluloid tubes inside tumours, which were used to introduce radium sources. Alexander Graham Bell, in a 1903 letter to the editor of *Archives of Roentgen Ray* (Figure 9.1) suggested the use of interstitial radiation therapy.[1] Duane in Boston, and Janeway in New York, described the use of radon encapsulated in glass capillary tubing, which was inserted into tumours.[2,3] Not surprisingly, the unfiltered beta and soft gamma radiation resulted in necrosis in many of the cases. In 1915, Regaud and Debierne from Paris suggested the use of platinum sheathing for the glass capillaries, in order to filter the soft radiation and reduce the likelihood of necrosis.[4] Gold capillary tubing filled with radon was used by Failla in New York in 1926, and these so-called 'gold seeds' were extensively used at Memorial Hospital for interstitial implants.[5] A landmark in brachytherapy was the standardization of the rules of radium implantation by Paterson and Parker from Manchester in 1930.[6] Even today

their guidelines are followed by many radiotherapists around the world in the performance of radioactive implants.

In the period immediately following the Second World War there was a decline of interest in brachytherapy. This was brought about partly by increasing awareness of the possible hazards of radium or radon, and also by the availability of megavoltage cobalt 60 units for external radiation therapy. Until that time radiotherapists had been severely constrained in external radiation therapy by the poor depth dose, poor penumbra, and the preferential absorption in bone and cartilage that is characteristic of X-rays in the orthovoltage range.[7] Megavoltage therapy was a significant advance in its ability to irradiate relatively uniformly sizeable tumour masses to higher doses than had previously been possible. The physical and biological advantages of brachytherapy, however, have led to a resurgence of interest in this modality in the last 20 years or so. This interest has been greatly aided by three developments: (1) the technique of afterloading; (2) the development of newer and safer radionuclides; and (3) the application of the computer to dosimetry.

Afterloading

The introduction of afterloading by Henschke

121

ʻAUGUST 15, 1903]

(AMERICAN MEDICINE   **261**

THE USES OF RADIUM.

To the Editor of American Medicine:—It has occurred to me that perhaps you would care to publish the enclosed letters, and thus start some one experimenting with the radium rays in the manner suggested.

Z. T. SOWERS.

DEAR DR. SOWERS:

I understand from you that the Röntgen rays, and the rays emitted by radium, have been found to have a marked curative effect upon external cancers, but that the effects upon deep-seated cancers have not thus far proved satisfactory.

It has occurred to me that one reason for the unsatisfactory nature of these latter experiments arises from the fact that the rays have been applied externally, thus having to pass through healthy tissues of various depths in order to reach the cancerous matter.

The Crookes' tube, from which the Röntgen rays are emitted, is of course too bulky to be admitted into the middle of a mass of cancer, but there is no reason why a tiny fragment of radium sealed up in a fine glass tube should not be inserted into the very heart of the cancer, thus acting directly upon the diseased material. Would it not be worth while making experiments along this line?

[Signed]   ALEXANDER GRAHAM BELL.

[REPLY.]

DEAR DR. BELL:

The suggestion which you make in regard to the application of the radium rays to the substance of deep-seated cancer I regard very valuable. If such experiments should be made I have no doubt they would prove successful in many cases in which we now have failures.

[Signed]   Z. T. SOWERS, M.D.

Figure 9.1 Correspondence between Alexander Graham Bell and Dr Z.T. Sowers (Editor, *Archives of Roentgen Ray*) about the principle of brachytherapy, published in *American Medicine*, volume 261, 15 August, 1903.

in 1955, and its subsequent widespread use, not only greatly decreased radiation exposure to radiotherapists during the performance of implants, but has also led the way for much more precise positioning of radioactive sources in tumours for better dose distributions.[8] The basic idea behind afterloading is a simple one, and was applied as early as 1903 by Strebel. It consists of the introduction of non-radioactive hollow applicators of some sort (such as needles or plastic tubes) in and around the tumour as the initial step in the implant (Figure 9.2). Proper positioning, so crucial for success, can therefore be performed without fear of radiation exposure, and implants are more often technically satisfactory. Localization studies and dosimetry may be performed with non-radioactive 'dummy' sources loaded into these applicators. When the radiotherapist is satisfied with the dose distribution, then radioactive sources may be loaded into the hollow applicators. After the sources have

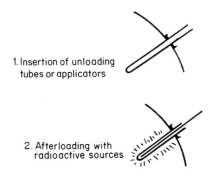

1. Insertion of unloading tubes or applicators

2. Afterloading with radioactive sources

Figure 9.2   Principle of afterloading: (1) Insertion of hollow tubes, (2) insertion of radioactive sources. (Reproduced with permission from Henschke, U.K., Hilaris, B.S., and Mahan, G.D. (1963). Afterloading in interstitial and intracavitary radiation therapy, *Am. J. Roentgenol.*, **90**, 387; copyright American Roentgen Ray Society, 1963.)

stayed in place for the desired period of time (in the case of temporary implants) they may be removed first, leaving the hollow applicators. The applicators may then be removed at leisure with appropriate precautions. In the case of a pre-loaded radioactive implant, one might sometimes encounter haemorrhage when only part of the implant has been removed, and one is faced with the unpleasant prospect of trying to control haemorrhage, and of applying other supportive measures while the patient is still radioactive.

Artificial Radionuclides

With the great progress made during and after the Second World War in nuclear technology a number of 'artificial' or 'man-made' radionuclides became available, some of which had physical characteristics preferable to radium and radon. These include caesium-137, iridium-192 and iodine-125. It is interesting to contrast the post-war developments in external radiation therapy with those in brachytherapy. In external radiation therapy this period has seen the development of megavoltage and supervoltage machines capable of delivering higher and higher photon energies, so that these photons might deposit their energy in the region of the tumour without excessive dose to the intervening normal tissues. In the field of brachytherapy, on the contrary, the newer radionuclides have lower energy; the energy of photons emitted by radium and radon can be as high as 2000 keV, where as that of caesium-137 is 660 keV, that of iridium-192 is 350 keV and that of iodine-125 is only 28 keV. Unlike in external therapy, the source of radiation is situated within the tumour, and low photon energies (with a short range in tissues) are desirable so that relatively little radiation might escape from the tumour into the adjacent tissues, and even less from the patient's body into the surroundings. Thus the patient benefits from a better dose distribution, while medical personnel are protected because a lower amount of radiation escapes from the patient's body, and also because low-energy photons can be stopped much more effectively by protective shields than the high-energy photons emitted by radium or radon.

Computerized Dosimetry

While guidelines and tables, such as those of the Manchester system, have value in the planning and performance of radioactive implants, in practice implants are rarely technically perfect. What is predicted by tables in terms of dose to tumour and to normal tissues might therefore be significantly different from what actually obtains in the patient. Computerized dosimetry allows radiotherapists to calculate accurately the actual dosimetry after the implant for every individual patient.[9,10] They can therefore make the necessary adjustments, leading to better tumour control and fewer complications.

BASIC PRINCIPLES

With modern megavoltage external radiation therapy and sophisticated treatment planning we are able to irradiate fairly large volumes to relatively high doses. However, since the radiation often has to traverse considerable normal tissue before reaching the target volume, the dose outside the target volume can be considerable and can limit the dose of radiation that can be delivered safely to the target volume.

An interstitial implant is an invasive procedure requiring insertion or application of radioactive sources within the target volume. It is generally feasible only for relatively small and well circumscribed lesions, and carries the risks of haemorrhage, sepsis and anaesthesia. The implant has, however, at least three advantages over external beam therapy; these are: (1) better dose distribution, (2) high tumour dose, and (3) the dose rate effect.

Dose Distribution

The dose of radiation at a point is inversely proportional to the square of the distance from the radiation source to that point. What this means, for an external therapy machine (where the tissues being irradiated are situated at a distance typically of 1 metre from the source of radiation) is that there is a very small change in dose delivered as the radiation passes from the target volume to the surrounding tissues or vice-versa. In the case of an implant, however, the sources of radiation are situated very close to the tissues irradiated; therefore the dose decreases dramatically every centimetre away from the sources (Figure 9.3). Thus the adjacent normal structure receive far less radiation than the tumour, within which the sources are physically located. Of course it can also lead to a markedly lower dose in one part of the tumour than another. The elaborate guidelines of the Manchester System for implants[6] (and more recent versions, such as the Paris system)[11] are aimed at preventing this inhomogeneity within the target volume, while maintaining the advantage of a sharp gradient in dose between the target volume and the adjacent structures. One is thereby able to deliver a dose to the tumour which is considerably higher than that which surrounding normal structures receive, to a degree not generally feasible with external beam therapy.

Tumour Dose

The term 'tumour dose' does not mean quite the same thing in brachytherapy as it does in external therapy. In external therapy sharp

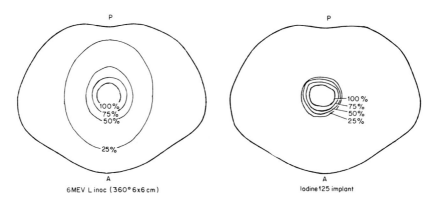

Figure 9.3   Comparison of idealized dose distributions around a small, deep-seated tumour: *left*: megavoltage photons with rotational technique; right: permanent interstitial implant. The radiation dose to tissues outside the tumour volume (100% isodose) is clearly lower with the implant. (Reproduced with permission from Hilaris, B.S., and Henschke, U.K. (1975). General principles and techniques of interstitial therapy. In B.S. Hilaris (Ed.), *Handbook of Interstitial Brachytherapy*, Publishing Sciences Group, Inc., Acton, Massachusetts; copyright Memorial Sloan–Kettering Cancer Center, 1975.)

variations in dose across the volume being irradiated are uncommon, because of the large distance of the target tissues from the source of radiation. The target volume generally receives a dose no less than 90% and no greater than 110% of the prescribed tumour dose. In the case of brachytherapy, however, the prescribed tumour dose usually means the minimum tumour dose, calculated at the periphery of the target volume, and virtually all of the tissues within this volume actually receive a dose higher than the minimum tumour dose. There is no denying the fact that 'hot spots' exist even within the most technically perfect implant, and indeed this might be one of the reasons for the success of brachytherapy in eradicating tumours. Immediately adjacent to the radioactive sources the doses are very high indeed. In summary, while in external therapy all parts of the tumour receive a dose close to the prescribed tumour dose, in brachytherapy most of the tumour receives a dose higher than the prescribed dose.

Dose Rate

Megavoltage external radiation therapy is usually delivered at doses of 100–200 rads per minute. A typical treatment lasts for a few minutes per day, and the patient is treated on several days per week for a period of several weeks (say to a tumour dose of 7000 rad over a period of 6–7 weeks). In the case of a temporary implant, the same total dose will be delivered over a period of only about 1 week, continuously, at a dose rate of around 40 rads per hour. Thus the actual dose rate is considerably lower than what is the case in external therapy, while the total dose is delivered in a substantially shorter time than in external therapy. It is well recognized that the same dose of radiation delivered in a shorter overall time is more efficient at cell killing than when given over a longer period of time.[12] One might therefore reasonably expect a greater likelihood of destroying tumour by delivering the total tumour dose in 1 week than in 7. This would be of no value whatsoever if the normal

tissues were also subject to the same enhanced radiation damage but, as we have seen above, the corresponding dose to the adjacent normal tissues with an implant is considerably less and therefore is more capable of being tolerated.

The fact that the actual dose rate is only about 40 rads per hour might also contribute to an improved therapeutic ratio. It has been shown experimentally that the oxygen enhancement ratio decreases as the dose rate decreases.[13] Normal tissues are well oxygenated; therefore the decrease in dose rate would not make them more susceptible to radiation damage. However, malignant tissues are believed to contain significant numbers of hypoxic cells,[14] which might be more efficiently killed by radiation at the lower dose rate of brachytherapy than the higher dose rates of external beam therapy. It is also possible that the lower dose rate allows some repair and repopulation to proceed even while the tissues are being irradiated, but that this happens much more efficiently in normal tissues with their preserved homeostatic capabilities than in malignant tissues with their impaired homeostatic mechanisms.

Just as the radiation dose outside the target volume of an implant is markedly lower than the inside, the dose rate outside is also markedly lower than in the inside. This can be expected to further contribute to the relative sparing of the surrounding structures from radiation damage.

In the case of permanent implants with iodine-125 the dose rate is even lower, i.e. 10 rad per hour or less.[15] The total dose, delivered over a period of 1 year, is of the order of 12 000–15 000 rad. One-half of this dose (6000–7500 rad) is delivered during the first 8 weeks (the half-life of iodine-125) and one-half is delivered during the next 44 weeks. The biological implications of these features of permanent iodine-125 implants are even less clearly understood than those of temporary implants.

The interaction of the total dose, the dose distribution, and the dose rate is complex and not well understood. Also, there are marked differences between what happens inside the target volume and the outside. This interaction, however, is what determines the therapeutic efficacy and further studies are needed to determine the relative importance of each of these factors. This is particularly important when external therapy and brachytherapy are increasingly being employed together in planned combinations.

TECHNIQUES

Only afterloading techniques will be described. In recent years our preferred radionuclide for temporary implants has been iridium-192 and for permanent implants iodine-125. Recently we have started a study of higher-intensity iodine-125 for temporary implants, because of its superiority with regard to radiation protection considerations. Until the results of this study are available, however, we intend to continue using iridium-192 as the standard radionuclide for temporary implants.

Temporary Implants

Implants for lesions which are relatively small and situated in easily accessible sites such as the face, lips, nose, and the anterior portion of the oral cavity can frequently be performed under local anaesthesia and mild sedation. For larger lesions, or for those situated more posteriorly, general anaesthesia is required. For lesions in the oropharynx or the hypopharynx tracheostomy is often necessary; implants in these areas produce considerable swelling of the pharyngeal structures which might result in an inadequate airway. Furthermore, there is the risk of pharyngeal haemorrhage during the performance or the removal of the implant, and in such an event a tracheostomy can be life-saving.

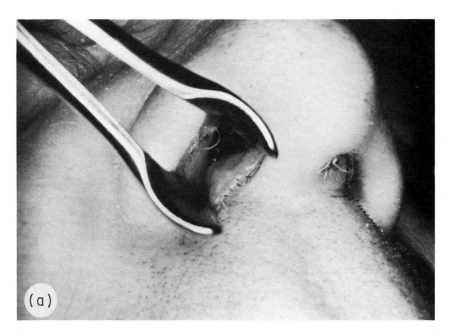

Figure 9.4   This 60-year-old male presented with a 1 cm lesion on the right side of his columella in November 1980. Biopsy revealed epidermoid carcinoma. He was treated with a temporary iridium-192 implant in angiocaths, which delivered 6000 rads in 5 days. He remained free of recurrence until his death from another cancer in May of 1983.

(a) Appearance of the lesion prior to implant;

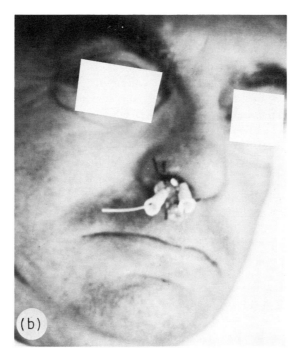

(b) Implant in place;

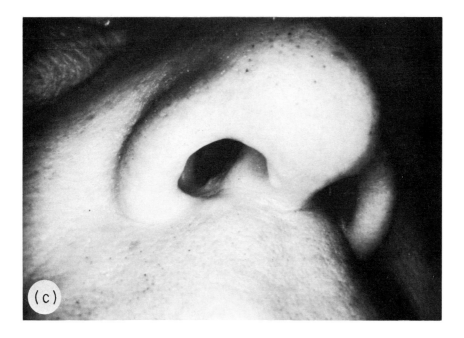

(c) Appearance 1 year later.

For small, superficial lesions we perform the implant with the help of 16-gauge, 5 cm long angiocaths.[16] Single-plane implants are usually adequate. The angiocaths are inserted through the lesion nearly parallel to the surface and are secured on the surface by means of commercially available plastic and metallic buttons, and silk sutures. The angiocath stylet is withdrawn and iridium-192 in ribbons can then be afterloaded into the sleeve (Figure 9.4).

For most lesions in the oral cavity, oropharynx, and hypophyarynx we have generally employed the plastic tube technique of Henschke[17]: hollow 14- or 16-gauge, thin-walled, stainless steel needles are inserted through the area of the tumour. Through these needles hollow, polyethylene afterloading tubes are inserted in place. The needles are then withdrawn and the tubes are secured by means of plastic and metallic buttons and silk sutures. A single-plane, multi-plane, or volume implant can be performed as appropriate, depending upon the size of the lesion.

Oral Cavity

A popular technique for intraoral implants is the 'loop' technique.[18] In this technique the tumour is sandwiched between the two limbs of a loop and thus receives cross-fire radiation from the two limbs, while irradiation to the dorsum of the lesion is ensured by the top of the loop (Figure 9.5). The tubes are anchored not inside the mouth but on the skin, and can be loaded almost up to the skin if necessary. This allows more adequate irradiation of the deeper portion of a tumour when compared with intraoral radioactive needle implants. In the postoperative period, as the implanted tissues become oedematous, the implant tends to rise due to oedema. In an intraorally anchored radioactive needle implant this might mean that the deeper portions of the tumour are no longer in the high-dose region, even though they were to start with. This, however, is not a problem with the loop technique.

The simple loop technique is adequate for many lesions of the floor of the mouth and the

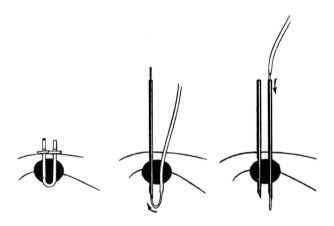

Figure 9.5 The 'loop' technique for temporary afterloading implants. *Left*: insertion of hollow needles; *center*: formation of loop with afterloading plastic tubes; *right*: completed loop after removal of needles. (Reproduced with permission from Hilaris, B.S., and Henschke, U.K. (1975). General principles and techniques of interstitial therapy. In B.S. Hilaris (Ed.), *Handbook of Interstitial Brachytherapy*, Publishing Sciences Group, Inc., Acton, Massachusetts; copyright Memorial Sloan–Kettering Cancer Center, 1975.)

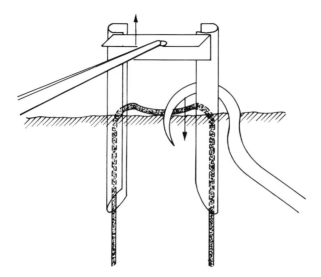

Figure 9.6 The 'hairpin' technique for afterloading temporary implants. A non-radioactive hairpin guide is inserted first and through this a radioactive wire (in the shape of a hairpin) is introduced, with the aid of a hook, as the guide is withdrawn. (Reproduced with permission from Pierquin, B. *et al.* (1978). The techniques. In B. Pierquin, D.J. Chassagne, *et al.* (Eds), *Brachytherapy*, Warren H. Green Inc., St. Louis Missouri; copyright Warren H. Green, Inc. 1978.)

oral tongue. Modifications have been developed for special situations. For relatively large lesions we add a third or sometimes even a fourth limb in the centre of the loop. The additional limbs are secured to the arch of the loop by a 3 – O silk sutures. The suture pierces the tip of the tube forming the additional limb and is then tied loosely around the tube forming the loop.

Pierquin has described the use of hairpin guides and hairpin shaped radioactive iridium-192 wires (Figure 9.6) for the implantation of small superficial lesions.[19] Due to restricted availability of iridium-192 wire in the United States we have very limited experience with this technique, but it appears to be useful for the implant of small lesions.

Pharynx

Lesions in the pharynx are much less easily accessible than those in the oral cavity. The considerable difficulty in performing technically satisfactory implants with radioactive needles in inaccessible sites has greatly limited the applications of brachytherapy in the pharynx. In recent years, however, a number of newer afterloading techniques permit much more adequate implants to be performed with a greater expectation of local control. When adequate delineation of the tumour is difficult otherwise, we have even found it worthwhile to expose the tumour surgically prior to implantation by techniques such as median mandibulotomy or lateral pharyngotomy. It cannot be emphasized too strongly that adequate delineation of the tumour is mandatory for a technically satisfactory implant.

For implants in the base of the tongue we have employed a 'non-looping loop' technique (Figure 9.7) which allows most of the work to be performed outside the patient's mouth,

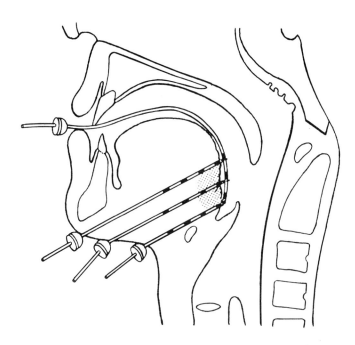

Figure 9.7   Non-looping afterloading technique for base of tongue implants, which eliminates the need for making loops in the cramped anatomy of the pharynx. (Reproduced with permission from Vikram, B., and Hilaris, B.S. (1981). A non-looping afterloading technique for interstitial implants of the base of the tongue, *Int. J. Radiat. Oncol. Biol. Phys.*, **7**, 421; copyright Pergamon Press, Inc., 1981.)

without the constraints imposed by the cramped anatomy of the oropharynx.[20] Recently Peters and Karolis have suggested a modification of this technique which permits the radioactive sources to extend superiorly beyond the dorsum of the tongue by bringing out the afterloading tubes through the nose instead of through the mouth.[21]

Pierquin has described the use of hairpin guides and radioactive wire for small superficial lesions arising from the soft palate,[19] but the plastic tube technique may also be used for lesions arising in the palate.[22] Lesions of the pharyngeal wall can also be implanted by this technique. We generally use a lateral approach, taking care to avoid trauma to the major blood vessels. The afterloading tubes may be looped over the lesion and brought back out through the same side of the neck when feasible, or they may be threaded across

the lesion and be brought out through the contralateral neck, especially in the case of posterior pharyngeal wall lesions.

Permanent Implants

The basic technique of afterloading permanent implant is shown in Figure 9.8. Local or general anaesthesia may be used. Hollow 16- or 17-gauge thin-walled stainless steel needles are inserted into the tumour up to the desired depth. Radionuclide sources are afterloaded into the tumour through these needles as the needles are withdrawn. One source at a time can be inserted, or one of many applicators which are available for inserting several sources in rapid sequence can be employed (Figure 9.9).

For many decades radon-222 encapsulated in gold 'seeds' was used as the radionuclide for permanent implants at Memorial Hospital.

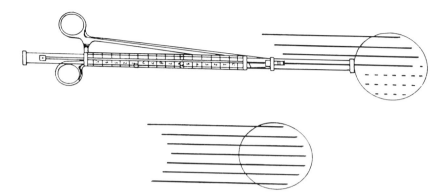

Figure 9.8   Technique of permanent interstitial implantation. *Left*: hollow stainless steel afterloading needles are introduced up to the desired depth in tumor; *right*: through the needles radioactive 'seeds' are introduced with an applicator as the needles are withdrawn. (Reproduced with permission from Hilaris, B.S., and Henschke, U.K. (1975). General principles and techniques of interstitial therapy. In B.S. Hilaris, (Ed.), *Handbook of Interstitial Brachytherapy*, Publishing Sciences Group, Inc., Acton, Massachusetts; copyright Memorial Sloan–Kettering Cancer Center, 1975.)

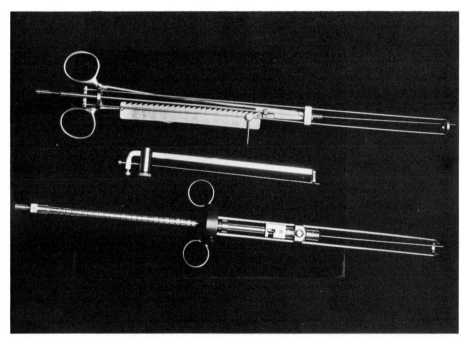

Figure 9.9   Applicators for permanent iodine-125 implants. From top to bottom: Henschke applicator, Scott applicator, Mick applicator.

Others have used radioactive gold-198 for this purpose. Since 1965 we have almost exclusively employed encapsulated sources containing an average of 0.5 mCi of iodine-125 as the radionuclide for permanent implants at Memorial Hospital.[23] The photon energy of iodine-125 is much less than, and its half-life is much longer than, that of radon-222. These two factors dramatically decreased the radiation exposure to hospital staff.[24]

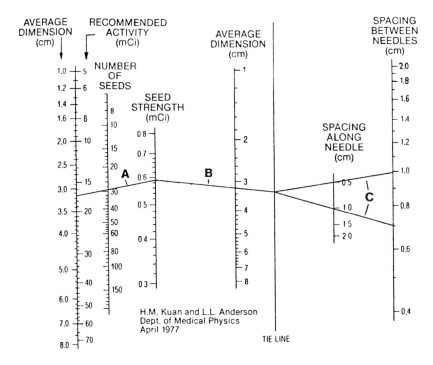

Figure 9.10 Nomogram for calculation of the total activity and the spacing of iodine-125 sources for permanent implantation. (Reproduced with permission from Anderson, L.L. *et al.*, Memorial Hospital methods of dose calculations for iridium-192. In F.W. George, (Ed.), *Modern Interstitial and Intracavitary Cancer Management*, Masson Publishing USA, Inc., New York, NY; copyright Masson Publishing USA, Inc., 1981.)

The activity of iodine-125 to be implanted is calculated as follows: the tumour to be implanted is measured in its three dimensions, and the average of the three dimensions is calculated. In the past the average dimension (in cm) was multiplied by 5 to arrive at the activity in millicuries to be implanted (rule of five). The appropriate number of seeds was then distributed throughout the tumour volume.

Computerized dose calculations on implants performed in this manner have revealed that the matched dose at the periphery of the tumour (which one might loosely regard as the minimum tumour dose) decreased considerably as the size of the tumour increased.[25] Clinical experience has also indicated that local control is less likely with large tumours than with smaller tumours treated by iodine-125 permanent implants.[26]

The incidence of serious complications following permanent iodine-125 implants has been low. We have therefore attempted to increase the matched peripheral dose by increasing the implanted activity, especially for larger tumours. We now use a nomogram incorporating this feature in order to calculate the required activity (Figure 9.10) instead of the rule of five.[27] It is as yet too early to state if this has significantly improved the local control; however no unusual toxicity has so far been observed.

By far the commonest indication for permanent iodine-125 implants in the head and neck area has been in the treatment of metastatic tumour masses in the neck. However, permanent implants for lesions in the oral cavity have also been performed, often through the mouth. For lesions in the base of the tongue we prefer a submental approach with bimanual palpation, so as to provide more adequate coverage of the tumour in its depth. Similarly, for lesions in the parapharyngeal space we use a retromandibular approach. Lesions of the nasopharynx can often be implanted through the nasal cavity, and this has been greatly facilitated by performing the implant under direct vision with the Storz nasopharyngoscope. We started using this technique for nasopharynx implants 3 years ago and since then we have not had to resort to fenestration of the palate for access to the nasopharynx. A technique for implanting the tonsillar region with iodine-125 sources in absorbable vicryl sutures has been described by Goode et al.[28]

Radiation Safety Considerations

Exposure rate measurements on patients undergoing temporary iridium-192 implants to the head and neck region have revealed that the exposure rate at 1 metre ranges usually between 15 and 50 mR per hour. These patients are therefore kept in a single room until removal of the radioactive sources.

With permanent iodine-125 implants the measured exposure rate at 1 metre has ranged usually between 0.1 and 1 mR per hour. These patients are generally allowed to go home on the same day, or the next day after the implant.

Tumour Bed Implants

Postoperative external radiation therapy is a valuable adjunct for improved local–regional control when the initial management of advanced head and neck cancer is by surgical excision.[29,30] When, however, adequate resection is not feasible the local recurrence rate remains very high. We have also found that postoperative radiation therapy is considerably less effective when for one reason or another its start is delayed beyond 6 weeks after the resection.[30,31]

We are exploring intraoperative tumour bed implants in high-risk patients in an effort to (1) deliver irradiation to residual tumour within a few days following resection; (2) deliver doses considerably higher than what is possible (without excessive toxicity) with external postoperative radiation therapy, to the area with the maximum tumour infestation; and (3) deliver postoperative irradiation to those patients who have received radical external radiation therapy in the past and therefore cannot receive further external radiation.

When the tumour mass is bulky and has indistinct margins, the area at risk of harbouring residual cancer is large; for example in soft-tissue sarcoma[32,33] or in carcinoma infiltrating the soft tissues of the neck. In such cases we generally employ single-plane or two-plane temporary iridium-192 implants of the tumour bed by the plastic tube technique. We deliver a dose of 3000–4000 rads at a depth of 0.5–1 cm if postoperative external radiation therapy is also planned, and 5500–6500 rads if no postoperative external radiation therapy is feasible.

In some patients the area of residual tumour is limited in extent but is unresectable by virtue of its intimate relation to major blood vessels, base of skull, etc. In such cases we have used permanent implants with iodine-125, either with single seeds or with seeds in absorbable vicryl sutures. Iodine-125 delivers its dose over several months, and if postoperative external radiation therapy is also given within a few weeks the local toxicity might be excessive; besides, it is usually difficult to shield the implanted region when external therapy is given. For these reasons we have been reluctant to employ permanent iodine-125 implants when postoperative external radiation therapy is also planned.

It is worth emphasizing that we do not recommend intraoperative implants as an alternative to wide-field external radiation therapy in the combined management of advanced head and neck cancers by surgery and radiotherapy. Rather, intraoperative implants are being investigated as a supplement to external radiation therapy in selected high-risk cases, or when external radiation therapy is not feasible or is likely to be unduly delayed postoperatively.

RESULTS

In 50 patients with carcinoma of the lower lip treated with temporary implants only one instance of local recurrence was reported by Pierquin.[34] For T_1 and T_2 carcinomas of the oral tongue and floor of the mouth he reported eight local recurrences (5%) among 153 patients, and for T_3 and T_4 cases 22 recurrences (25%) among 86 patients. Ten per cent of his patients developed necrosis. Ghossein and Decroix reported local recurrence in 14% of 94 cases with T_1 carcinoma of the oral tongue, 22% of 288 cases with T_2, and in 29% of 220 cases with T_3 or T_4 cancer.[35] They used interstitial implant in 97% of their T_1 and T_2 cases and external radiation therapy in 16%. In T_3 and T_4 cases they used interstitial implant in 72% and external radiation in 78% of the patients. Several other authors have concluded that the use of interstitial implant alone, or in combination with external radiation therapy, gave better local control compared with external radiation therapy alone.[36-40] Fu observed that the minimal optimal dose for local control with implant alone was 6000 rads, but when external radiation therapy and implant were used in combination the minimal optimal dose was 7500 rads.[41]

Pierquin has also reported the results of brachytherapy for several other sites in the oral cavity and oropharynx.[34] For T_1 or T_2 carcinoma of the hard palate he reported one recurrence in nine patients (11%) and for the soft palate five recurrences in 51 patients (10%). He observed 21 local recurrences in 111 patients (19%) with T_1 to T_4 carcinomas of the base of the tongue. In carcinoma of the tonsillar region he reported six recurrences in 75 patients (8%) with T_1 or T_2 lesions and 17 recurrences in 68 patients (25%) with T_3 or T_4 lesions.

It would appear that local eradication of small, accessible lesions can be accomplished rather consistently with temporary interstitial implant. Local failures are more frequent, however, in the case of larger lesions. Cervical nodal metastases are another frequent site of failure. For these reasons we generally employ interstitial implants in combination with external therapy, or surgery if indicated. External radiation therapy of 5000–6000 rads, directed to the primary site and to the cervical region, is expected to sterilize areas of microscopic tumour, and to shrink gross tumour masses down to a size where an implant is more likely to produce local control. We are investigating both temporary and permanent implants in this manner, but as yet the number of patients so treated, and the length of follow-up, are inadequate for meaningful statistical analysis.

Previously Treated Patients

The management of patients whose cancer has recurred following a full course of external radiation therapy is difficult, to say the least. Further radiation therapy is generally considered to be contraindicated because the risk of radionecrosis is regarded as prohibitive. Some workers, however, convinced of the unique properties of brachytherapy (see 'Basic Principles' above), have defied this conventional wisdom and re-treated these patients by interstitial irradiation. Pierquin reported on 124 patients with recurrent cervical adenopathy (only excluding patients with ulcerated lesions) who had been previously treated with one or more courses of external radiation therapy to doses of 6000–10,000 rads.[34] He gave them doses of 6000–7000 rads by temporary implant, and found complete disappearance of adenopathy in 30 patients (24%) and partial regression in another 40 patients (32%).

Syed treated 64 patients with persistent or recurrent cancer of the head and neck after prior treatment by external radiation therapy to about 6000 rads.[42] He delivered a further 4500–6000 rads in 3–5 days by temporary iridium-192 implant. Complete regression of the tumour occurred in 31 patients (48.5%) and partial regression in another 22 (34.5%). In 11 patients (17%) there was no regression; 17 of the responders subsequently developed local recurrence. Thus 28 out of 64 (44%) had either locally persistent or recurrent cancer following implant, while 28 patients (44%) remained alive without local recurrence for 18–36 months. The remaining eight patients died of metastases or intercurrent disease without local recurrence. Nineteen patients (30%) developed necrosis. The author considered the necrosis rate acceptable in view of the poor prognosis of the patients involved.

We have reported on 124 patients with head and neck cancer recurrent following previous radiation therapy, treated with permanent iodine-125 implant.[43] Complete regression was seen in 71%, and partial regression in another 18%. In 11% there was no regression and 28% of the responders subsequently had local recurrence. The magnitude of the response decreased and the likelihood of local persistence or recurrence increased as the size of the tumour increased. Necrosis developed in 9% but healed in 3.5%.

It is interesting to compare Syed's results with our own, even though the two groups are not strictly comparable (the majority of our patients had had surgery in addition to radiation therapy previously, while the majority of Syed's patients had been treated only by external radiation therapy without surgery). The incidence of patients not responding to implants is similar in both series (17% vs 11%) and the proportion of patients having persistent or recurrent cancer after implant is also very similar (44% vs 39%). The incidence of local necrosis, however, appears to be higher in Syed's series (30%) than in ours (9%). It is conceivable that this difference is related to the differences in the photon energies of the two radionuclides employed (350 keV for iridium-192 versus 28 keV for iodine-125), and/or to their dose rates (over 40 rads per hour with iridium-192 versus less than 10 rads per hour with iodine-125). Further experimental and clinical trials to study, and perhaps to exploit, these differences are indicated.

REFERENCES

1. Bell, Alexander Graham (1903). Letter to the Editor. *Archives of Roentgen Ray*, **8**, 64.

2. Duane, W. (1915). On the extraction and purification of radium emanation. *Phys. Rev.*, **5**, 311–314.

3. Janeway, H.H. (1917). *Radium Therapy in Cancer*, Paul B. Hober, New York.

4. Regaud, C. (1925). Quelques fondements radiobiologiques de la radiotherapie des neoplasmes malins. *Paris Med.*, **15**, 113–125.

5. Failla, G. (1920). Radium technique at the Memorial Hospital, New York. *Arch. Radiol. Electrother.*, **24**, 3.

6. Paterson, R. and Parker, H.M. (1934). A dosage system for gamma ray therapy. *Br. J. Radiol.*, **7**, 592–612.

7. Johns, H.E. (1961). *The Physics of Radiology*, Charles C. Thomas, Springfield, Illinois, chapters 5 and 6.

8. Henschke, U.K. (1956). Interstitial Implantation with Radioisotopes. In F. Hahn (Ed.), *Therapeutic Use of Artificial Radioisotopes*, New York. John Wiley and Sons, Inc., pp. 375–397.

9. Shalek, R.J., and Stovall, M. (1961). The calculation of isodose distributions in interstitial implantation by a computer. *Radiology*, **76**, 119–120.

10. Laughlin, J.S. (1963). A dose description system for interstitial radiation therapy – seed implant. *Am. J. Roentgenol. Radium Ther., Nucl. Med.*, **89**, 470–490.

11. Pierquin, B., and Dutreix, A. (1967). Towards a new system in curietherapy. *Br. J. Radiol.*, **40**, 184–186.

12. Bedford, J.S., and Mitchell, J.B. (1973). Dose rate effects in synchronous mammalian cells in culture. *Radiat. Res.*, **54**, 316–327.

13. Kal, H.B., and Barendsen, G.W. (1976). The oxygen enhancement ratio at low dose rate. *Br. J. Radiol.*, **49**, 1049–1051.

14. Gray, L.H., Conger, T.D., *et al.* (1953). The concentration of O_2 dissolved in tissues at the time of irradiation as a factor in radiotherapy. *Br. J. Radiol.*, **26**, 638.

15. Hilaris, B.S. *et al.* (1968). Clinical experience with long half life and low energy encapsulated sources in cancer radiotherapy. *Radiology*, **91**, 1163–1167.

16. Daly, N.G., Malisard, L. *et al.* (1978). Technique d'endocurietherapie Par Fil Dans Les Epitheliomas Cutanes a L'aide de Catheters a Ponctoin Vasculaire. *J. Radiol. Electrol.*, **59**, 361–364.

17. Henschke, U.K., Hilaris, B.S., and Mahan, G.J. (1963). Afterloading in interstitial and intracavitary radiation therapy. *Am. J. Roentgenol., Radium Ther., Nucl. Med.*, **2**, 386–395.

18. Hilaris, B.S., and Henschke, U.K. (1975). In

B.S. Hilaris (Ed.), *Handbook of Interstitial Brachytherapy*, Memorial Sloan-Kettering Cancer Center, New York, pp.75–76.

19. Pierquin, B. (1978). In Pierquin B. *et al.* (Eds), *Brachytherapy*, Warren H. Green, Inc., St Louis, Mo., pp.22–27.

20. Vikram, B., and Hilaris, B.S. (1981). A non-looping afterloading technique for interstitial implants of the base of the tongue. *Int. J. Radiat. Oncol. Biol. Phys.*, **7**, 419–422.

21. Karolis, C., and Peters, L.J. (1982). Implantation of tumors of the base of the tongue. Letter to the Editor. *Int. J. Radiat. Oncol. Biol. Phys.*, **8**, 1463–1464.

22. Syed, A.M.N., and Feder, B.H. (1978). Technique of afterloading interstitial implants. *Front. Radiat. Ther. Oncol.*, **12**, 119–135.

23. Kim, J.H., and Hilaris, B.S. (1975). Iodine-125 sources in interstitial tumor therapy. *Am. J. Roentgenol. Radium Ther. Nucl. Med.*, **123**, 163–169.

24. Hilaris, B.S. (1968). Techniques of interstitial and intracavitary radiation. *Cancer*, **22**, 745–751.

25. Anderson, L.L., and Ding, I.V. (1975). Dosimetric concentrations for iodine-125. In B.S. Hilaris (Ed.), *Afterloading – 20 Years of experience*, Memorial Sloan-Kettering Cancer *Center, New York, pp.63–72.*

26. Hilaris, B.S. (1978). I-125 implantation of the prostate: dose–response considerations. In J.M. Vaeth (Ed.), *Renaissance of Interstitial Brachytherapy*, S. Karger, San Francisco, California, pp.82–90.

27. Anderson, L.L. *et al.* (1981). Memorial Hospital method of calculation for iridium 192. In F.W. George (Ed.), *Modern Interstitial and Intracavitary Irradiation Cancer Management*. Masson Publishing, New York, pp.9–15.

28. Goode, R. *et al.* (1979). Radioactive suture in the treatment of head and neck cancer. *Laryngoscope*, **89**, 349–354.

29. Fletcher, G.H. (1979). The role of irradiation in the management of squamous cell carcinoma of the mouth and throat, *Head Neck Surg.*, **1**, 441–457.

30. Vikram, B., Strong, E.W. *et al.* (1980). Elective post-operative radiation therapy in stages III and IV epidermoid carcinoma of the head

and neck. *Am. J. Surg.*, **140**, 580–584.

31. Vikram, B. (1979). Importance of the time interval between surgery and post operative radiation therapy in the combined management of head and neck cancer, *Int. J. Radiat. Oncol. Biol. Phys.*, **5**, 1837–1840.

32. Ellis, F. (1975). Tumor bed implants at the time of surgery. In B.S. Hilaris (Ed.), *Afterloading – 20 Years of Experience*, Memorial Sloan-Kettering Cancer Center, New York, pp.125–132.

33. Ellis, F. (19). Soft tissue tumors: surgery and simultaneous implantation, *Front. Radiat. Ther. Oncol.*, **12**, 162–178.

34. Pierquin, B. *et al.* (1978). In Pierquin, B. *et al.* (Eds), *Brachytherapy*, Warren H. Green, Inc., St Louis, Mo., pp.93–146.

35. Decroix, V., and Ghossein, N.A. (1981). Experience of the Curie Institute in the treatment of cancer of the mobile tongue. *Cancer*, **47**, 496–502.

36. Fu, K., Ray, J.W. *et al.* (1976). External and interstitial radiation therapy of carcinomas of the oral tongue: a review of 32 years of experience. *Am. J. Roentgenol. Radium Ther. Nucl. Med.*, **127**, 107–115.

37. Benak, S., Buschke, F. *et al.* (1970). Treatment of carcinoma of the oral cavity. *Radiology*, **96**, 137–143.

38. Campos, J., Lampe, I., and Fayos, J.V. (1971). Radiotherapy of carcinoma of the floor of the mouth. *Radiology*, **99**, 677–682.

39. Fletcher, G.H., and Stovall M., (1962). *Radiology*, **78**, 766.

40. Pierquin, B., Chassagne, D. *et al.* (1971). The place of implantation in tongue and floor of mouth cancer. *JAMA*, **215**, 961–963.

41. Marcus, R.B., Million, R.R. *et al.* (1980). A preloaded, custom-designed implantation device for Stage T1 T2 carcinoma of the floor of the mouth. *Int. J. Radiat. Oncol. Biol. Phys.*, **6**, 111–113.

42. Syed, A.M.N. (1978). Iridium-192 afterloading implant in the re-treatment of head and neck cancers. *Br. J. Radiol.*, **51**, 814–820.

43. Vikram, B., Hilaris, B.S. *et al.* (1983). Permanent iodine-125 implants in head and neck cancer. *Cancer*, **51**, 1310–1314.

Chapter **10**

Hypoxic Cell Radiation Sensitizers

George A. Alexander and
David A. Pistenmaa
*Radiation Research Program, Division of
Cancer Treatment, National Cancer
Institute, National Institutes of Health,
Bethesda, Maryland, USA*

INTRODUCTION

A neoplastic tumour is believed to contain at least three populations of malignant cells. These include rapidly proliferating well-oxygenated cells, non-proliferating oxygenated cells, and hypoxic cells. Experimental and some clinical data[1,2] suggest that hypoxic cells may limit the curability of certain types of human cancers by conventional fractionated radiotherapy. In head and neck cancer the incidence of primary recurrence as the first site of failure in patients treated by radiotherapy alone ranges from 9.5% for hypopharyngeal cancers to 41.5% for cancers of the paranasal sinus.[3] The most commonly suspected cause for radiotherapy failures is the presence of tumour cells which are hypoxic and therefore resistant to the cytotoxic effect of radiation. Peters *et al.*[4] have recently discussed the problem of tumour radioresistance in clinical radiotherapy. Several factors which may make a tumour radioresistant are summarized in Table 10.1. The objective of the present discussion is to review the progress to date in investigations of hypoxic cell radiation sen-

sitizers in the treatment of head and neck cancer and to discuss the rationale for future studies with hypoxic radiosensitizers.

TABLE 10.1   CAUSES OF CLINICAL
RADIORESISTANCE[4]

Tumour-related factors
  Number of clonogenic cells
  Hypoxia
  Tumor kinetics
  Intrinsic radioresistance
  Reseeding of irradiated sites
  New primary tumour

Host-related factors
  The 'volume effect'
  Dose-limiting normal tissues
  Pathophysiological factors
  Host defences

Technical factors
  Geographical miss
  Errors in dose delivery

Probabilistic radioresistance

THE EXISTENCE OF HYPOXIC CELLS

It is well established that solid tumours contain deficient vascular beds, areas of severe vascular insufficiency, and, frequently, regions of frank necrosis.[5-7] Therefore these tumours would be expected to contain hypoxic cells. In their classic study Thomlinson and Gray[8] analysed the distribution of blood vessels, viable tumour tissue, and necrosis in pathological specimens from human lung carcinoma with respect to the distribution and utilization of oxygen within the tissue. They observed that the areas of necrosis generally occurred at a distance of about 150–200 microns from the nearest capillary. These authors concluded that the viable cells on the periphery of necrotic regions in the tumours were severely hypoxic. The existence of hypoxic cells in solid tumours was first demonstrated radiobiologically by Powers and Tolmach,[9] using a transplantable mouse lymphosarcoma. Over the years investigations of experimentally transplanted tumours in rodents have shown that the majority of these tumours contain 10–20% hypoxic cells.[10-12]

In addition, it is now also established that hypoxic cells in solid murine tumours limit the response of these neoplasms to treatment with large single doses of radiation and lead to regrowth of tumour cells *in vitro*.[13-17] A fractionated course of radiation in animal tumours permits 'reoxygenation' of hypoxic cells between treatments. As a result of reoxygenation the sensitivity of the formerly hypoxic cells to future irradiation is increased. It should be emphasized however, that the patterns of reoxygenation in animal tumour models vary with the dose of radiation, the conditions of irradiation, and with the particular tumour line studied.[18-20] If reoxygenation occurs slowly, then hypoxic cells may still present a problem even with fractionated radiotherapy.

The evidence for the presence of hypoxic cells in human tumours is only indirect. Nevertheless, for more than 20 years since hypoxia was first recognized as a problem in radiotherapy, several methods of overcoming the problem have been proposed and tested clinically. These include the administration of hyperbaric oxygen during radiotherapy, the use of high linear-energy transfer radiations, and the use of hypoxic cell radiation sensitizers. Although clinical experience with hyperbaric oxygen during radiotherapy has shown improved local control rates in head and neck cancer,[1,21,22] improvement in survival has not reached statistical significance in the majority of trials. The encouraging observations in studies of hyperbaric oxygen administration suggest that hypoxic cell radiosensitizers may offer some benefit.

HYPOXIC CELL RADIATION SENSITIZERS

Sensitizers from five functional categories have been used to investigate the radiosensitization of mammalian cells *in vitro* and *in vivo* (Table 10.2). Oxygen is the most efficient radiation sensitizer known. For nearly 20 years researchers have worked on identifying chemical substances which mimic the sensitizing effect of oxygen and allow the preferential radiosensitization of hypoxic cells within tumours without causing any significant

TABLE 10.2   CLASSIFICATION OF RADIATION SENSITIZERS BASED ON MECHANISM OF ACTION[46]

Suppression of intracellular SH groups
Formation of toxic radiation products
Inhibition of post-irradiation cellular repair processes
Structural incorporation of thymine analogues into intracellular DNA
Oxygen-mimetics*

* Electron-affinic sensitizers are included in this group.

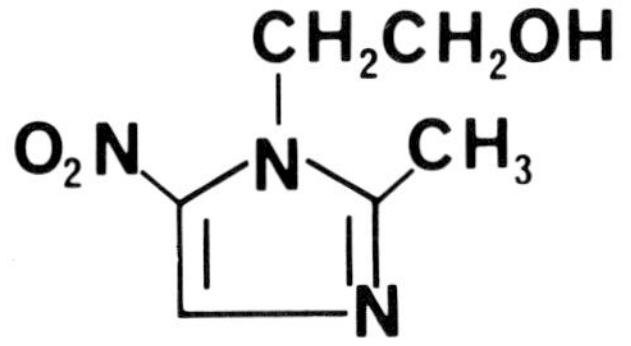

$$O_2N \overset{CH_2CH_2OH}{\underset{N}{\bigvee}} CH_3$$

Figure 10.1 Chemical structure of the 5-nitroimidazole, metronidazole

increase in normal tissue toxicity. The initial experiments with anoxic bacteria were designed to see if their radiosensitivity could be altered. Adams and Cooke[23] suggested in early studies that electron affinity was the dominant feature that conferred radiosensitizing potential on chemicals. Subsequently, many compounds were found to sensitize hypoxic cells *in vitro*, but most of these agents showed little or no effect *in vivo*. In 1973 Foster and Willson[24] reported that the well-known antitrichomonal drug metronidazole (Figure 10.1), or Flagyl, was an effective hypoxic cell sensitizer. When Chinese hamster fibroblasts were irradiated *in vitro* under anoxic conditions the cell survival

curve was shallow, whereas in the presence of metronidazole the curve became steeper and was displaced to the left. With respect to *in vivo* sensitization by metronidazole, Begg *et al.*[25] observed a direct relationship between tumour cure and X-ray dose for the C3H mouse mammary carcinoma. A single dose of about 40.00 Gy was required to control 50% of the tumours (TCD_{50}). When the mice were treated with a high-dose metronidazole prior to the same radiation dose the tumour control rate increased from 50% to about 90%. Table 10.3 summarizes the enhancement ratios of misonidazole and metronidazole in several different mouse tumour systems *in vivo*.

Stone and Withers[27] studied the modification of the response to irradiation of C3H mouse mammary carcinoma, mouse skin, and mouse jejunum by metronidazole. A dose of 2.5 mg of metronidazole per mouse had no effect on tumour growth rate and toxic effects were not observed. The single dose required for tumour control (TCD_{50}) was reduced from 63.60 Gy in control animals to 53.10 Gy in drug-treated animals. Since the drug alone had no effect on tumour growth, the authors

TABLE 10.3   EXPERIMENTAL TUMOUR ENHANCEMENT RATIOS *IN VIVO**

Tumour	Doubling time (days)	Hypoxic cells (%)	Enhancement with misonidazole (1 mg/g)	Enhancement with metronidazole (1 mg/g)
CBA fast sarcoma F	1	> 10	1.6	1.3
CBA carcinoma NT	3	6	1.9	1.6
CBA fast sarcoma F	1	> 10	2.2	
WHT intradermal squamous carcinoma G	1	0.3	1.8	
C$_3$H sarcoma KHT	2	6	1.8	1.5
C$_3$H 1st-generation transplant of spontaneous mammary carcinoma	6	10	1.8	1.3
WHT anaplastic carcinoma MT line transplant	1.5	50	2.0	1.5
WHT bone sarcoma 2	2.5		1.8	
MDAH-MC$_A$-4 mammary carcinoma	2.5	20−25	2.3	1.5
MDAH-MC$_A$-4 mammary carcinoma	4	20−25	2.3	1.3
EMT6 tumour	3.5	30	2.9	2.1

* Modified from Phillips[26]
  Enhancement ratio equals the ratio of two X-ray doses required to cause a given level of biological effect, with and without the stated radiosensitizing agent.

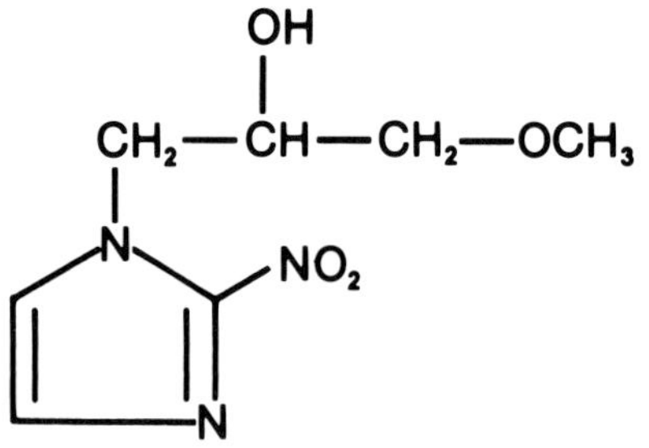

Figure 10.2 Chemical structure of the 2-nitroimidazole, misonidazole

concluded that the effect shown was one of sensitization of hypoxic cancer cells. It was not long before a clinical trial was established to evaluate the sensitizing capability of metronidazole. Urtasun et al.[28] reported the results of a controlled prospective trial of 36 patients irradiated for grade 4 astrocytomas. Patients were randomized to radiation alone or to radiation and high-dose metronidazole. A dose of 30.00 Gy in nine fractions over 3 weeks was used in both groups of patients. Although the radiation dose was inadequate, this study did show that the probability of survival was greater in the metronidazole-treated patients.

In 1974, Asquith et al.[29] described a nitroaromatic drug that had radiosensitizing potential superior to that of metronidazole and also had better pharmacological properties. This drug, misonidazole (Figure 10.2), was shown to be more effective than metronidazole in several animal tumours irradiated with single- as well as with multiple-fraction schedules.[30] Additional studies with multiple doses[31] revealed that neurological toxicity, primarily peripheral neuropathy, was dose-limiting and that the maximum tolerated dose for multiple dose schedules was between 10 and 12 g/m^2.

In 1972 Adams reportedly[32] demonstrated that another nitroimidazole, the Roche experimental drug Ro-07-0582, was a much more effective sensitizing agent than metronidazole. Adams and associates[33] have made determinations of the radiosensitizing

efficiencies in hypoxic Chinese hamster cells of seven different 2-nitroimidazoles including Ro-07-0582 (misonidazole), and two 5-nitroimidazoles, including metronidazole. All of these chemical agents were found to be active hypoxic cell radiosensitizers with the sensitization proportional to drug concentration.

Metronidazole and misonidazole are being investigated clinically in a number of countries for a variety of malignant tumours.

SUMMARY OF CLINICAL TRIALS IN HEAD AND NECK CANCER

Initial Clinical Trials

A summary of available clinical data on the treatment of head and neck cancer by irradiation with radiosensitizers is shown in Table 10.4. Sealy[34] reported results of irradiation and misonidazole in 38 patients with advanced cancer of the head and neck. Twenty-three of the 38 patients received misonidazole. Of these 23 patients, 13 received misonidazole, as part of a randomized study, seven were given misonidazole with radiation after previous treatment, and three were irradiated with both misonidazole and hyperbaric oxygen. A total tumour dose of 36.00 Gy using cobalt-60 gamma rays was delivered to the tumour in six fractions over 17 days. Misonidazole 2 g/m^2 was administered orally 4 hours before treatment. Local control was achieved in four of 13 patients who received misonidazole and was indeterminate in three patients. Six patients developed recurrence of their tumours. Four of the seven patients treated previously were locally free of disease while two of three patients who received misonidazole, radiation, and hyperbaric oxygen developed metastatic disease outside of the irradiated volume. The results of the randomized study failed to show any clinical advantage of the combination of misonidazole and irradiation. Sealy et al.[35] have updated this limited series and reported no difference in local control rate (42%) at 1 year in patients who received misonidazole and those who did not.

Thirty-two patients were entered into a pilot study of combination hyperbaric oxygen and misonidazole.[35] Among a subgroup of 19 patients with previously untreated squamous carcinoma 13 patients (68%) achieved local control, whereas four patients had local treatment failure. A more recent analysis of these studies[36] using life-table methods has shown no significant differences between groups in terms of time to death or relapse. There were no

TABLE 10.4   SUMMARY OF CLINICAL TRIALS OF HYPOXIC CELL SENSITIZERS AND RADIATION IN HEAD AND NECK CANCER

Author	Primary site	No. of patients	Study design	Radiation schedule	Sensitizer schedule	Summary of results
Sealy[34]	All sites, T_{3-4}	38	R	36.00 Gy/6 fx/ 17 days	MISO 12 g/m^2 in six doses	No clinical advantage of MISO and radiation
Arcangeli et al.[37]	All sites, N_{2-3}	25	P	$\geqslant$50.00 Gy/ MDF^b	MISO 12 g/m^2 in 10 doses	Enhancement of local tumour control
Paterson et al.[38]	All sites, advanced	29	P	40.00–45.00 Gy/ 10 fx/22 days	MISO 12 g/m^2 in 10 doses	60% local control at 9 months
Orr et al.[39]	Oral cavity, recurrent	23	P	45.00–60.00 Gy in 65–120 hours with iridium-192	Metronidazole 12–18 g/m^2 in two or three doses	43% NED^c at 25 months median follow-up
Fazekas et al.[40]	Oral cavity, oropharynx, hypopharynx, T_{3-4}	50	P	66.00–72.00 Gy/ 33–46 fx/7–8 weeks	MISO 15 g/m^2 in six doses; modified to 12 g/m^2 in six doses	47% NED at 18 months median follow-up^d
Overgaard et al.[41]	Larynx, pharynx, Stages II–IV	202	R	64.00 Gy/34 fx/ 10 weeks in split course	With or without MISO 11.0 g/m^2 in 20 doses during 1st course	Statistically significant difference in tumour regression in MISO group (76.5% vs. 53.4%); Difference in disease-free survival (67% vs. 56%)
				57.04 Gy/22 fx/ 10 weeks in split course	With or without MISO 11.0 g/m^2 in 8 doses during 1st course	
Karim and Njo[42]	All sites, T_{2-4} Stages III–IV	70	P	65.00–78.00 Gy/ 5 fx/wk/7–8 weeks with shrinking fields	Metronidazole 2.5 g/day/five doses/week; total dose 72–92 g	54% local control rate at 30 months minimum follow-up
Van den Bogaert et al.[43]	All sites, Advanced stages	179	P	48.00 Gy/3 fx a day/5 days a week/2 weeks followed by rest period, then boost for total of 67.20–72 Gy/5–7 weeks	MISO 1 g/m^2/ day/five doses/ week; total dose 13–14 g/m^2 in 53 patients	No statistically significant difference in local tumour control (57% vs. 48%) at 20 months

^{a} R = Randomnized controlled study; P = Pilot study
^{b} MDF, multiple daily fractionation (200 + 150 + 150 rad/day, 5 days/week)
^{c} NED, no evidence of disease
^{d} Survival among 36 patients who completed the sensitizer schedule.
   MISO = misonidazole

significant differences in prognosis based on age, T-stage, N-stage, or histology.

Arcangeli et al.[37] reported the preliminary results of a pilot study employing multiple daily fractionation (MDF) radiotherapy combined with hyperthermia and/or misonidazole for the treatment of 25 patients with single or multiple ($N_2 - N_3$) neck node metastases from head and neck cancer. Patients were irradiated with 5.7 MeV photons up to a total dose of 40.00 – 70.00 Gy with either MDF alone (2.0 + 1.5 + 1.5 Gy/day, 5 days each week), or MDF plus hyperthermia (500 MHz, 42 – 43 °C for 45 minutes after the second daily fraction of radiotherapy, 3 days each week), or MDF plus misonidazole (1.2 g/m² daily, 2 hours before the first fraction, for a maximum dose of 12 g/m²) or MDF, hyperthermia, and misonidazole at the above schedules. These groups of patients were compared to a historical series of patients treated with conventionally fractionated photon irradiation (2.0 Gy/day, 5 days each week). By the end of treatment complete regression of palpable tumour had occurred in 47% (9/19) of lesions treated by MDF alone, in 85% (17/20) of lesions treated by MDF plus hyperthermia, in 54% (6/11) of lesions treated by MDF plus misonidazole, in 80% (8/10) of lesions treated by MDF, hyperthermia and misonidazole but in only 30% (14/46) of lesions treated with conventional radiotherapy. These preliminary results suggested to the authors that radiation combined with hyperthermia alone, or with hyperthermia and misonidazole, enhanced local tumour control.

Paterson et al.[38] reported the results of a pilot study of 29 patients with locally advanced squamous cell carcinoma of the upper aerodigestive tract treated by radiotherapy and misonidazole. Depending on field size the tumour dose ranged from 40.00 to 45.00 Gy in 10 fractions (three fractions each week) over 22 days. Misonidazole was administered to a total dose of 12 g/m² divided into 10 doses given 3 – 4 hours before irradiation. Twenty-four of the 29 patients (83%) had complete regression

of tumour following treatment. Seven of the 24 patients developed local recurrence within the irradiated volume within nine months. Three patients died without evidence of tumour in the treated volume: two of intercurrent disease and one of metastases. The local tumour control rate at 9 months was 60%. The results of this pilot study suggested improvement in local control with misonidazole.

Orr et al.[39] reported the results of a pilot study of 23 patients with recurrent or persistent squamous cell carcinoma of the oral cavity treated by iridium-192 interstitial implantation in conjunction with metronidazole. The tumour dose ranged from 45.00 to 60.00 Gy in 65 – 120 hours. All patients received metronidazole 6 g/m² orally 6 hours before the implant and every 48 hours for the duration of the implant. Of 23 patients receiving treatment, 16 (69.5%) had complete regression of local disease generally within 12 weeks. Ten of the 23 patients (43%) were alive and disease-free at an average follow-up of 25 months. Nausea, mild diarrhoea, and radiation-induced mucositis were the principal side-effects. Within the limitations of this pilot study the results suggested to the authors that enhanced local tumour control and improved survival among responding patients was achievable using the metronidazole-implant technique.

Fazekas et al.[40] have reported the results of a Radiation Therapy Oncology Group (RTOG) pilot study in which 50 patients with T_3 and T_4 squamous cell carcinomas of the oral cavity, oropharynx, and hypopharynx were treated with misonidazole and definitive radiotherapy. Misonidazole was given orally once per week 4 hours before radiotherapy at a dose of 2.5 g/m² to the first 30 patients and at a dose of 2.0 g/m² to the remainder of the patients. A 2.5 Gy tumour dose was delivered to the patient and 4 hours later a second dose of 2.1 Gy was delivered. On 3 other days each week patients received daily tumour doses of 1.8 Gy. This scheme was continued for 5 weeks with the cumulative misonidazole dose not exceeding 12.5 g/m^2 or 24 grams. The total tumour dose was 50.00 Gy in 5 weeks. Afterwards, a radiation boost of 1.8–2.0 Gy per day was given to the primary tumour and any originally palpable nodes. The total tumour dose was 66.00–72.00 Gy in 7–8 weeks. Forty-six of 50 patients were evaluable. Thirty-six of the 46 (78%) received a minimum tumour dose of more than 60.00 Gy and three doses of misonidazole. Complete tumour responses were observed in 25 of 50 patients (50%) overall and in 24 of the 36 patients (67%) completing both radiotherapy and misonidazole. Seventeen of the 36 patients (47%) were alive without evidence of disease ranging from 9 to 24 months with a median disease-free survival of 18 months. Peripheral neuropathy was the most frequent side-effect and occurred in 16 patients. Central nervous system toxicity (encephalopathy) occurred in five patients, two of whom lapsed into coma and died from complications. Nausea, vomiting, and rash were noted in five patients. These data suggested to the authors that the local control and survival with misonidazole and radiotherapy may be superior to radiotherapy alone.

Overgaard *et al.*[41] have reported the preliminary results of a double-blind randomized multi-institutional trial of misonidazole combined with split-course radiotherapy in the treatment of 202 patients with Stage II–IV carcinoma of the larynx and Stage I–IV carcinoma of the pharynx. Patients were randomized to four treatment schedules as shown in Figure 10.3. In arm I patients received radiation on a split course schedule consisting of 2 Gy fractions five times each week for a tumour dose of 40 Gy. Misonidazole, 0.55 g/m^2, was given before each of the 20 doses to a cumulative dose of 11 g/m^2. After a 3-week interval an additional 24 Gy was given in 14 fractions (five fractions each week) for a total tumour dose of 64 Gy. In arm II the radiotherapy fractionation schedule was exactly the same as in arm I, but misonidazole was not given. In arm III a split-course radiation schedule using a higher dose per fraction was employed. Patients received 4.13 Gy fractions twice each week for 4 weeks to a tumour dose of 33.04 Gy. Misonidazole, 1.4 g/m^2, was given prior to each of the eight doses not to exceed a cumulative dose of 11 g/m^2. Following a 3-week interval an additional 24 Gy was given in 14 fractions (five fractions each week) for a total tumour dose of

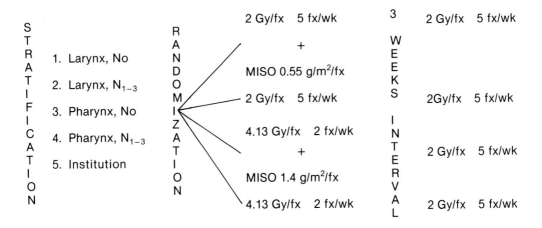

Figure 10.3   Treatment schedule for the Danish Head and Neck Cancer Study Protocol 2. Adapted from Overgaard *et al.*[41]

57.04 Gy. In arm IV patients were treated with the same radiotherapy fractionation schedule as in arm III – however, misonidazole was not administered. The complete tumour regression rate at 2 months after treatment in both groups of patients treated with misonidazole was 76.5% compared to 53.4% in those patients given a placebo. This difference was statistically significant ($P<0.01$) and was independent of the radiation schedule. At 15 months following treatment the disease-free survival rates in the misonidazole and placebo groups were 67% and 56%, respectively (not statistically significant). The main side-effect of misonidazole was peripheral neuropathy. There was no relationship between the severity of symptoms and the different radiation fractionation schedules. The incidence and severity of peripheral neuropathy was related to total misonidazole dose. There was significantly less neuropathy at doses less than or equal to 11.0 g/m^2 than with doses greater than 11.0 g/m^2 ($P<0.05$) which some patients received early in the study. These same authors also found that moderate to severe oedema and/or epithelitis occurred more frequently in the misonidazole-treated group (56.2%) compared to the placebo group (38.3%). This difference was statistically significant ($P<0.005$) and is of interest inasmuch as radiosensitizers should not sensitize normal tissues.

Karim and Njo[42] reported the results of a non-randomized study of 70 patients with advanced head and neck cancers (Stages III and IV) treated with metronidazole and high-dose protracted radiotherapy. The total tumour dose ranged from 65.00 to 78.00 Gy and was administered in 2 Gy fractions, five fractions a week over 7–8 weeks using megavoltage radiation. Metronidazole 2.5 g was given each treatment day in divided doses in the morning (0.75 g), 2 hours before radiotherapy (1.0 g) and in the evening (0.75 g). The total cumulative dose ranged between 72 and 94 g. The dose schedule of metronidazole was chosen in order to maintain steady serum and tissue levels of the drug while delivering a high cumulative dose but a low daily dose. Thirty-eight of 70 patients (54%) had local control of their disease with a minimum follow-up of 30 months. Gastrointestinal intolerance was the most frequent side-effect, occurring in 34 patients (48%). Peripheral neuropathy was noted in four patients (5.7%) and central nervous system toxicity in one patient. It has been speculated that prolonged and continuous exposure of tumour to metronidazole may have a selective cytotoxic effect on hypoxic cells in addition to a radiation dose-modifying effect.[42] Protracted radiotherapy may have been a contributing factor to local tumour control since the hypoxic cells surviving an individual radiation fraction may possibly have reoxygenated before the subsequent radiation dose.

Van den Bogaert *et al.*[43] have recently reported the results of a pilot study of the Radiotherapy Group of the EORTC (European Organization for Research on Treatment of Cancer) investigating high-dose multiple daily fractionation (MDF) combined with misonidazole in the treatment of 179 patients with advanced head and neck cancers. Patients were irradiated three times daily in 1.6–2.0 Gy fractions at 3–4 hour intervals. A total tumour dose of 48 Gy was given over 2 weeks. After a 2–4-week interval a boost was given, using the same irradiation scheme, to a total dose of 67.2–72 Gy in 5–7 weeks. Misonidazole 1 g/m^2 was given to 53 patients 2 hours before the first radiation session on every treatment day to a total dose of 13–14 g/m^2. The complete tumour regression rate in 179 patients after 2 or 3 months was 86%. At 20 months the actual survival and local control rates were 31% and 48%, respectively. In the 53 patients treated with misonidazole the local control rate at 20 months was 57% compared to 44% for the 126 patients not given the drug. This difference was not significant. In this series nine patients died from treatment-related causes: four patients died from haemorrhage, three from necrosis, one from postoperative complications, and one from misonidazole toxicity. In this study the addition of misonidazole did not appear to affect the degree of skin or mucosal reactions.

Ongoing Clinical Trials

The clinical evaluation of misonidazole in Phase II and Phase III trials is going on in a number of countries. However, there are only a few studies where this hypoxic cell radiosensitizer is being investigated for the treatment of head and neck cancer. In the United Kingdom the Medical Research Council conducted a randomized double-blind study of the role of misonidazole given in combination with radiotherapy for the treatment of patients with squamous carcinoma of the upper aerodigestive tract.[44] In one arm, patients receive supervoltage irradiation and misonidazole while in the other arm patients receive the same radiotherapy and a placebo. One of two dose-fractionation schemes is used. Patients receive a total tumour dose of 50.00–57.50 Gy in 20 fractions (five fractions per week) or 40.00–45.00 Gy in 10 fractions (three fractions per week). Misonidazole is administered orally 4–5 hours before each radiation fraction with the total cumulative dosage not to exceed 12 g/m^2. Patient entry into this trial has been stopped because of peripheral neuropathy from misonidazole treatment (40–70%) and the unlikelihood that a minimum improvement of 15% in local tumour control could be achieved with misonidazole to justify continued use of the drug.[45]

In the United States the RTOG has two ongoing randomized clinical trials of radiotherapy with or without misonidazole for advanced squamous cell carcinoma of the head and neck. The first, RTOG 79–04, is a Phase I/II study of high fractional dose radiotherapy in patients with non-resectable Stage III or IV, or recurrent, carcinomas. In the radiotherapy-alone arm patients receive 44.00 Gy in 11 fractions (five fractions per week) plus 4.0 Gy on the day following the eleventh fraction if clinically indicated. In the misonidazole-plus-radiotherapy arm, patients receive the same radiation treatment plus misonidazole, 1.5 g/m^2 orally, 4–6 hours prior to three of the radiation doses each week to a total cumulative dosage of 10.5 g/m^2.[44] The second study, RTOG 79–15, is an ongoing Phase III trial of radiotherapy with or without misonidazole in patients with inoperable head and neck cancer. Patients are randomized to receive 66.00–73.80 Gy in 6½–8 weeks to the primary and surrounding structures alone or with misonidazole, 2 g/m^2 orally, once weekly (12 g/m^2 maximum cumulative dose) 4–6 hours prior to radiotherapy.[44]

In view of the encouraging preliminary results of high-dose MDF combined with misonidazole in the treatment of head and neck cancers, a three-arm randomized clinical study is under way in the EORTC Radiotherapy Group comparing single daily fraction radiotherapy with multiple daily fractionation with or without misonidazole.[43]

DEVELOPMENT OF NEW HYPOXIC CELL SENSITIZERS

At present the ideal hypoxic cell radiosensitizer has not been found.[42] Hypoxic cell radiosensitizers should selectively sensitize only hypoxic cells and not well-oxygenated tissues. Adams[46] has described the criteria for selecting a drug to fulfil this requirement. These criteria are:

(1)   the sensitizer must be non-toxic to normal tissues at therapeutic doses;
(2)   sensitizing activity on oxygenated cells must be minimal or non-existent;
(3)   the sensitizer must be capable of penetrating poorly vascularized tumours and of diffusing through non-vascularized regions;
(4)   the sensitizer must not be subject to rapid metabolic breakdown.

Although these were rigid requirements, drugs have been developed which meet these criteria. The electron-affinic sensitizers are examples.

The higher the electron affinity of the sensitizer, the lower the concentration required for sensitization.[46] High lipophilicity (lipid solubility) is a property which allows these sensitizers to penetrate tumours, governs the plasma half-life of the drugs, and at the same time is responsible for peripheral and central neuropathy.

For the nitroimidazole compounds the ring structure determines the electron-affinity and ultimately the degree of radiosensitization, while the aliphatic side chain at the 1-position of the ring largely determines the lipophilicity and, in turn the pharmacokinetics and toxicity of the drugs.[47]

In the US the development of hypoxic cell radiosensitizers is part of the comprehensive drug development effort of the Division of Cancer Treatment, National Cancer Institute.[48] Because of basic differences between cytotoxic chemical agents and radiosensitizers and radioprotectors, the criteria for selecting radiation sensitizers are significantly different from those for cytotoxic agents. The treatment linear array allows for timely and systematic testing of new compounds. Compounds are selected which:

(1) have high electron affinity;
(2) have measurable lipid/water partition coefficients;
(3) show *in vitro* sensitization of hypoxic mammalian cells to radiation;
(4) show no significant sensitization of aerated mammalian cells *in vitro* to radiation;
(5) have a cell kill that is limited at active levels *in vitro* for brief periods of exposure;
(6) have a structure indicative of reasonable stability in solution;
(7) have measurable LD_{50} in the animal to be used for *in vivo* testing; and
(8) have sensitizing activity in at least one *in vivo* model tumour at doses below the drug LD_{50}.[49]

Wasserman *et al.*[50] have recently reported the results of a RTOG Phase I trial of the sensitizer desmethylmisonidazole (Figure 10.4) in patients with advanced cancer. Desmethylmisonidazole, a metabolite of misonidazole, is presumed to have therapeutic advantages over misonidazole which include lower lipophilicity, improved renal clearance, shorter half-life, less penetration into neural tissues, and good peak serum levels. Desmethylmisonidazole was administered by intravenous infusion using an escalating number of doses per week and the size of individual doses for either a 3-or 7-week dose schedule. Individual doses up to 4 g/m^2 and total doses up to 18.9 g/m^2 have been given. Ten per cent of patients had nausea and vomiting which was not dose-limiting. Grade 1–2 peripheral neuropathy was observed in 34 patients and occurred only in patients who received total doses greater than 9 g/m^2. The

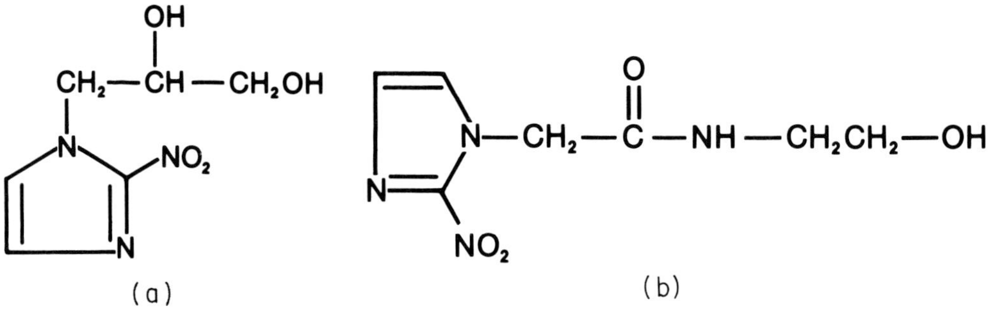

Figure 10.4   Chemical structures of the 2-nitroimidazoles, (a) desmethylmisonidazole and (b) SR-2508

absence of central neurotoxicity and the lower incidence of ototoxicity at the doses studied were features distinctly different from misonidazole. However, the incidence of peripheral neuropathy with desmethyl-misonidazole limits its administration to doses only 10–15% greater than can be given with misonidazole. Therefore, the investigators recommended that desmethylmisonidazole not be used in any efficacy trials at the present time.

SYNTHESIS OF NEW COMPOUNDS

It has now become evident that the neurological side-effects of misonidazole are the major limitations to achieving drug levels that would provide adequate radiosensitization. Ideally, a compound should have radiosensitizing capacity equal to mison-idazole but should be less neurotoxic. A wide variety of 2-nitroimidazoles with electron-affinity similar to misonidazole have been synthesized.[51] They have been tested with tumours *in vivo* and with hypoxic cells *in vitro* and gave equivalent levels of radiosensitization.[47] Two such compounds are SR-2508 and SR-2555. The degree of radiosensitization produced by the latter is less than that produced by the former. With respect to neurotoxicity in mice, the relative amounts of the drug on a molar basis for the same toxicity are 1, 2.3, 3.1, and 3.9 for misonidazole, desmethyl-misonidazole, SR-2508, and SR-2555, respectively. Both SR-2508 and SR-2555 have significantly shorter plasma half-lives in mice. Recent data from Stanford University have shown that SR-2508 is the optimal compound among the 2-nitroimidazoles with an electron-affinity similar to misonidazole,[47] and markedly lower toxicity. Phase I clinical testing of SR-2508 (Figure 10.4) has begun in the US.

The search continues in a number of laboratories for the identification of compounds which are superior to misonidazole in their radiosensitizing ability. Studies by Astor *et al.*[52] have shown that newly synthesized 4-and 5-substituted nitroimidazoles,

SK-21981 and MJL-1-191-V11, are much more effective than misonidazole as radiosensitizers in Chinese hamster cells in culture. Their data suggested that the MJL compound sensitizes by two completely different mechanisms, the first resulting from its electron affinity and the second involving the removal of endogenous thiols (primarily glutathione) which are naturally occurring radioprotective substances. Because gluta-thione competes with electron-affinic radiosensitizers for radiation-induced radicals in cells, any significant depletion of intracellular glutathione might make hypoxic tumour cells more prone to radiosensitization by electron-affinic compounds.[53] Bump *et al.*[53] showed that depletion of glutathione in Chinese hamster ovary cells *in vitro* by diethyl maleate enhanced the radiosensitization of hypoxic cells by misonidazole.

Under contracts with the National Cancer Institute, the Stanford Research Institute and the Institute of Cancer Research in Sutton, England, have been synthesizing and testing new compounds with radiosensitizing poten-tial.[49] Since 1977 about 400 compounds have been evaluated.[54] At the Stanford Research Institute current efforts are being focused on classes of compounds other than nitroimidazoles including quinones, 1,2-dicarbonyl compounds, aminoxides, alpha–beta-unsaturated carbonyls, maleic acid derivatives, and diamide analogues. Investigators at the Institute of Cancer Research are concentrating on the development of nitroimidazoles and other nitro compounds as well as electron-affinic non-nitro compounds.

PROSPECTS FOR HYPOXIC CELL RADIATION SENSITISERS

For those head and neck cancers where hypoxic cells may be a problem for radiotherapy, hypoxic cell sensitizers, particularly electron-affinic compounds, represent one of the more promising areas of research. Although the results of initial clinical trials[34,37,38] using radiation sensitizers in head and neck cancer have not been as rewarding as was originally hoped, they provide some basis for expecting that more effective sensitizer compounds will be more successful. Some improvement was suggested in the local control rates of patients with advanced head and neck cancers. Disease-free survivals of 43–47% have been reported in patients with median follow-up of 18–25 months.[39,40] Long-term follow-up (30 months minimum) of patients has shown local control rates as high as 54%.[42] Moreover, statistically significant differences in tumour regression in patients receiving misonidazole have been noted.[41] The main disadvantage of misonidazole is its neurotoxicity; thus, new compounds are needed which have the same sensitizing capacity as misonidazole but have less toxicity so that larger doses can be given.

The preliminary results of a Phase I trial of desmethylmisonidazole in patients with advanced cancers indicate that neurotoxicity remains a problem.[50] At present it is not planned to evaluate this drug in Phase II/III clinical trials because a more promising electron-affinic compound, SR-2508, is currently in Phase I clinical trials.

Although some data[55,56] are available for estimating the proportion of hypoxic cells in human cancers, there is a lack of practical techniques to detect the presence or absence of hypoxic cells and to measure the rates of reoxygenation in human cancers. Recent studies of sensitization ratios suggest that knowledge of the degree of tumour reoxygenation may obviate the need for the perfect radiosensitizer.[57]

Finally, there is much which remains to be done in the development and clinical evaluation of hypoxic cell radiation sensitizers, particularly in head and neck cancer. It is reasonable to expect that within a few years a number of more effective radiosensitizers will be available for clinical evaluation. Whether such compounds will improve the results of treatment of cancer with radiotherapy needs to be determined in well-designed randomized studies.

CONCLUSIONS

(1) Major advances in the development of hypoxic cell radiation sensitizers have been made in the last 20 years as demonstrated in both *in vitro* and *in vivo* experimental tumour systems.

(2) Misonidazole and metronidazole have been the principal hypoxic cell radiosensitizers evaluated for the treatment of patients with head and neck cancer. The major limitation of these agents has been neurotoxicity.

(3) To date, neither misonidazole nor metronidazole has been shown to give a statistically significant improvement in disease-free survival in a prospective randomized study. However, the results of studies to date do show improvements in local control rates.

(4) Further development and clinical testing of hypoxic cell radiation sensitizers in patients with head and neck cancer are needed and ultimately may improve the effectiveness of radiation therapy in the treatment of these neoplasms.

ACKNOWLEDGEMENTS

The authors acknowledge the assistance of Mr Alex Abraham in preparation of this manuscript, and Mrs Nancita Lomax, Developmental Therapeutics Program, NCI in supply chemical structures.

REFERENCES

1. Henk, J.M. (1975). *Laryngoscope*, **85**, 1134.
2. Bush, R.S., Jenkin, R.D.T., Allt, W.E.C., Beale, F.A., Bean, H., Dembo, A.J., and Pringle, J.F. (1978). *Br. J. Cancer*, **37**, Suppl. III, 302.
3. Lindberg, R.D. (1983). *Cancer Treat. Symp.*, **2**, 21.

4. Peters, L.J., Withers, H.R., Thames, Jr., H.D., and Fletcher, G.H. (1982). *Int. J. Radiat. Oncol. Biol. Phys.*, **8**, 101.

5. Vaupel, P. (1977). *Microvascular Res.*, **13**, 399.

6. Vaupel, P., and Thews, G. (1974). *Oncology*, **30**, 475.

7. Mottram, J.C. (1936). *Br. J. Radiol.*, **9**, 606.

8. Thomlinson, R.H., and Gray, L.H. (1955). *Br. J. Cancer*, **9**, 539.

9. Powers, W.E., and Tolmach, L.J. (1963). *Nature (London)*, **197**, 710.

10. Kallman, R.F. (1972). *Radiology*, **105**, 135.

11. Kallman, R.F., and Rockwell, S. (1977). In F.F. Becker (Ed.), *Cancer*, vol. 6, Plenum Press, New York, p.225.

12. Steel, G.G. (1977). *Growth Kinetics of Tumors*, Clarendon Press, Oxford, p.147.

13. Rockwell, S., and Kallman, R.F. (1973). *Radiat. Res.*, **53**, 281.

14. Suit, H.D., and Shalek, R.J. (1963). *J. Natl. Cancer Inst.*, **31**, 479.

15. Suit, H.D., and Maeda, M. (1966). *Am. J. Roentgenol.*, **96**, 177.

16. Fowler, J.F., Morgan, R.L., and Wood, C.A.P. (1963). *Br. J. Radiol.*, **36**, 77.

17. Barendsen, G.W., and Broerse, J.J. (1969). *Europ. J. Cancer*, **5**, 373.

18. Van Putten, L.M. (1968). *Europ. J. Cancer*, **4**, 173.

19. Howes, A.E. (1969). *Br. J. Radiol.*, **42**, 441.

20. Moulder, J.E., Fisher, J.J., and Milardo, R. (1976). *Int. J. Radiat. Oncol. Biol. Phys.*, **1**, 431.

21. Sause, W.T., and Plenk, H.P. (1979). *Int. J. Radiat. Oncol. Biol. Phys.*, **5**, 1833.

22. Berry, G.H., Dixon, B., and Ward, A.J. (1979). *Clin. Radiol.*, **30**, 591.

23. Adams, G.E., and Cooke, M.S. (1969). *Int. J. Radiat. Biol.*, **15**, 457.

24. Foster, J.L., and Willson, R.L. (1973). *Br. J. Radiol.*, **6**, 234.

25. Begg. A.C., Sheldon, P.W., and Foster, J.L. (1974). *Br. J. Radiol.*, **47**, 399.

26. Phillips, T.L. (1981). *Semin. Oncol.*, **8**, 65.

27. Stone, H.B., and Withers, H.R. (1974). *Radiology*, **113**, 441.

28. Urtasun, R., Band, P., Chapman, J.D., Feldstein, M.L., Mielke, B., and Fryer, C. (1976). *N. Engl. J. Med.*, **294**, 1364.

29. Asquith, J.C., Watts, M.E., Patel, K. (1974). *Radiat. Res.*, **60**, 108.

30. Fowler, J.F., Adams, G.E., and Denekamp, J. (1976). *Cancer Treat. Rev.*, **3**, 227.

31. Dische, S., Saunders, M.I., Lee, M.E., Adams, G.E., and Flockhart, I.R. (1977). *Br. J. Cancer*, **35**, 567.

32. Dische, S., (1977). *Clin. Otolaryngol.*, **2**, 403.

33. Adams, G.E., Flockhart, I.R., Smithen, C.E., Stratford, I.J., Wardman, P., and Watts, M.E. (1976). *Radiat. Res.*, **67**, 9.

34. Sealy, R. (1978). *Br. J. Cancer*, **37**, Suppl. III, 314.

35. Sealy, R., Williams, A., Levin, W., Blair, R., Flockhart, I., Stratford, M., Minchinton, A., and Cridland, S. (1980). In L.W. Brady (Ed.), *Radiation Sensitizers: their Use in the Clinical Management of Cancer*, Masson, New York, p.361.

36. Sealy, R., Williams, A., Cridland, S., Stratford, M., Minchinton, A., and Hallet, C. (1982). *Int. J. Radiat. Oncol. Biol. Phys.*, **8**, 339.

37. Arcangeli, G., Barocas, A., Mauro, F., Nervi, C., Spano, M., and Tabocchini, A. (1980). *Cancer*, **45**, 2707.

38. Paterson, I.C.M., Dawes, P.J.D.K., Henk, J.M., and Moore, J.L. (1981). *Clin. Radiol.*, **32**, 225.

39. Orr, L.E., Puthawala, A., Nisar Syed, A.M., and Fleming, P.A. (1981). *Cancer*, **48**, 43.

40. Fazekas, J.T., Goodman, R.L., and McLean, C.J. (1981). *Int. J. Radiat. Oncol. Biol. Phys.*, **7**, 1703.

41. Overgaard, J., Anderson, A.P., Jensen, R.H., Hjelm-Hansen, M., Jørgensen, K., Petersen, M., Sandberg, E., and Sand Hansen, H. (1982). *Acta Otolaryngol.*, Suppl. **386**, 215.

42. Karim, A.B.M.F., and Njo, K.H. (1982). In K.H. Kärchner *et al.* (Eds), *Progress in Radio-Oncology*, vol. II, Raven Press, New York, p.263.

43. Van den Bogaert, W., van der Schueren, E., Horiot, J.C., Chaplain, G., Arcangeli, G., Gonzalez, D., and Svoboda, V. (1982). *Int. J. Radiat. Oncol. Biol. Phys.*, **8**, 1649.

44. International Cancer Research Data Bank (1982). *Compilation of Experimental Cancer Therapy Protocol Summaries*, 6th edition, US Department of Health and Human Services, Public Health Service, National Institutes of Health, NIH Publication No. 82–1116, p.505.

45. Adams, G.E. (1982). *Br. J. Radiol.*, **55**, 464.

46. Adams, G.E. (1973). *Br. Med. Bull.*, **29**, 48.

47. Brown, J.M. (1982). *Int. J. Radiat. Oncol. Biol. Phys.*, **8**, 1491.

48. DeVita, V.T., Oliverio, V.T., Muggia, F.M., Wiernik, P.W., Ziegler, J., Goldin, A., Rubin, D., Henney, J., and Schepartz, S. (1979). *Cancer Clin. Trials*, **2**, 195.

49. Schwade, J.C., Pistenmaa, D.A., and Phillips, T.L., (1982). In A. Breccia *et al.* (Eds), *Advanced Topics on Radiosensitizers of Hypoxic Cells*, Proceedings of Advanced Topics on Radiosen-

sitizers of Hypoxic Cells, Cesenatico, Italy, 27 August–7 September 1980, Plenum Press, New York, p.239.

50. Wasserman, T.H., Coleman, C.N., Uratsun, R., Phillips, T.L., and Strong, J. (1982). *Int. J. Radiat. Oncol. Biol. Phys.*, **8**, (Suppl. 1), 76.

51. Brown, D.M., Parker, E., and Brown, J.M. (1982). *Radiat. Res.*, **90**, 98.

52. Astor, M., Hall, E.J., Biaglow, J.E., and Parham, J.C. (1982). *Int. J. Radiat. Oncol. Biol. Phys.*, **8**, 75.

53. Bump, E.A., Yu, N.Y., and Brown, J.M. (1982). *Science*, **217**, 544.

54. Narayanan, V.L. and Lee, W.W. (1982). *Adv. Pharmol. Chemother.*, **19**, 155.

55. Dische, S., Gray, A.J., and Zanelli, G.D. (1976). *Clin. Radiol.*, **27**, 159.

56. Thomlinson, R.H., Dische, S., Gray, A.H., and Errington, L.M. (1976). *Clin. Radiol.*, **27**, 167.

57. Denekamp, J., and Joiner, M.C. (1982). *Br. J. Radiol.*, **55**, 657.

Chapter 11

Radiotherapy with Pi Mesons

Steven E. Bush
*St. Joseph Hospital, 400 Walter NE,
Alberquerque, New Mexico, USA.*

The therapeutic challenges of advanced neoplasia of the head and neck persist despite increasing knowledge of the biological behaviour of these tumours and the availability of an expanding variety of treatment modalities. Although head and neck tumours of early stage are generally amenable to effective management by conventional therapy with surgery or irradiation, more advanced neoplasms arising in the same sites present often insurmountable difficulties in eradication of the primary tumour or regional nodal metastases.

Long-term cure rates of less than 30% are frequently reported for advanced tumours of the hypopharynx, larynx, oropharynx, oral cavity, and nasopharynx. Other anatomical sites of the head and neck region, including the paranasal sinuses and salivary glands, less commonly affected by neoplasia, also have unacceptably low rates of cure by conventional therapy.[1-3]

Megavoltage radiation therapy has been the primary form of treatment available for advanced tumours unsuitable for surgical excision. Unfortunately, such treatment has been of palliative benefit only in the majority of cases, indicating the necessity of new modalities of treatment. Various observations regarding the biology, physics, and techniques of radiotherapy explain, in part, the failure of conventional treatment methods to eradicate such neoplasms. Hypoxic tumour cells are known to be relatively radioresistant and the abundance of such cells in large, necrotic lesions may be one source of local failures. The variability of cell sensitivity to X-irradiation during the cell cycle, with relative insensitivity of cells in late G_1 and S phases, may also be a contributing factor. Finally, repair of radiation injury is a well-documented phenomenon which may result in failure of tumour eradication with fractionated radiotherapy.[4-6]

In addition to such biological considerations, technical and physical problems with delivery of adequate tumour doses and prevention of overdose of sensitive normal tissues, including the spinal cord, eyes, brainstem, cartilage, salivary glands, and mucosa have impeded efforts to control advanced tumours with radiation alone. Over the last decade the development and evaluation of new radiation modalities had been a major effort in clinical radiation research. The field of particle radiotherapy encompasses the study of the physical and biological properties and clinical applicability of radiation beams including neutrons, protons, heavy charged ions and negative pi mesons (pions).

Physics of Pi Meson Radiotherapy

In 1961 Fowler and Perkins predicted potential therapeutic advantages for pion irradiation based largely on the favourable dose distribution which obtains during the absorption of charged particles in matter.[7] The negative pi meson has a mass 273 times that of the electron with an identical electrical charge and comprises, in particulate form, a part of the energy that binds protons and neutrons together in atomic nuclei. When it impinges upon matter the pion initially behaves much like an electron and has characteristic interactions with orbiting electrons within the absorbing medium. As it decelerates, however, it comes under the influence of positively charged nuclei within the material. As the pion is

absorbed into a nucleus, there is initially emission of short-range, pi-mesic X-rays as the particle cascades through the electron shells of the atom. When the pion combines with the nucleus, the ensuing energetic instability leads to the destruction of the nucleus in a shower of densely ionizing particles including neutrons, protons, deuterons, and light nuclei, the so-called 'star'. The characteristic depth dose distribution of a monoenergetic pion beam is shown in Figure 11.1, and is contrasted with that of megavoltage X-rays. The two most conspicuous differences are the abrupt decline in dose at the depth determined by the initial momentum of the pion and the large increase in absorbed dose at the termination of its track, the 'Bragg peak'. The potential therapeutic advantages of these properties include the possibility of sparing normal tissue in the low-dose entrant portion of beam while concentrating the highest dose on a tumour at depth. At the same time, sensitive tissues distal to the

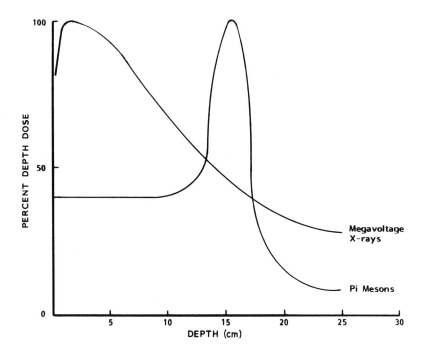

Figure 11.1   Schematic representation of depth–dose distributions of negative pi mesons and megavoltage X-rays.

treatment volume can be spared by appropriate selection of pion momenta and use of beam shaping filters.

Radiobiology of Pi Meson Radiotherapy

In addition to the dose-shaping benefits inherent in the Bragg peak absorption of pions, the characteristics of the radiation in the peak region confer increased biological effect for a given dose. Pions in the entrant region or 'plateau' of the absorption spectrum have biological properties indistinguishable from those of X-rays or gamma rays, i.e. a relative biological effectiveness (RBE) of 1. RBE is defined as the ratio of the doses of a test radiation and a reference radiation, usually 250 kV X-rays, producing equal biological effects in a given system.

Pions in the Bragg peak region of absorption have an RBE of approximately 1.2 for single-exposure irradiation of CHO cells in suspension and 1.6 for acute skin reactions in mice and pigs receiving fractionated radiotherapy with more than 10 treatments.[8] Similar results have obtained for human skin and mucosa irradiated in 35 fractions over 7 weeks.[9] The increased RBE of peak pions results from the accumulation of dose from densely ionizing, sub-atomic particles released from disintegrating nuclei in this region. This portion of the dose represents so-called high linear energy transfer (LET) radiation which directly damages biological macromolecules and produces more injury for a given dose than do low LET radiations such as X-rays and plateau pions. Thus, the potential therapeutic advantages of pions include both the favourable distribution of dose at depth and the increased biological effect of radiation in the region where dose is maximal.

Previously mentioned biological characteristics which may render tumours incurable by radiation include hypoxia, cell cycle variability in radiosensitivity, and repair of radiation injury. The high LET characteristics of peak pions may be expected to overcome these potential impediments. High LET radiations show a reduced oxygen enhancement ratio (OER), i.e. the ratio of doses of radiation necessary to produce a given biological effect in the presence or absence of oxygen. The OER for X-rays is approximately 3.0 while that of pions[10] is around 2.2. Thus, a portion of those cells in the hypoxic core of a large tumour which is relatively insensitive to X-rays may be destroyed by high LET radiation. Cell cycle variability in radiation sensitivity is also reduced with high LET radiation as is repair of sublethal and potentially lethal radiation damage.[5,6]

Pi Meson Radiotherapy at the Los Alamos Meson Physics Facility

Between 1974 and 1982 a group of 230 patients with locally advanced and metastatic neoplasms from a variety of primary sites and histologies received pion radiotherapy at the Los Alamos Meson Physics Facility (LAMPF). Of these, 43 patients received treatment for advanced neoplasms of head and neck sites, excluding primary brain tumours.

All patients in this series were treated at LAMPF, a dedicated, 1 kilometre linear accelerator designed to produce an 800 MeV proton beam with current of 1 millampere. Pions with momenta producing penetration from 12 to 23 cm in water are collected from a water-cooled graphite target through a channel of quadrapole and bending magnets as described by Paciotti *et al.*[11] The channel produces a fixed, vertical, minimally divergent beam with a dose rate of approximately 5 rad per minute in a volume of 2 litres. Channel characteristics and treatment techniques appear in detail in previous publications.[12,13] In brief, each patient receiving pion irradiation for head and neck neoplasia had fabricated an immobilizing body case, followed by computerized axial tomographic scanning of the treatment volume at 0.9–1.0 cm intervals. The data obtained were used in determination of the depth of penetration of the treatment beam and the calculation of the proper thickness and configuration of a compensating filter, or bolus,

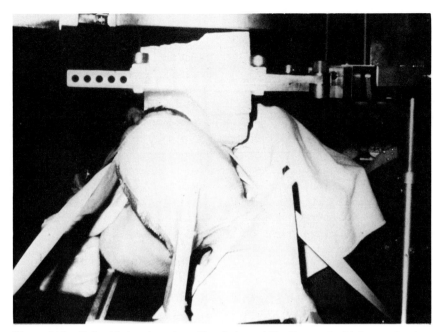

Figure 11.2   Patient in treatment position in immobilization cast with beam-shaping wax bolus and collimator above.

individually designed to assure appropriate distribution of the high-dose, Bragg peak zone of irradiation within the patient. Finally, individualized collimators were fabricated for shaping of the beam in transverse and axial dimensions. Figure 11.2 shows a patient in treatment position with cast and beam shaping devices.

A population of 43 patients with advanced neoplasms of the head and neck received pion radiotherapy alone, or in combination with other conventional therapy. All patients have been followed for a minimum of 30 months and maximum of 74 months. Thirty-nine patients had locally advanced squamous cell carcinomas of the oral cavity, larynx, pharynx, and sinuses, Stage III and IV according to AJC staging criteria. All patients were free of known metastases at the start of therapy. One patient had an unstageable recurrent squamous carcinoma of the facial skin with invasion of the maxilla, two had advanced minor salivary gland tumours, and one has esthesioneuroblastoma. Four patients were female and 39 male, with an age range for the entire group of 41–75 years at diagnosis.

Patients received daily irradiation with maximum doses ranging from 100 to 150 pion rads per day, with five fractions weekly to total doses of 1000–5400 pion rad. Most patients were treated with opposed lateral fields, although occasional single-field treatments were employed either primarily or for cone-down volumes. The dose of pion irradiation, deliberately minimized during early clinical trials to avoid unanticipated normal tissue reactions, was gradually increased as experience was gained. Additional surgery or conventional irradiation implant or external beam techniques followed pion treatment in patients with incomplete tumour regression following planned pion irradiation. The lowest dose at which complete tumour regression occurred and long-term local control obtained was 2700 pion rad, a dose received by all but three patients in this series.

Table 11.1 shows statistics regarding local control and survival according to T and N stage. Thirty-six of 39 patients with stageable squamous cell carcinomas had stage T_3 or T_4

TABLE 11.1 LOCAL CONTROL AND SURVIVAL
BY T AND N STAGE

Stage	Local Control	Survival
T_{1-2}	1/3	1/3
T_3	6/14	3/14
T_4	3/22	4/22
N_0	2/10	3/10
N_1	1/6	2/6
N_{2-3}	7/23	3/23
NA*	4/4	4/4

* Tumours not appropriately staged.

TABLE 11.2 LOCAL CONTROL AND SURVIVAL
BY SITE OF DISEASE

	Local control	Survival
Oral cavity	0/6	0/6
Oropharynx	7/17	5/17
Nasopharynx	2/7	2/7
Hypopharynx	0/1	0/1
Larynx	1/6	1/6
Other	4/6	4/6
Total	14/43	12/43

TABLE 11.3 LOCAL CONTROL AND SURVIVAL
FOR GROUPS OF PATIENTS
RECEIVING PION RADIOTHERAPY
ALONE OR IN COMBINATION
WITH ADDITIONAL
CONVENTIONAL TREATMENT

	Local control	Survival
Pions only	8/23	6/23
Pions + Conventional Therapy	6/20	6/20
Total	14/43	12/43

primaries and 23 patients had cervical node disease staged N_{2-3}. All patients with unstaged tumours, including those with salivary gland tumours, esthesioneuroblastoma, and recurrent skin cancer survived with local control of disease from 36 to 62 months. Only three of 22 patients with T_4 primaries had local control, although seven of 17 patients with lesser disease remained free of local recurrence.

Unexpectedly, seven of 23 patients with advanced nodal metastasis, stage N_{2-3}, had local control after pion irradiation, with or without additional therapy. Four patients with local control of tumour expired; two had distant metastases and two had fatal complications of therapy. Two patients remain long-term survivors after surgical salvage of local recurrence. The median survival for all patients in this series was 14 months.

Table 11.2 summarizes local control and survival statistics according to site of disease. The largest group of patients had carcinomas of the oropharynx with five of 17 surviving free of disease from 49 to 74 months. Two others expired with locally controlled disease. Only two of eight patients with carcinomas arising elsewhere in the pharynx survive and none of the six patients with oral cavity primaries are alive. Four of six patients with tumours in random sites including salivary gland, sinuses, skin, and nasal cavity survive with local control.

Table 11.3 compares a group of 23 patients treated with pions alone to a group of 20 receiving additional conventional irradiation or surgery with respect to survival and local control of disease. The groups are comparable in proportions of patients with T_4 primaries, advanced neck disease, and squamous cell histology. No apparent differences emerge between these groups regarding treatment outcome.

A major goal in the evaluation of a new medical treatment is the definition of therapy-related toxicity and its determinants. All patients in this study group have been systematically followed and radiation-related complications have been recorded according to the late effects scoring system of the Radiation Therapy Oncology Group (RTOG). This system assigns numerical scores from 0 (no detectable injury) to 5 (lethal complication related to radiation) for individual tissues and organs. Pertinent tissues in the head and neck region include the skin, subcutis, mucosa, salivary gland, larynx, central nervous system, and eye. In order to quantify levels of normal

TABLE 11.4   DEGREE OF CHRONIC NORMAL TISSUE REACTIONS
ACCORDING TO TREATMENT MODALITY

Treatment	No. of patients	Chronic Reactions		
		Minimal	Moderate	Severe
Pions Only	23	12	8	3
Pions + X-ray therapy				
External Beam	6	3	3	0
Implant	4	1	1	2
External + Implant	2	0	2	0
Pions + Surgery	7	0	4	3
Pions + Surgery + Implant	1	0	0	1

tissue injury related to pion irradiation, a value for average normal tissue reaction was calculated for each patient by summing the total scores for chronic reactions in all tissues irradiated and dividing the sum by that number of tissues exposed to pions in the high-dose, Bragg peak region. Numbers of tissues scored varied according to the site and size of the disease and typically included three to five sites. Average normal tissue reactions were arbitrarily classified as minimal (0.0–0.5), moderate (0.51–1.5) and severe (1.51–2.5). Table 11.4 shows the distribution of normal tissue reactions according to severity and type of treatment received. The most impressive finding is the disproportionate increase in moderate and severe reactions with supplementary conventional therapy. While 11 of 23 patients receiving pions alone developed moderate to severe injury, 16 of 20 receiving additional treatment had significant late effects of therapy. All seven patients who had surgery subsequent to pion irradiation sustained such normal tissue damage.

Figures 11.3 and 11.4 show the relationship of treatment volume and total dose to the pattern of late normal tissue effects for those groups of patients receiving pions alone or pions combined with other treatment. These data include only those 37 patients surviving more than 6 months after treatment. It is apparent that both treatment volume and dose are important determinants of late normal

tissue effects. Of 11 patients receiving pions alone in doses of 4500 pion rad or less, eight had minimal, and three had moderate reactions, while all eight receiving higher doses had moderate to severe late effects. Only one of eight patients receiving less than 4500 pion rad to a volume less than 1500 cc experienced moderate late injury; the remaining seven had minimal effects. As shown in Figure 11.4, the combination of pion radiotherapy with other treatment greatly increased the chance for normal tissue damage. Three of five patients receiving doses greater than 4500 pion rad had severe late effects, as did four of eight patients treated to volumes greater than 1500 cc and subsequently subjected to additional therapy. Two patients expired as a result of treatment-related complications. One developed a tracheal–innominate artery fistula approximately 2 weeks after attempted composite resection for salvage of locally persistent tonsillar carcinoma treated to 5100 pion rad. A second patient received 4740 pion rad in 140 pion rad fractions and developed pharyngeal necrosis 5 months post-treatment. He expired despite multiple attempts at surgical repair of the lesion.

The minimum follow-up for patients in this series is 30 months and all clinical activities at LAMPF were concluded in 1981. Analysis of this group of patients indicates the pion irradiation may eradicate locally advanced tumours of the head and neck in approximately

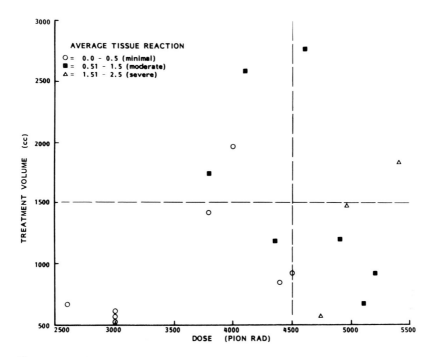

Figure 11.3   Chronic normal tissue reactions by treatment volume and tumor dose in 18 patients treated with pions alone and surviving at least 6 months.

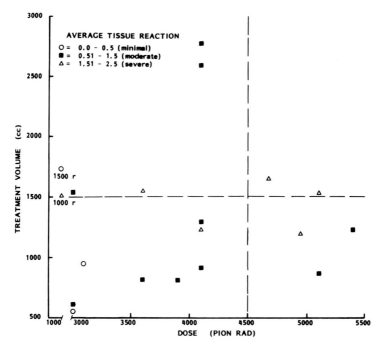

Figure 11.4   Chronic normal tissue reactions by treatment volume and tumor dose in 19 patients treated with pions and additional conventional therapy and surviving at least 6 months.

one-third of patients treated. As anticipated, pion radiotherapy is more effective for smaller primary tumours (stages T_1 to T_3) with local control of disease in 41% of cases compared to only 14% of T_4 tumours. Advanced cervical node metastases (N_2–N_3) were controlled in 30% of cases. Acute treatment-related morbidity was qualitatively indistinguishable from that anticipated with conventional radiation therapy and resulted in anticipated delays in therapy in only four patients. Chronic normal tissue reactions were within acceptable limits in the majority of the group of patients treated with pions alone, but tended to increase markedly with additional conventional treatment. Chronic reactions were minimal to moderate in all patients but one treated to tumour doses less than 4500 pion rad and volumes less than 1500 cc regardless of additional therapy.

Clinical research with pion radiotherapy continues at the TRIUMF accelerator in Vancouver, Canada and at the Schweizersches Institut für Nuklearforschung in Villigen, Switzerland. While the data presently available are insufficient for definitive conclusions regarding the promise of pion radiotherapy, and randomized clinical trials have yet to be accomplished, additional gains may be anticipated from further research with pions, other types of particle radiation such as protons or heavy ions, and high LET radiation including neutrons.

REFERENCES

1. Fletcher, G.H. (1977). *Semin. Oncol.*, **4**, 375.
2. Million, R.R., Cassisi, N.J., and Wittes, R.E. (1982). In V.T. DeVita *et al.* (Eds), *Cancer, Principles and Practice of Oncology*, J.B. Lippincott Co., Philadelphia, pp.320–377.
3. Wang, C.C. (1983). *Radiation Therapy for Head and Neck Neoplasms*, John Wright–PSG, Inc., Boston, pp.73–221.
4. Gray, L.H., Conger, A.D., Ebert, M., Hornsey, S., and Scott, O.C.A. (1953). *Br. J. Radiol.*, **26**, 638.
5. Withers, H.R., Mason, K., Reid, B.O., Dubraysky, N., Barkley, H.T., Brown, B.W., and Smathers, J.B. (1974). *Cancer*, **34**, 39.
6. Hall, E.J., and Kraljevic, U. (1976). *Radiology*, **121**, 731.
7. Fowler, P.H., and Perkins, D.H. (1961). *Nature*, **189**, 524.
8. Skarsgard, L.D., Palcic, B., Douglas, B.G., and Iam, G.K.Y. (1982). *Int. J. Radiat. Oncol. Biol. Phys.*, **8**, 2127.
9. Bush, S.E., Smith, A.R., and Zink, S. (1982). *Int. J. Radiat. Oncol. Biol. Phys.*, **8**, 2181.
10. Raju, M.R., Amols, H.I., Bain, E., Carpenter, S.G., Cox, R.A., and Robertson, J.B. (1979). *Br. J. Radiol.*, **52**, 494.
11. Paciotti, M., Bradbury, J., Huston, R., Knapp, E., and Rivera, O. (1977). *IEEE Trans. Nucl. Sci., NS-24*, 1058.
12. Hogstrom, K.R., Smith, A.R., Kelsey, C.A., Simon, S.L., Somers, J.W., Lane, R.G., Rosen, I.I., VonEssen, C.F., Kligerman, M.M., Bernardo, P.A., and Zink, S.M. (1979). *Int. J. Radiat. Oncol. Biol. Phys.*, **5**, 875.
13. Kligerman, M.M., Hogstrom, K.R., Lane, R.G., and Somers, J. (1977). *Int. J. Radiat. Oncol. Biol. Phys.*, **2**, 1141.

Chapter **12**

Fast Neutrons

Thomas W. Griffin
Radiation Oncology Department, University of Washington Hospital, Seattle, Washington, USA

Advances in the field of radiation oncology have, over the last two decades, resulted in a substantial improvement in the outlook for patients with carcinomas of the head and neck region. This improvement has been largely due to an increased understanding of the biology of the disease process and to the development of machines capable of optimizing radiation dose distributions. Nevertheless, there still remains a substantial number of patients in whom failure to control local disease contributes materially to their death. For the reasons outlined in the following paragraphs, particle beam radiation therapy might be expected to offer a therapeutic gain, as compared to conventional photon and electron beam therapy, in the management of these patients.

Currently, the following particle beams are being clinically tested: fast neutrons; protons; alpha particles; heavy ions (carbon, neon, argon); and negative pions. Fast neutrons are being investigated because they have radiobiological properties that are potentially superior to those of conventional X- and gamma rays. Protons and alpha particles are being studied because the dose distributions which may be achieved with these particles are superior, in many clinical situations, to those obtainable with photons or electrons. Heavy

ions and pions have both a potential biological advantage and a dose distribution advantage.

BIOLOGICAL CHARACTERISTICS OF PARTICLE BEAMS

The biological effects of a radiation beam are dependent on the spatial distribution of the ionizing events produced in tissue. The rate at which charged particles deposit energy per unit distance is known as the linear energy transfer (LET), expressed in keV/µm. Protons, electrons and photons are sparsely ionizing and are characterized by a low linear energy transfer. Fast neutrons, heavy ions, and pions are densely ionizing and are referred to as high LET radiations.

In reviewing the possible causes of treatment failure in head and neck cancer with conventional radiation therapy, the major areas in which neutrons and other high LET radiations offer a potential biological advantage are:

Tumour Cell Hypoxia

Numerous studies in many biological systems have shown that hypoxic cells are significantly more resistant to the effects of X- and gamma irradiation than are well-oxygenated cells. While cells in most normal tissues are well oxygenated, most solid tumours are thought to

159

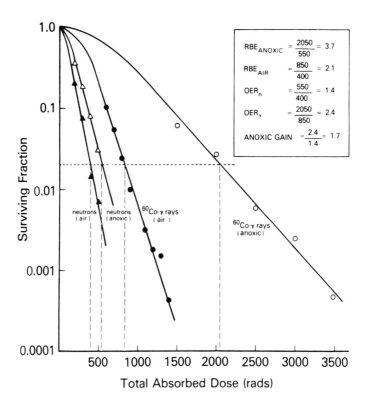

Figure 12.1 Survival curves for Chinese hamster ovary (CHO) cells irradiated with ^{60}Co gamma rays or 50 MeVd→Be fast neutrons under aerated and anoxic conditions. At the survival level illustrated, the oxygen enhancement ratio (OER) for neutrons is 1.4 compared to 2.4 for ^{60}Co gamma rays.

have hypoxic regions which have outgrown their vascular supply. It has been postulated that these cells remain viable and provide a focus for local tumour recurrence.[1]

The oxygen enhancement ratio (OER) is defined as the ratio of the dose of radiation required to produce a specified biological effect under anoxic conditions to the dose required to produce the same effect under well-oxygenated conditions. With photons, the OER for most mammalian cells is 2.5–3.0. With neutrons, heavy charged particles, or pions, the OER is significantly smaller (1.4–1.7), and therefore the protection conferred on tumour cells by hypoxia is diminished. Figure 12.1 illustrates survival curves for Chinese hamster ovary cells irradiated with ^{60}Co gamma rays or 50 MeVd→Be neutrons. The OER for neutrons

is 1.4, appreciably improved over the value of 2.4 for ^{60}Co gamma rays.

In practice, the clinical advantage of high LET radiation may be less than that suggested by this difference in OER. Not all tumour cells are severely hypoxic, and reoxygenation occurring during intervals between dose fractions diminishes the influence of hypoxic cells on tumour recurrence.

Relative Biological Effectiveness

The relative biological effectiveness (RBE) of an ionizing radiation is the ratio of the dose of that radiation compared to the dose of a reference radiation required to produce a specific endpoint in a specific tissue.

Another potential area of therapeutic gain from high LET radiation exists when tumour

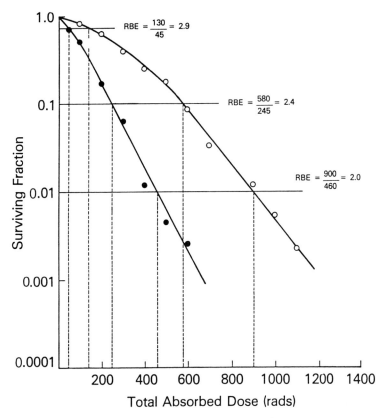

$$RBE = \frac{130}{45} = 2.9$$

$$RBE = \frac{580}{245} = 2.4$$

$$RBE = \frac{900}{460} = 2.0$$

Figure 12.2   Survival curves for CHO cells exposed to ^{60}Co gamma rays or 50 MeVd→Be fast neutrons illustrating the increase in relative biological effectiveness (RBE) with decreasing dose per fraction. With fast neutron irradiation, most cell killing results from single-hit lethal events leading to survival curves with little or no shoulder.

cells are relatively radioresistant because of an increased capacity to accumulate sublethal radiation injury. This is reflected in a wide shoulder for the tumour cell survival curve. With neutrons and other high LET radiation most cell killing results from single lethal events, leading to survival curves that are almost exponential in the range of clinical relevance (Figure 12.2). Tumours characterized by a large capacity to accumulate and repair sublethal radiation injury, such as some salivary gland tumours, should have a higher RBE for neutrons than normal tissue. It should be noted, however, that Howlett *et al.*[2] have shown that RBEs of neutrons for different experimental tumours vary considerably, and no general statement about which types of tumours are best treated with high LET radiation can be made at present.

Tumour Cell Kinetics

Because of the variation in radiosensitivity between cells in different stages of the cell cycle, redistribution between dose fractions results in an effective sensitization of proliferating cells that is not shared by non-proliferating normal cells. The latter are probably responsible for late radiation sequelae, which are the usual dose-limiting factors in radiation therapy. The cell-cycle-dependent variation of radiosensitivity is similar for neutrons and gamma rays, but the magnitude of the difference is

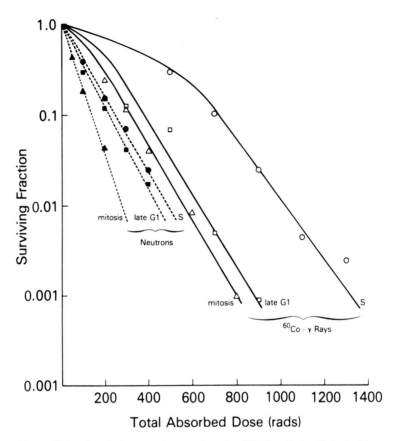

Figure 12.3   Survival curves for synchronized CHO cells irradiated with
^{60}Co gamma rays or 50 MeVd → Be fast neutrons illustrating the variation
in radiosensitivity with the position in the cell cycle. The cells were
irradiated in three different positions in the cell cycle – mitosis, late
G_1/early S, and mid-to-late S phase. The cell-cycle-dependent variation in
radiosensitivity is qualitatively similar for neutrons and gamma rays, but
the magnitude of the variation is reduced by a factor of 4 for neutrons.

smaller for neutrons[3] (Figure 12.3). Whether
this property constitutes a therapeutic advantage for high LET radiation cannot be
predicted. Tumours whose cells redistribute
poorly, or whose spectrum is demonstrated by
cells in resistant phases, would be more effectively treated with neutrons.

Repair of Potentially Lethal Damage

The recovery from potentially lethal damage
(PLD) occurs over a period of hours in cells
irradiated *in vitro* when the post-irradiation
conditions are suboptimal for growth. Repair
of PLD occurs following X- and gamma
irradiation, but is less frequently observed

following neutron irradiation[4] (Figure 12.4).
If, as has been suggested by Hall and
Kraljevc,[5] PLD repair after X- and gamma
irradiation occurs in nutritionally deprived
tumour cells, but not in normal tissue cells,
then the use of high LET beams would be
therapeutically advantageous.

PHYSICAL CHARACTERISTICS OF PARTICLE BEAMS

Fast neutron beams can be generated for
radiation therapy either by bombarding a
target containing tritium (T) with accelerated

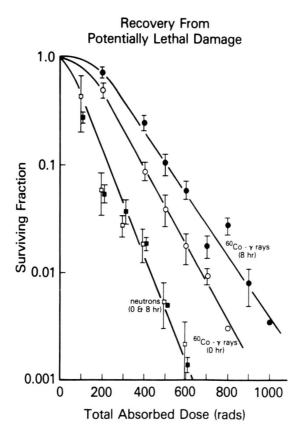

Recovery From Potentially Lethal Damage

Figure 12.4   Potentially lethal damage (PLD): survival curves for plateau-phase CHO cells irradiated with ^{60}Co gamma rays (circles) or 50 MeVd→Be fast neutrons (squares) and plated either immediately (open symbols) or 8 hours after irradiation (closed symbols). Repair of PLD occurs following irradiation with gamma rays, but is not observed following neutron irradiation.

deuterium (D) ions in a D–T generator or by bombarding a suitable target such as beryllium (Be) with protons (p) or deuterons (d) accelerated in a cyclotron or linear accelerator. The D–T generator produces a monoenergetic 14 MeV neutron beam, whereas the proton-on-beryllium (p → Be) and deuteron-on-beryllium (d → Be) reactions produce neutron beams with a spectrum of energies.

While protons, alpha particles, pions, and heavy ions all have dose-distribution advantages over conventional photons, neutrons do not. In fact, with the current limitation of physics-based machines with fixed horizontal treatment beams, the dose distributions achieved with neutrons are somewhat inferior to those achievable with modern megavoltage isocentric equipment. In 1983, new hospital-based neutron generators began operation at the University of Washington, UCLA, M.D. Anderson, and the University of Pennsylvania Hospitals. These new machines will allow dose distributions equivalent to modern 6 MeV linear accelerators.

CLINICAL STUDIES

Fast neutron radiotherapy of head and neck cancer in the United States dates back to the 1940s when Stone and co-workers[6] used a neutron beam to treat patients having various advanced malignancies. Almost all of the long-term survivors had severe radiation sequelae in the normal tissue surrounding the tumour sites. This was initially interpreted as due to an increased relative biological effectiveness (RBE) for late effects as compared to acute effects, and deterred further clinical investigation for approximately 20 years. In the 1950s mammalian cell culture techniques were developed and it became apparent that the shapes of post-irradiation cell survival curves were very different for high-energy photons and fast neutrons. This meant that the clinically used neutron fraction sizes corresponded to much higher RBEs than were extrapolated from the large-dose increment animal model studies prior to Stone's clinical work. Hence, nearly all of Stone's patients with serious radiation sequelae had inadvertently received extremely high radiation doses as reflected by calculated nominal standard doses (Ellis NSD formula) of 2000–3200 rets.[7]

Clinical trials were first resumed at Hammersmith Hospital, London, England, in the 1960s. After several hundred patients with extensive cancers were treated, it was concluded that fast neutron radiotherapy was well tolerated, and that many advanced malignancies responded amazingly well to fast neutron irradiation.[8] Based upon these very optimistic results, various centres throughout the world again began clinical trials with fast neutrons.

In the United States, patient treatments were started in 1972 at the M.D. Anderson Hospital, utilizing the Texas A&M University variable energy cyclotron (50 MeV d $\rightarrow$ Be reaction). Clinical trials were next instituted at the University of Washington utilizing a fixed energy cyclotron (22 MeV d $\rightarrow$ Be reaction) in 1973. Significant numbers of patients have also received neutron radiotherapy at the MANTA facility (35 MeV d $\rightarrow$ Be reaction) centred at George Washington University in Washington, DC, at the GLANTA facility (25 MeVd $\rightarrow$ Be reaction) in Cleveland, Ohio, and at the Fermi Laboratory facility (66 MeV p $\rightarrow$ Be reaction) in Batavia, Illinois. Initially, Phase I clinical trials were carried out utilizing patients with advanced head and neck tumours who were felt to have less than a 10% 5-year survival with conventional forms of treatment. This work yielded considerable information about the RBEs for different tissues and about the variation of the neutron RBEs from facility to facility. More recently, the majority of patients receiving fast neutron radiotherapy have been entered into randomized, prospective clinical trials designed to compare neutron irradiation with the best available photon control arm for a given tumour histology and site. Approximately 2500 patients have been treated in all, resulting in a fairly extensive patient data base.

The earliest clinically significant results treating head and neck cancer with fast neutrons were reported from the Hammersmith Hospital, London, by Dr Mary Catterall.[9] In a randomized trial of 133 patients with advanced cancers of the head and neck, neutron therapy showed a statistically significant superiority over photons for control of local-regional disease (Table 12.1). Neutrons were given in 12 fractions over 4 weeks to a total dose of 15.60 Gy_n. (Since Hammersmith investigators report only the neutron component of the beam and US investigators report total radiation delivered, this is equivalent to 17 $Gy_{n\gamma}$.) Pilot studies using both neutrons alone and 'mixed beam' radiation therapy were started in the US in 1972. Treatment with 'neutrons only' irradiated the primary tumour site and any region of clinically involved cervical adenopathy to 17–22 $Gy_{n\gamma}$ according to one of the following three fractionation schemes: (a) 1.5 $Gy_{n\gamma}$ on Mondays and Fridays, (b) 1.0 $Gy_{n\gamma}$ on Mondays, Wednesdays and Fridays, or (c) 0.75 $Gy_{n\gamma}$ on Mondays, Tuesdays, Thursdays, and Fridays. The term '$Gy_{n\gamma}$' refers to the *total* measured radiation dose and

TABLE 12.1   RESULTS FROM THE HAMMERSMITH HOSPITAL-MRC CLINICAL TRIAL OF FAST NEUTRON THERAPY OF HEAD AND NECK CANCER (ALL SITES OF HEAD AND NECK REGION)

Modality	Number of patients	Permanent local control		Complications	Survival at 2 years
Neutron	70	53	(76%)*	10/70†	28‡
Photon	63	12	(19%)	2/63	15‡

* 53/70 > 12/63, $P < 0.001$.
† 10/70 > 2/63, $P < 0.05$.
‡ Actuarial percentages; difference is not significant.

TABLE 12.2   TWO-YEAR LOCAL CONTROL RATES (PERCENTAGES) AT THE PRIMARY SITE AND ACTUARIAL SURVIVAL RATES FOR PATIENTS WITH ADVANCED HEAD AND NECK CANCERS TREATED WITH FAST NEUTRON TELETHERAPY

	Local control of primary (2-year actuarial)	Survival (2-year actuarial)
Hammersmith (Catterall *et al.*) Neutrons only (70 patients)	76	28
Amsterdam (Batterman and Breuer) Neutrons only (59 patients)	61	17
M.D. Anderson (Maor *et al.*) Neutrons only (48 patients) Mixed beam (25 patients)	43 35	20 25
University of Washington (Laramore *et al.*) Neutrons only (62 patients) Mixed beam (38 patients)	20 30	10 40

includes the gamma ray contaminate produced by neutron–nuclei interactions ($< 10\%$ at a depth of 10 cm). These three treatment schemes were 'normalized' to deliver 3.0 Gy$_{n\gamma}$ per week over 7 weeks. The 'mixed beam' treatment consists of combined neutron and photon irradiation according to the following scheme: 0.6 Gy$_{n\gamma}$ on Mondays and Fridays and 1.8 Gy$_\gamma$ on Tuesdays, Wednesdays, and Thursdays. Assuming an RBE = 3, this corresponded to 9 Gy equivalent per week, as did the 'neutrons only' form of treatment. The 'mixed beam' patients received between 65 and 70 Gy equivalent to the primary site and any region of clinically involved cervical adenopathy. Table 12.2 summarizes the results from two US pilot studies,[10,11] the Catterall trial,[9] and studies accomplished by Drs Batterman and Breuer in Amsterdam.[12] Patients in the Amsterdam trial received between 18 and 24 Gy$_{n\gamma}$ given in five fractions per week over 4 weeks. Although caution must be used when comparing results from different studies, there seems to be a trend favouring neutrons alone over mixed beam, and a trend favouring 12 fractions in 4 weeks over a more prolonged fractionation scheme.

Studies using fast neutrons to treat salivary gland tumours have also been carried out in the US and Europe. In a group of advanced tumours, often recurrent after multiple prior operations, the local control rates varied between 72% and 94%.[9,12-14] This control rate was felt by most of the investigators involved in the studies to be superior to that obtained with historical photon controls.

Currently, the role of fast neutron beam radiation therapy is being investigated with Phase III randomized studies both in the US and in Europe. The preliminary results of these studies have been somewhat disappointing. Until randomized controlled trials are completed using the new hospital-based isocentric neutron generators, the place of fast neutron beam radiation therapy in the armamentarium of head and neck cancer physicians will remain to be defined.

REFERENCES

1. Gray, L.H., Conger, A.D., Ebert, M., Hornsey, S., and Scott, O.C.A. (1953). Concentration of oxygen dissolved in tissues at time of irradiation as factor in radiotherapy. *Br. J. Radiol.*, **26**, 638.

2. Howlett, J.F., Thomlinson, R.H., and Alper, T. (1975). A marked dependence of the conformative effective causes of neutrons on tumor line and its implications for clinical trials. *Br. J. Radiol.*, **48**, 40.

3. Gragg, R.L., Humphrey, R.M., Thomas, H.T., and Meyn, R.E. (1978). The response of Chinese hamster ovary cells to fast neutron radiotherapy beams. I. Variations in RBE with position in the cell cycle. *Radiat. Res.*, **76**, 283.

4. Gragg, R.L., Humphrey, R.M., and Meyn, R.E. (1977). The response of Chinese hamster ovary cells to fast neutron radiotherapy beams. II. Sublethal and potentially lethal damage recovery capabilities. *Radiat. Res.*, **71**, 461.

5. Hall, E.J., and Kraljevic, J. (1976). Repair of potentially lethal radiation damage: comparison of neutron and X-ray RBE and implications for radiation therapy. *Radiology*, **121**, 731.

6. Stone, R.S. (1948). Neutron therapy and specific ionization. *Amer. J. Roentgenol.*, **59**, 771.

7. Brennan, J.T., and Phillips, T.L. (1971). Evaluation of past experience with fast neutron teletherapy and its implications for future applications. *Europ. J. Cancer*, **7**, 219.

8. Catterall, M. (1974). The treatment of advanced cancer by fast neutrons from the Medical Research Council's cyclotron at Hammersmith Hospital, London. *Europ. J. Cancer*, **10**, 343.

9. Catterall, M., Bewley, D.K., and Sutherland, J. (1977). Second report on a randomized clinical trial of fast neutrons compared with X- or gamma rays in treatment of advanced cancers of the head and neck. *Br. Med. J.*, **1**, 19.

10. Maor, M.H., Hussey, D.H., Fletcher, G.H., and Jesse, R.H. (1981). Fast neutron therapy for locally advanced head and neck tumors. *Int. J. Radiat. Oncol. Biol. Rhys.*, **7**, 155.

11. Griffin, T., Blasko, J., and Laramore, G. (1979). Results of fast neutron beam pilot studies at the University of Washington. *Europ. J. Cancer*, **23**.

12. Battermann, J.J., and Breuer, K. (1981). Results of fast neutron teletherapy for locally advanced head and neck tumors. *Int. J. Radiat. Oncol. Biol. Phys.*, **7**, 1045.

13. Henry, L.W., Blasko, J.C., Griffin, T.W., and Parker, R.G. (1979). Evaluation of fast neutron therapy for advanced carcinomas of the major salivary glands. *Cancer*, **44**, 814.

14. Kaul, R., Hendrickson, F., Cohen, L., Rosenberg, I., Ten Haken, R., Awschalom, M., and Mansell, J. (1981). Fast neutrons in the treatment of salivary gland tumors. *Int. J. Radiat. Oncol. Biol. Phys.*, **7**, 1667.

Chapter **13**

The Potential Role of Hyperthermia

N. M. Bleehen
University Department, and Medical Research Council Unit of Clinical Oncology and Radiotherapeutics, Cambridge, England

A failure to control locoregional disease in head and neck cancer is a major contributing factor to eventual patient death in unsuccessful treatments. It is for this reason that any other therapeutic modality that might be employed in addition to the conventional ones of surgery, radiation therapy, and chemotherapy might be advantageous. Hyperthermia has recently been attracting a considerable degree of attention as such a method, although it must be stated at this time it still remains of more experimental than routine clinical value.

The use of elevated temperatures of between 40 and 45 °C as therapy has been advocated for cancer for many years. Observations in the latter half of the last century produced evidence of its efficacy in the occasional patient. Thus Busch in 1866 described the disappearance of a histologically confirmed facial sarcoma in a patient after two attacks of erysipelas associated with high fever.[1] Coley subsequently artificially induced erysipelas and the repeated infections produced some tumour regressions.[2] Numerous other workers over the first half of the twentieth century also advocated the use of various forms of hyperthermia but none were

really successful or attracted very much attention. It is only in the last decade that a major interest has revived in the subject, with a veritable explosion in both laboratory and clinical work.

This chapter will briefly review the background of the experimental interest in hyperthermia and discuss its relevance to head and neck cancer. The reader is referred to more detailed references cited in this paper and the reviews on historical aspects,[3] biological considerations,[4] and the heating methods[5,6] and thermometry techniques[7,8] which discuss various aspects in greater detail. There have also been several symposia recently containing both reviews and original presentations which may be consulted.[9-13] Individual references to particular aspects of work will not therefore be quoted in this text.

REASONS FOR THE POTENTIAL VALUE OF HYPERTHERMIA

Biological reasons why hyperthermia might be of clinical value as an additional treatment modality are numerous. The evidence for

TABLE 13.1 EXPERIMENTALLY DERIVED
REASONS FOR THE POTENTIAL
VALUE OF HYPERTHERMIA IN
MAN

1. Tumour cells are no less sensitive to heat than normal cells.
2. Poorly oxygenated cells remain at least as sensitive to heat as well-oxygenated ones, in contrast to conventional X-ray therapy.
3. Tumour cells in an altered metabolic environment, such as nutritional deprivation and at low pH such as might be expected at a distance from a capillary, are more sensitive to heat than normal cells.
4. The resistance to heat and X-rays differs at comparable stages through the cell cycle.
5. Heat usually enhances the effect of X-rays but normal tissues are also affected so that time relationships can be important to obtain therapeutic gain.
6. Heat may enhance the cytotoxicity of some commonly used anti-cancer drugs but normal tissue effects may be critical in determining therapeutic gain.
7. The altered blood flow in tumours may result in higher tumour than normal tissue temperatures when localized heating techniques are employed.
8. The microvasculature may be more sensitive to heat in tumours than in normal tissues.

these reasons has been gained from a variety of experimental *in vitro* and *in vivo* work. Unfortunately, as yet, there still are few critically evaluable clinical data to put the possible therapeutic gain to man in perspective.

The possible reasons for potential clinical value are listed in Table 13.1. It can be seen that the value of hyperthermia depends on several different biological properties. Its ability to kill cells, both tumour and normal, with a varying degree of efficiency is dependent on many factors. In particular the location of tumour cells in abnormally vascularized, poorly nourished areas largely predicates towards selectivity for tumours. The interactions with radiation and drugs are more difficult to optimize because of enhanced toxicities on normal tissues as well, but selective scheduling may help in this situation. These various aspects of the problem are discussed in the next section.

BIOLOGICAL ASPECTS

Heat Alone

Numerous workers have documented, both *in vitro* and *in vivo*, the efficacy of moderately raised temperatures in killing cells from a variety of animal and human tumour and normal tissue sources. The effect is both temperature-and time-dependent, and various relationships have been determined by different workers. In general, for short heat exposure times of minutes up to 1 or 2 hours the survival curves closely resemble those of radiation survival curves. An initial shoulder representing an accumulation of sublethal damage is followed by an exponential slope. The size of the shoulder decreases, and that of the slope becomes steeper, as temperatures increase. Above about 42.5 °C, for unit time there is approximately a doubling of cell kill for every degree centigrade temperatures rise, or conversely at a constant temperature above 42.5 °C cell kill doubles for every doubling of the treatment time. Below this temperature a different relationship obtains where data are available. This rather simplistic rule only applies as a general working basis. There are also considerable quantitative differences over a 10-fold range in the sensitivity of various cell lines whose heat response has so far been investigated. Further discussion of this is beyond the scope of this review and readers should refer to the reviews[3,4] and the symposia already quoted.[9-13] Following long heating times or fractionated heat doses, the phenomenon of thermal tolerance may reduce the degree of cell killing and alter heat dose (time/temperature). This phenomenon is discussed further later.

An important consequence of the observation of the relationship between temperature and time of exposure is the question of 'units' of hyperthermia dose. It is clearly of importance in any treatment to specify as accurately as possible the temperature achieved and the time for which those tissues or tumours are exposed to that temperature. Even so, precision in these measurements will not be as easily defined as, for example, in radiation therapy. Inhomogeneities of energy deposition and physiological parameters will result in both variable rates of heating and the final temperatures achieved, even in a relatively small tissue volume. Consequent differences in cell kill, and thermal tolerance to a subsequent heat shock, or optimal interaction with drugs or radiation will all reduce the significance of precision in the original time/temperature measurements.

Initially, reports suggested that tumour cells were more sensitive to heat than normal cells. However this concept is now questioned and it remains an open issue. It would not be surprising if there were differences in heat sensitivity associated with the differences in membrane structure or metabolic pathways in cells. However the most important factors relating to selective tumour response are those relating to environmental differences.

The presence of radiobiologically hypoxic cells has long been thought to be of importance for locoregional failure of radiation treatment. In addition to the very considerable body of experimental data in favour of this are the data from hyperbaric oxygen studies,[14] and fast neutron therapy in the treatment of head and neck cancer.[15] It is still a matter of debate whether or not hypoxia *per se* confers increased heat sensitivity on tumour cells. This may be dependent on the cell type. However there is, in contrast to ionizing radiation, no evidence that it confers resistance.

Of considerable importance are the differences in pH that may occur at different levels of oxygenation and nutrition. There is a uniformity of opinion confirming that at low pH (<6.8) cells are much more sensitive to heat than at normal pH. This reduced pH is thought to occur in tumours as a result of lactic acid production, and the increase in this anaerobic metabolism consequent upon hypoxia in localized areas of tumour, together with the decreased removal of acid metabolic products as a result of impaired vascularization. Some workers have advocated infusion of glucose as a means of increasing anaerobic

glycolysis with further reduction in tumour pH. A poor metabolic environment may also confer increased heat sensitivity for reasons other than hypoxia and pH changes. These are less well understood but may relate to metabolic depletion of essential growth products altering either the membrane integrity or repair capacity of the cells.

Hyperthermia has an additional advantage in that cells in the S-phase of the mitotic cycle, shown to be more resistant to X-rays than at other stages of the cell cycle, are still relatively sensitive to heat. There is also the suggestion that plateau phase cells may be more sensitive to heat. Both such differences in sensitivity would confer an advantage when one is combining therapies. Heat treatment is associated with a considerably greater mitotic delay than X-rays for comparable levels of cell kill together with a marked heat-induced redistribution of cells throughout the cell cycle. Such effects could modify subsequent treatment with X-rays, drugs, or further heat exposure.

The response of tumours in general follows that observed in cells in culture, with the additional effects of tumour dependence on blood supply that have already been discussed. A further important phenomenon is the apparent greater sensitivity to heat of the microvasculature of tumours than that of normal tissues. After a critical time–temperature exposure there may be very profound changes in the capillary circulation resulting in a rapid necrosis of tumour. This necrosis may show geographical arrangement and be greatest in the central parts of a tumour whilst the periphery is relatively protected. The latter effect may be related to the protective effect of normal circulation keeping the periphery at a cooler temperature than that in the centre, and particularly applies to treatments where external heat sources are applied. The heat imparted by such an external source, as for example microwaves, will be more rapidly dissipated in the better-vascularized areas and retained in a poorly vascularized situation. This once again could be advantageous in providing a method of selectively heating hypoxic areas of tumour more than adjacent normal tissue.

The response of normal tissues is obviously very important. Clinical hyperthermia attempts to achieve therapeutic gain rather than indiscriminate damage to both normal tissue and tumour. Several groups have studied this experimentally, and much data have been accumulated. Data for man are relatively sparse but indicate a somewhat similar situation, as in the few well-documented clinical tumour curve experiments; where both normal tissue and tumour responses have been documented, there does appear to have been some increased effect on the tumour. Normal tissue necrosis is a rare event. However this once again may be due not so much to selectivity on the part of the tumour cells, as to more advantageous conditions within the tumour. These are the physiological reasons already discussed and also the frequent use of surface cooling to protect normal tissues.

If ever hyperthermia is to take its place in routine clinical practice, it will probably be employed as part of a fractionated course of treatment. It is in this situation that thermal tolerance, that is the reduced efficacy of a second dose following on soon after a first dose of heat, can occur. The diminished effect of hyperthermia as a result of thermal tolerance may also be seen during prolonged single exposure, that is in excess of 3–4 hours at temperatures below about 43.5 °C. This type of situation may occur in prolonged whole-body heating when the upper temperature achieved is limited to about 42 °C. The magnitude of thermal tolerance varies in different experimental systems. However it is a clinically significant phenomenon as its occurrence can increase the time required for an isoeffect from a second heat treatment by several-fold.

The time course of thermal tolerance is clearly important as it will influence the frequency with which heat treatment may usefully be given. It develops very rapidly after even short treatment times and may be maximal at times ranging between 1 and 2 days after the first heat treatment. In most experimental systems investigated it has largely disappeared after about 96 hours. Fortunately the magnitude of thermal tolerance does not appear to be cumulative in following subsequent treatments.

Tolerance has been seen not only in normal tissues but in tumours as well. As a result it is proposed that most clinical schedules should employ heat treatments at intervals of at least 3 or more days if the occurrence of thermal tolerance is not to interfere with efficacy. The situation is complicated even further when one considers the interaction of heat and drugs, as seen later.

MECHANISM OF CELL KILL

Many mechanisms have been proposed for the thermal inactivation of cells. These include direct damage to cell, nuclear, and lysosomal membranes, the latter with consequent release of lytic enzymes; direct or indirect effects on DNA and RNA; and damage to mitotic spindle formation as a result of effects on spindle protein. In addition, in organized tissue there is the specific effect on tumour microvasculature already discussed. There are also other associated phenomena such as the generation of heat shock proteins coincident with the induction of thermal tolerance, the exact role of which remain to be elucidated.

None of the above mechanisms can be clearly implicated in all the direct effects of heat damage. It is likely that one or more of these mechanisms are effective and of varying relevance under different conditions. In addition other factors come into play when one considers the interaction of heat with either radiation or drugs.

HEAT WITH RADIATION

A synergism between the actions of heat and ionizing radiation has been demonstrated in a variety of model systems and in man. *In vitro*, there is a change in the slope of the radiation cell survival curve (D_0) indicating radiosensitization. Frequently there is a reduction in the magnitude of the initial shoulder of the curve, indicating an impairment of the ability of cells to accumulate and possibly repair sublethal radiation damage. These effects may also be seen in the heat treatment of tumours and normal tissues. Therapeutic gain will therefore depend on maximizing differences between tumour and normal tissue response.

An effect seen *in vitro* which might be therapeutically advantageous is the inhibition of recovery from potentially lethal damage by hyperthermia. This has been demonstrated in plateau phase cells. It is likely that the nutritionally deprived and proliferation-limited cells in tumours might similarly be affected, although there is no clear experimental evidence of this. Secondly, the differing sensitivities at various phases in the mitotic cycle to heat and X-rays have already been discussed. When both modalities are combined it is likely to be advantageous in terms of cell kill because of the increased effect of heat on the relatively radioresistant S phase cells. However the situation is somewhat more complex than this because of the varying degrees of mitotic delay induced by both treatments in fractionated courses and the differing response to radiation of oxic and hypoxic cells. Nonetheless it is likely that tumour cells in well-oxygenated zones will respond better to radiation while cells in the hypoxic zones are likely to be more responsive to heat. Provided normal tissue effects can be modulated in favour of therapeutic gain this should result in increased tumour control.

A considerable body of experimental work using model systems has confirmed that in general heat will potentiate the damaging effect of radiation on tissues in a very similar manner to that of its potentiation on tumours. When the two modalities are given at the same time or very close together the enhancement ratios remain approximately the same, and therapeutic gain is nil. However, data from mouse experiments show that if the heat treatment is given at approximately 4 hours after the radiation a greater response will be seen in tumour than in normal tissue, with consequent therapeutic gain.

At present there are no good clinical data to support the concept of an optimum time for the combination of the two modalities of treatment. This has resulted in two different viewpoints on treatment strategy. some proponents advocate simultaneous or near-simultaneous treatment by the two modalities in order to optimize the enhancement ratio. They combine this with attempts to minimize normal tissue damage by devices such as surface cooling, improved localization of heat distribution, and the reliance on selective heating of tumour because of its altered vascular supply. Others have proposed that it would be better to treat with radiation first and follow this by heat 4 hours later as suggested by the data from animal model systems. In theory, this should result in maximum therapeutic gain. With radiation treatment given first, then nutritionally deprived and hypoxic clonogenic cells surviving radiation treatment would be sensitive to the subsequent heat treatment. Also there would be enhancement of the sublethal and potentially lethal effects of radiation.

HEAT WITH DRUGS

The cytotoxicity of some chemotherapeutic agents is enhanced by hyperthermia. Thermal synergism can be seen with several groups of drugs, notably the alkylating agents and some antibiotics and nitrosoureas. Those which have commonly been used in clinical hyperthermia include melphalan, cyclophosphamide, doxorubicin, bleomycin, CCNU, and BCNU. In addition to these conventional anti-cancer drugs certain other agents, such as alcohols, and hypoxic cell sensitizers such as misonidazole, will interact with heat.

The modes of action of anti-cancer drugs vary considerably and it is therefore not surprising that several different mechanisms are likely to be involved in their interaction with heat. An increased reaction with target DNA is a likely mechanism for the alkylating agents, based on simple thermodynamic grounds. However with others such as cyclophosphamide or thiotepa there may be additional factors involved such as increased activation of the drug itself.

A different mechanism for enhanced cytotoxicity may be a change in access of the drug to the cellular target. This is seen with doxorubicin, where heat treatment is shown to increase permeability of the cell to the drug. However, this phenomenon is complex; with more prolonged periods of heat resulting in thermal tolerance, there is a reversal of this permeability change. No such change in cellular drug concentration is seen with bleomycin. In this case it is thought that heat inhibits the recovery from bleomycin-induced potentially lethal damage.

As might be expected the thermo-chemotherapeutic interactions may be complicated by alterations in drug pharmacokinetics and metabolism. With doxorubicin, for example, there is a change in the proportion of aglycone production observed. Alterations in blood flow and vascular pattern with repeated heat treatments will have an effect on drug access. The temperature at which combined treatment may be useful will also differ with different drugs. For the alkylating agents, useful enhancements are seen both above and below 42 °C, whilst with the antibiotics temperatures in excess of 42 °C are necessary. This temperature limitation has implications for their value in whole-body techniques which are limited to a maximum of around 42 °C.

Potential clinical advantages of hyperthermia include the spatial cooperation between locoregional treatment modalities such as surgery or radiation and the systemic drug treatment. The prime disadvantage is likely to be increased normal tissue toxicity. This has been demonstrated in several experimental systems, suggesting possible negative therapeutic gain. However it does not appear to have been a major problem in whole-body clinical treatments that have been reported. Systemic treatment by chemotherapy of metastases, both occult and overt, could be advantageously managed in this way, provided that the toxicity is not enhanced greatly.

POTENTIAL HAZARDS

The major hazard of hyperthermia is normal tissue damage and this has already been discussed. Less well documented are effects on the host immune system and an increased risk of metastasis.

The effects of hyperthermia on the immune system are complex and have not been documented in an unequivocal way. In experimental systems increased immunity to tumour has been noted but experiments have usually been with a highly immunogenic tumour. Some clinical workers believe that heat treatment may provoke an advantageous response to the tumour but others have questioned this concept.

Even more controversial is the effect of hyperthermia on metastasis. An increased metastasis rate following local treatment of a tumour with hyperthermia has been reported by some workers but the majority of experimental work has not confirmed this. There is also no evidence from clinical data, but most treatments have been carried out on patients with advanced disease making it difficult to assess this question. In view of the profound effects of hyperthermia on the microvasculature it is difficult to see why there should be any risk of increased metastasis. Finally it should be pointed out that there is no evidence for any carcinogenic effect of hyperthermia. This is clearly an advantage over radiation treatment and the action of some drugs. Whether or not there is an increased risk of cancer induction following the combination of heat and radiation or drugs is unknown.

HEATING TECHNIQUES

It has already been stressed how important it is to obtain accurate delivery of heat in order to obtain therapeutic gain. Unfortunately at this time the methods available for heating a localized tumour volume, and also for the non-invasive measurement of the temperatures achieved, remain imperfect. Current methods are still relatively crude. Precision of heat delivery is also complicated by local physiological variables such as blood flow and tumour vascularization. Local patho-physiological differences such as pH changes and levels of hypoxia will also complicate the issue in terms of net biological gain.

The various methods used to induce hyper-thermia include whole-body techniques; regional techniques, usually by perfusion or infusion of heated blood; or those suitable for more localized volumes using ultrasound, microwaves, or radiofrequency radiation. The physical requirements for these heating techniques include reliability of equipment with reproducibility of its heat output; the availability of non-interactive thermometry; and sufficient power output to attain temperatures required in a reasonably short heating time. The thermal dosimetry requirements are such that the techniques should heat at depth and possess an ability to overcome tissue inhomogeneities such as bone, fat, and air cavities. Ideally it should be possible with the technique selected to define a suitable treatment volume and use suitable

TABLE 13.2   METHODS FOR INDUCING CLINICAL HYPERTHERMIA

Technique	Uniformity of tumour temperature	Heating at depth ($>$ 4cm)	Principal advantages	Problems
Whole-body wax bath; hot suit; hot blanket; heated cabinet; heated perfusion	Good	Good	Systemic treatment which is not site- or tissue-dependent; may be combined with chemotherapy	42 °C limit. Systemic complications which are enhanced by chemotherapy. Superficial burns. Very cumbersome and requires anaesthesia. No temperature difference between tumour and normal tissue
Isolated perfusion	Good	Good	Localizes heat to region; may be combined with chemotherapy	Invasive, cumbersome and requires anaesthesia. Applications limited to regions such as limbs. No difference in temperature between tumour and normal tissue
Infusion bladder peritoneum	Poor	Poor	Treats a large volume; may be combined with chemotherapy	Normal tissue damage because of poor heat distribution
Ultrasound (0.5–5 MHz)	Good	Good	Cheap; can focus single beams or arrays	Reflection at tissue interfaces, particularly air and bone. Poor transmission in air
Microwave (300–2450 MHz)	Fair	Poor	Phased arrays may heat at depth; coaxial applicators can be used for implantation	Interact with conventional thermometry. Limited depth of heating. Stray microwaves may need shielding
Radiofrequency (10–30 MHz), capacitive and inductive	Poor	Fair	Localization poor	Interact with thermometry. Overheating of fat with capacitive coupling dependent on frequency

thermometry to define minimum tumour and maximum normal tissue temperatures. Optimally, thermometry should be non-invasive, but such techniques are not yet available. Finally it is important that there is reasonable temperature homogeneity in the treatment volume as this may critically affect both the cure of tumour and the risk of adverse effects in normal tissue.

All of the techniques described and currently available are appropriate for the treatment of head and neck cancer although not all have been so used. A summary of the various heating methods, together with their main advantages and disadvantages, is given in Table 13.2. These can only be discussed briefly in this section. For more information readers are referred to several recent reviews.[5-8]

Whole-Body Hyperthermia

Whole-body hyperthermia may be achieved by heating the body through the skin with external heat sources or by perfusing blood in an extracorporeal circulator. External sources are provided by radiant heat and sometimes boosted by hot air or radiofrequency heating. Immersion in a hot bath of wax may achieve total heating, as can covering with blankets or space suits heated with water. Temperatures of around 42 °C have been achieved and maintained for periods of time up to 21 hours.

These techniques are all cumbersome, require anaesthesia, and are potentially very time-consuming. Complications vary in different reports, but in general superficial burns are the only major problem, with a low incidence of a few per cent. Various other complications have been reported, including disseminated intervascular coagulation, pulmonary oedema, transient cardiac arrhythmias, fibrosing alveolitis (when the lungs are used as a heat exchanger), and altered hepatic serum enzymes. However the incidence of fatalities at around 1% has been surprisingly low in view of the very advanced nature of the disease in the patients so treated. Except for the extracorporeal heating method

the rate at which the body's temperature can be raised tends to be somewhat slow. A build-up time of 90–120 minutes is usually required to reach the maximum temperature of 42 °C.

The advantages of whole-body hyperthermia include generalized heating which is of potential value in diseases which are widely metastatic. This is perhaps not quite so relevant to the usual clinical situation in head and neck cancer. Temperature measurements are also relatively easy as core temperatures can be taken to approximate those in tumour. The results of over 600 patients collected from the literature with a variety of stages of disease show a tumour response rate of around 30%, of which around 5% are reported as complete responders. This includes a very motley collection of patients with extensive tumours, and it is difficult to know how valid these results are in terms of overall clinical value of the treatment. There are no reports of its use in head and neck cancer as far as this author is aware.

Whole-body hyperthermia is frequently used on its own but when combined with cytotoxic chemotherapy does not appear to have been associated with excess toxicity, which might have been expected from current laboratory data. Indeed the evidence would suggest that the treatment is well tolerated. The major problem with whole-body hyperthermia is that it is a laborious technique to apply, both for staff and patients, and the responses reported in the main appear to be transient.

Perfusion Techniques

Regional perfusion of isolated areas has been used by many groups, notably for melanoma and sarcoma of the limbs, using pump–oxygenator systems. Enthusiastic reports have been published by its advocates, although results from randomized studies are not available. There have also been brief reports of the treatment of brain and abdominal tumours. The method is not easily applicable to head and neck cancers and little more need be said about it in this context.

Intracavitary Infusion

Intracavitary infusions have been used for the treatment of cancer of the bladder and also carcinomatosis peritonei. Once again, in these situations results have not been very promising and the technique is clearly not applicable to head and neck cancer.

Ultrasound

The use of ultrasound to produce localised heating has many advocates and has been used for the treatment of head and neck cancer.[16-18] The physical and biological effects are complex. Ultrasound has advantages over microwave and radiofrequency radiation as the short wavelengths at which it is generated permit the treatment of smaller volumes of tissue than are possible with the other types of radiation.

Ultrasound is usually generated by a piezoelectric transducer crystal. The maximum surface area treated will depend on the size of this crystal. Currently these are about 5 cm in diameter. Ultrasound attenuates very rapidly in air and transducers are therefore coupled to the body surfaces with an aqueous gel or degassed water. Attenuation through the tissues in man will vary according to the tissue irradiated and depend on the frequency at which it is generated. Maximum attenuation will occur in bone, with muscle as an intermediate, and fat with the least amount of attenuation. Air cavities within the body, and particularly within the lungs, will also rapidly attenuate. Reflection of ultrasound from interfaces will also cause changes in energy distribution.

Ultrasound beams have a small angle of divergence and this permits the construction of focused transducers. Defined target volumes may then be treated by scanning the transducer. More sophisticated techniques employ groups of transducers activated either as annular of phased arrays.

A further advantage of ultrasound is the absence of interaction with the usual thermometry devices. Thus conventional metallic thermocouples will not be selectively heated by ultrasound, in contrast to radiofrequency and microwave methods.

Conventional ultrasound is therefore a relatively easy and inexpensive method of heating small volumes of tissue. Single transducers can be used to heat superficial tumours in the skin and head and neck region. For larger tumours at depth, bone may cause problems of differential heating, but this is perhaps less of a problem when the bone has been destroyed by tumour. It is an ideal method for use in the treatment of enlarged lymph nodes in the neck or superficial soft tissue cancers.

The most detailed reports of use of ultrasound in head and neck cancer are by Marmor, Hahn and their colleagues.[16,17] Heating was induced at frequencies of 1–3 MHz and tumour temperatures held at 43–45 °C for 30 minutes in each treatment. Each of the 12 lesions in patients with squamous cell carcinoma of the head and neck showed regression, including one complete responder. However most responses were partial and the median follow-up time was short because most of the patients had widespread metastatic disease and either died or were put on other treatments such as chemotherapy.[16] In another series the effects of adding hyperthermia given by a similar technique to radiation treatment was investigated in paired nodules including some in the head and neck region.[17] In 7/15 evaluable patients the tumours that received heat in addition to radiation had a greater objective response than those receiving radiation alone. However there was also some indication of sensitization of skin to the radiation reaction in two of the patients. This was perhaps not surprising as there was very little temporal separation between the heat and radiation treatments. More recently Corey and colleagues[18] have reported a further series of 28 patients with superficial tumours treated with ultrasound, including three with squamous cell carcinoma of the head and neck region. One of these showed a complete response and the other two were partial responders following the hyperthermia. Readers are referred to the original papers for further technical details of the heating methods. It is established, however, that ultrasound, even with single transducers, is capable of producing adequate local heating and it would seem likely that the focused ultrasound such as is being developed by Hahn and Marmor should be advantageous in producing good heat distribution in head and neck cancers. Further work with this type of technique is eagerly awaited.

Non-Ionizing Electromagnetic (EM) Radiation

The most commonly used methods for the localized heating of tissues employ microwave or radiofrequency radiation. These non-ionizing electromagnetic waves result in the generation of heat as a result of ionic movements and molecular rotations. The depths and the magnitude to which these interactions will occur in different tissues relate to the electrical properties of the latter, and these largely depend on their water content. Groups of tissues with high water content such as muscle, skin, and visceral organs will be heated differently from those which have a low water content, such as bone and fat. These effects will also vary with the frequency of the radiation. It is by selection of these various properties that it may be possible to obtain useful heating with localized hyperthermia at depth in tissues. For more detailed discussion of these physical aspects readers are referred to the recent review by Hand and Ter Haar.[6]

Thermometry

One problem that is common to the use of both microwave and radiofrequency heating results from the very different dielectric properties of most temperature detectors. For example, metallic thermocouples may selectively be heated by EM radiation giving both local hot spots and spurious temperature recordings.

Different techniques and designs of such detectors have been produced to try and overcome these problems. One method which helps to minimize the difficulty of monitoring with very fine thermocouples includes implanting them with their long axis as perpendicular to the incident field as possible so as to result in least interaction. The temperature is then recorded after a switch-off of the EM power for a few seconds. Non-perturbing probes that have been designed include optical fibres with liquid crystal detectors, small semiconductors or birefringent crystals. None of these are in fact anywhere near ideal, as they are still of rather large dimension and are probably sufficiently invasive to alter local circulation and thus heating patterns by their very presence.

There are also problems in placing the detector at a suitable site of measurement. This may not be too difficult with superficial tumours but may be insuperable when one is considering tumours deep in the thorax or even in the head and neck region. Such measurements are of importance, as phantom measurements in static non-perfused material cannot give a detailed thermal profile when heat is applied to perfused tissues *in vivo*. Some estimate may be made by making sensible assumptions about blood flow patterns, but ultimately, for safe hyperthermia, it is essential to have concurrent monitoring of tumour and normal tissue temperatures.

Most of the developed microwave and indeed RF heating techniques rely on averaging out of the temperature throughout the tissue volume and protection of normal tissue by their better heat dissipation. For safety's sake many of the systems carry a feed-back temperature monitoring system to the EM generator which will then maintain and control a reference maximum temperature at a safe level.

Radiofrequency (RF) Heating

The currently accepted ISM (industrial, scientific, and medical) frequencies are 13.56 and 27.12 MHz. These frequencies are not normally used for radio communication so that they have the advantage that they may be used in unscreened rooms. If other frequencies are used, then electrically screened areas are required.

Two principal methods are employed in RF heating known as capacitive or inductive coupling. Inductive coupling occurs close to a coil carrying an RF current. The alternating current in the coil produces a magnetic field and results in a flow of current into tissues. This is greater in tissues with a high water content such as muscles and viscera than in fat and bone, but rapid attenuation still means that heating can only occur in a relatively superficial few centimetres of tissue, and the heat deposition is not particularly uniform. Improved heat distribution at depth may be partially achieved using pairs of coils or more complex arrangements including ring arrays around the patient. For most superficial head and neck cancers a series of pancake coils for inductive heating may well be adequate.

Capacitive heating uses pairs of electrodes laid across a block of tissue through which the electrical fields produce current and consequent heating. A major problem is the possibility of excessive heating in subcutaneous fat. This is because fat has a high electrical resistance and dissipates heat rather poorly as a consequence of its low thermal conductivity and poor vascular perfusion. Burns in superficial fat are therefore a very real danger with capacitive RF heating. However once again in the head and neck region this is rarely a significant worry.

The use of a cooled saline solution in a bag between the electrodes and the skin will permit better contour matching and also reduces the risk of superficial overheating. A crossfire technique between a pair of electrodes will normally produce a reasonable degree of heating at a few centimetres below the surface. If greater precision and heating at depth is required, then crossfire techniques with more than one pair of electrodes can be used.

RF heating may also be achieved using needle electrodes inserted as arrays into tumours such as those in the head and neck. Alternatively metallic particles or seeds can be implanted into superficial tumours which are then selectively heated by external RF beams. Neither of these techniques have been used extensively because they are invasive. However both would seem to be particularly suitable for treating localized cancer volumes in the head and neck region.

Microwaves

Electromagnetic radiation in the microwave frequency range (300–3000 MHz) is perhaps the most commonly used method of heating tissues. Depths of penetration decrease with increasing frequency. Energy absorption as with RF is greatest in tissues with the highest water content. The standard ISM frequencies which may be used without shielding are 434, 915, and 2450 MHz. In practice the microwave radiation is delivered to tissues through direct-contact applicators. There are many different designs of such applicators as the heat distribution will very much depend both on frequency and the shape of the applicator and its dielectric loading. These are specifically employed to optimize treatment of a selected size and depth of target volume. As is to be expected, single applicators heat maximally near the surface. For this reason skin cooling is often built into such applicators, either with circulating cold water or cold air, in order to reduce the risk of superficial burns.

A particular problem is that it is not easy to produce clearly defined heated volumes. The use of opposed and synchronous phased arrays of applicators may ultimately prove able to heat selective volumes more uniformly, although these remain to be proved in practice. Other techniques include coaxial applicators which can be used over a range of frequencies. The diameter of these may be adjusted, and they may be sufficiently small to be implanted directly into cavities such as the oesophagus, or into recurrent tumour masses.

In the head and neck region most tumours outside the skull will be accessible by judicious selection of a range of frequencies, such as 2450 MHz for very superficial regions and down to 434 MHz for deeper lesions.

However, selective absorption may be a problem.

There have been few detailed reports on the use of microwave heating in head and neck cancer. Perhaps the largest series is by Arcangeli and his colleagues,[19] in which several modalities of treatment including microwave hyperthermia at 500 MHz have been used to treat nodal metastases. The randomization protocol was somewhat complex, as patients received multi-dose X-ray fractions per day with or without misonidazole and some received chemotherapy with doxorubicin or bleomycin. Analysis of the results in those groups where hyperthermia was added either to the multi-dose fractionation scheme or the multi-dose fractionation scheme with misonidazole and heat suggested an advantage to the addition of heat in terms of tumour response. Likewise in those patients who were treated with either doxorubicin or bleomycin the addition of heat to that treatment significantly improved the response rate. There did not appear to be any increase in normal tissue toxicity with these treatments.

Another report by Hornback and colleagues[20] on 70 patients with advanced histologically proven malignancies included several who had tumours in the head and neck region treated by a combination of 434 MHz microwave radiation together with ionizing radiation. Patients tolerated the treatment well. From the responses reported, however, it is difficult to assess results because tumour temperature measurements were not taken during the microwave therapy and treatments were not randomized. However considerable relief of symptoms was associated with tumour response in many of the patients. Responses of head and neck cancers are also reported in a series presented by Fazekas and Nerlinger,[21] in which hyperthermia was added to radiation treatment for superficially recurrent tumours. Perez and co-workers,[22] also using a combination of microwave treatment and external radiation noted that 9/12 recurrent squamous carcinomas of the head and neck region showed complete regression and a further one was a partial responder. These patients received between 2000 and 4000 rad total dose given as 400 rad fractions every 72 hours, followed by hyperthermia at 42–43 °C for 90 minutes every 72 hours.

CONCLUSIONS

The clinical experience with hyperthermia is not well documented. Different groups of workers have published the results on small series of patients with very mixed histologies and sites of origin, and often with incompletely documented treatment details and results. The reports are largely anecdotal and firm scientific conclusions about the clinical place of hyperthermia at any site and in particular in the head and neck region must await further evaluation. However the potential biological advantages of hyperthermia in cancer treatment are such as to make further investigation of its role worthwhile.

A major problem which affects all current studies is the difficulties in physical delivery of the heat and the unpredictability of the physiological variations from patient to patient. These physical and biological properties that have already been detailed in the previous sections make current clinical hyperthermia difficult. Further progress will undoubtedly be dependent on the development of better heating methods.

REFERENCES

1. Busch, W. (1866). *Verh. Naturh. Preuss, Rhein Westphal.*, **23**, 28.
2. Coley, W.B. (1893). *Am. J. Med. Sci.*, **105**, 487.
3. Har Kedar, I., and Bleehen, N.M. (1976). *Adv. Radiat. Biol.*, **6**, 229.
4. Field, S.B., and Bleehen, N.M. (1979). *Cancer Treat. Rev.*, **6**, 63.
5. Hand, J.W., and Ter Haar, G. (1981). *Br. J. Radiol.*, **54**, 443.
6. Bleehen, N.M. (1982). In *Lung Cancer 1982* (Eds S. Ishikawa, Y. Hayata, and K. Suemasu), Excerpta Medica, Amsterdam, p.73.
7. Cetas, T.C. (1982). In *Physical Aspects of Hyperthermia* (Ed G.H. Nussbaum), Am. Ass.

Physicists in Medicine Medical Physics Monograph No 8 New York, p. 231.

8. Christensen, D.A. (1979). *Cancer*, **29**, 2325.

9. *Cancer Therapy by Hyperthermia and Radiation* (1978). (Eds C. Streffer, D. Van Beuningen, F. Dietzel, E. Rottinger, J.E. Robinson, E. Scherer, S. Seeber, and D.R. Trott), Urban and Schwarzenburg, Baltimore – Munich, p.3.

10. Milner, J.W. (Ed.) (1979). *Conference on Hyperthermia in Cancer Treatment, 1979. Cancer Res.*, **39**, (2), 2235.

11. *Proceedings of the International Symposium on Cancer Therapy by Hyperthermia and Radiation* (1975). American College of Radiology, Washington, p.1.

12. *Proceedings of the 3rd International Symposium: Cancer Therapy by Hyperthermia, Drugs and Radiation* (1981). J. Nat. Cancer Inst. Monogr. **60**.

13. *British Journal of Cancer*, (1982). **45**, Suppl. V.

14. Medical Research Council Working Party, (1978). *Lancet*, 21 October, p.881.

15. Caterall, M., Bewley, D.K., and Sutherland, I. (1977). *Br. Med. J.*, **1**, 1642.

16. Marmor, J.B., Pounds, D., Postic, T.B., and Hahn, G.M. (1979). *Cancer*, **43**, 188.

17. Marmor, J.B., and Hahn, G.M. (1980). *Cancer*, **46**, 1986.

18. Corry, P.M., Barlogie, B., Tilchen, E.J., and Armour, E.P. (1982). *Int. J. Radiat. Oncol. Biol. Phys.*, **8**, 1225.

19. Arcangeli, G., Cividalli, A., Lovisolo, G., Mauro, F., Creton, G., Nervi, C., and Pavin, G. (1980). In G. Arcangeli and F. Mauro (Eds), *Proceedings of the 1st Meeting of European Group of Hyperthermia in Radiation Oncology*, Masson, Milan, p.257.

20. Hornback, N.B., Shupe, R.E., Shidnia, H., Joe, B.T., Sayoc, E., and Marshall, C. (1977). *Cancer*, **40**, 2854.

21. Fazekas, J.T. and Nerlinger, R.E. (1981). *Int. J. Radiat. Oncol. Biol. Phys.*, **7**, 1457.

22. Perez, C.A., Kopecky, W., Rao, D.V., Baglan, R. and Mann, J. (1981). *Int. J. Radiat. Oncol. Biol. Phys.*, **7**, 765.

Chapter **14**

The Current Status of Chemotherapy

Mario Eisenberger, Juan Posada,
William Soper, and Robert Wittes
*Cancer Therapy Evaluation Program,
Division of Cancer Treatment, National
Cancer Institute, Bethesda, Maryland,
USA*

Although head and neck cancer accounts for only 5% of all malignancies among males and 2% among females,[1] this group of diseases has traditionally excited more interest in the medical community than its incidence might suggest. Surgeons and radiotherapists have long regarded these tumours as major challenges and have been rewarded by substantial cure rates in early-stage disease, at least for certain sites. Because speech, alimentation, and appearance are so important to the functioning and self-image of a patient, the surgeon and radiotherapist must routinely elicit the assistance of the dentist, the maxillofacial prosthodontist, speech therapist, nutritionist, and reconstructive surgeon in a comprehensive approach to the patient.

The medical oncologist is the newest member of the team, and his contribution is still regarded in some quarters with a certain amount of scepticism. There is, of course, no serious disagreement that the standard local therapies of advanced (Stage 3 and 4) head and neck cancer are unsatisfactory; cure rates at nearly all sites are unacceptably low despite maximally vigorous use of surgery and radiation, either singly or in combination. Though much of the cause for this excessive mortality is failure of locoregional control, it is also true that a high proportion of these patients die with, if not of, distant metastases.[151] Whether failure is regional or distant, one might reasonably anticipate that active chemotherapy could well contribute to an improvement in end results.

Nevertheless one must admit that a good dose of healthy scepticism is justified. Until recently chemotherapy was used only in patients with far-advanced disease which had already resisted attempts at cure with surgery and/or radiation. The effect of chemotherapy in this clinical setting has been less than striking; although shrinkage of tumour occurred not uncommonly, durations of response were brief and the natural history of the disease was unaltered.

In this chapter we shall examine the current status of chemotherapy in head and neck cancer. We shall see that the progress made over the past several years has been substantial but the definitive demonstration that chemotherapy can improve the cure rate or even the total survivorship of the treated population still lies in the future.

CHEMOTHERAPY IN RECURRENT AND/OR METASTATIC DISEASE

A number of antitumour drugs have been tested in squamous cell carcinomas of the head and neck; many of these trials have been broad Phase II studies including a variety of other tumours (Table 14.1). Because of the lack of strict eligibility criteria, a high percentage of inevaluable cases, the variety of dose schedules, and imprecise response criteria, the extent of activity of many drugs is even now unclear.

TABLE 14.1   SINGLE AGENT ACTIVITY

Drug (Reference) and dose schedule	Evaluable patients	Response*
CTX[2]		
(a) 8–40 mg/kg IA *or* 4 mg/kg/d IV *or* 40–60 mg/kg single dose	56	2 CR 35 Improved
(b) 150–300 mg/d; then 100–200 mg/d PO	15	2 Improved
(c) 2 g in divided doses for 8 days; then 100 mg/d PO	6	3 PR 3 Improved
CTX[3]		
IV, PO, IP, or intra-pleural ranging from 100 mg daily PO to 8 g IV loading dose preceding PO therapy	4	2 excellent and 2 moderate responses
CTX[4]		
50–200 mg/d PO *or* 30 mg/kg IVP; then 10–15 mg/kg Q 1–2 wks	1	Improved

Drug (Reference) and dose schedule	Evaluable patients	Response*
CTX[5]		
Various IV and PO doses	4	1 Improved
CLB[6]		
0.2 mg/kg/d × 42 days PO	34	1 CR 4 PR
Nitrogen mustard[7,8]		
Total dose 0.5–0.8 mg/kg	2	None
or 0.6 mg/kg in 3 divided doses	41	5 Improved
5FU[9–13]		
15 mg/kg/d × 5 IV; then 7.1 mg/kg every other day until toxicity. Maximum loading dose per day, 1000 mg	84	1 CR 4 PR 20 Improved
5FU[14]		
1000 mg/d × 5; then 500 mg every other day until toxicity	2	2 Improved
5FU[15,16]		
4–8 mg/kg/d × 14–42 days	17	3 Improved
5FU[17]		
15–20 mg/kg/wk	12	1 CR 1 PR
Hydroxyurea[18,19]		
80-mg/kg Q 3 d × 6 wks	1	1 Improved
40 mg/kg PO in 2 divided doses per day × 21 days; escalated to 60 mg/kg/d after 21 days if not toxic	10	3 Improved
VLB[20]		
0.1 mg/kg/wk to a maximum of 0.3 mg/kg/wk IV	23	4 PR 7 Improved
PCZ[21]		
150–400 mg/d PO *or* 250–1250 mg single dose IV	31	3 Improved
Adriamycin[22]		
60–75 mg/m² IV Q 3 weeks	12	0

Drug (Reference) and dose schedule	Evaluable patients	Response*
Adriamycin[23]		
Review of various IV dose schedules, i.e.		
60–90 mg/m^2, Q 3 wks		
20–30 mg/m^2/d × 3, Q 3 wks	76	11 PR
0.4 mg/kg d 1, 2, 7, 8, 9, 10, Q 2 wks		
1 mg/kg/d, Q 7 D and, IA:		
75/mg/m^2 over 72 h		
Mitomycin C[24]		
50 mg/kg/d × 6; then 50 mg/kg every other day until toxicity	4	0

* Improvement – includes subjective, < 50% or unquantitated responses.

Among the bifunctional alkylating agents,[2–8] the widest experience has been with cyclophosphamide. Although currently accepted response criteria were not in use at the time of these studies, a careful reading of these papers suggests that only a small proportion of patients had significant objective responses. Similarly, 5-fluorouracil (5FU)[9–17] administered by rapid intravenous injection appears to have a rather low level of activity. Other agents with varying degrees of activity include hydroxyurea,[18,19] vinblastine,[20] procarbazine,[21] doxorubicin,[22,23] actinomycin D,[24] mitomycin C,[24] cytosine arabinoside,[25] BCNU,[26,27] CCNU,[28–31] and methyl-CCNU.[32,33]

Methotrexate

This agent has fascinated biochemists and clinicians alike since its discovery; it has been studied more intensively than any other drug in squamous cell carcinoma of the head and neck. Its cytotoxicity is largely attributable to inhibition of DNA synthesis[34] through tight binding of the drug and its polyglutamates to the enzyme dihydrofolate reductase (DHFR). This results in depletion of the pool of reduced folates and interruption of thymidylate and purine biosynthesis.[35,36]

The reversal of MTX cytotoxicity with the primary goal of enhancing the therapeutic index has been the focus of intensive investigations. The initial approach was through the use of calcium leucovorin as a source of reduced folates. Enhancement of the therapeutic index of MTX given at high doses in conjunction with leucovorin rescue (LR) has been documented in L1210 leukaemia cells.[37] Thymidine[38] can also prevent MTX-induced cell death, and the reversal of cytotoxicity apparently is independent of the drug concentration.[39] However, clinical studies have not shown that thymidine produces a clear-cut improvement in the efficacy of MTX and further studies are needed to explore optimal dose schedules of thymidine and MTX.[38]

Pharmacological studies indicate that MTX in doses below 30 mg/m^2 is completely absorbed from the gastrointestinal tract, but absorption of higher doses is incomplete and unpredictable.[40] The drug distributes in total body water and circulates loosely bound to serum albumin. Plasma pharmacokinetics indicate that the drug disappears from the plasma in two distinct phases, with half-lives of 2–3 hours and about 10 hours respectively. MTX is almost totally excreted in the urine in 12 hours, but changes in glomerular filtration and tubular excretion rates will increase the terminal elimination. Certain organic acids (probenecid, aspirin) may inhibit tubular excretion.

Methotrexate penetrates into third spaces such as pleural fluid and ascites, reaching equilibrium with plasma concentrations in approximately 6 hours. Subsequently, the slow re-entry of drug from third spaces into the systemic circulation results in prolongation of the terminal half-life in plasma. This effect should be carefully considered in planning for LR in patients with third space fluid collections who are receiving high dose MTX (HDMTX).[41]

During HDMTX administration precipitation of parent compound and metabolites in the renal tubules and collecting system may result in decreased excretion and increased toxicity. Precipitation can usually be prevented by administration of sodium bicarbonate and vigorous hydration to assure large volumes of alkaline urine.[42] Monitoring of plasma MTX levels plays a valuable role in avoiding toxicity and assessing the need for modifying schedules of LR.[43]

An extraordinary number of MTX regimens have been studied in head and neck cancer, both in conventional doses with and without leucovorin, and in high doses with LR (Table 14.2). Response rates have ranged from 25% to 80%, without obvious dependence on dose and schedule of drug, though this is a very difficult judgement to make when data are uncontrolled and sample sizes in individual studies are small. Disappointingly, regressions have been of very short duration (3–4 months) independent of schedule.[45]

A few controlled trials have sought to determine whether a dose–response relationship exists for MTX in head and neck cancer (Table 14.3). Levitt *et al.*[46] compared doses of $80-230$ mg/m^2 Q 2 w given in a 30-hour infusion *versus* $240-1080$ mg/m^2 Q 2 w in a 30–42-hour infusion with LR 36–42 hours after initiating the MTX. The study demonstrated a slightly superior response rate and less toxicity with the higher dose + LR, but response durations were similar in the two arms. Woods *et al.*[47] have explored the dose–response

characteristics of MTX over a 100-fold dosage range; they found a somewhat higher response rate at the highest dose, but at the cost of increased toxicity. There were no significant differences in survival among the three groups. DeConti and Schoenfeld[48] compared weekly MTX, biweekly MTX with LR, and biweekly MTX + LR with CTX and cytosine arabinoside (Ara-C). No treatment showed clear-cut superiority in response rate, duration of response, or survival. The combination regimen produced significantly more haematological toxicity.

These data suggest that high doses of MTX followed by LR, with monitoring of MTX levels, may be given safely to head and neck cancer patients. They do not establish, however, that higher doses of MTX with LR offer a therapeutic advantage over more conventional doses, with or without LR, in terms either of response rate or duration. The small sample sizes in most of these trials, however, severely limit the strength of any conclusions one might draw from them.

Bleomycin

Bleomycin has shown activity against a number of squamous cell carcinomas, including those of the head and neck. Cell kinetic studies *in vitro* indicate that the maximum cytotoxicity of the drug is exerted during the M and G2 phases of the cell cycle.[52] BLM

TABLE 14.2 MTX DOSE SCHEDULES*

	Dose	Route	Frequency
I.	Conventional dose		
	(a) $15-20$ mg/m^2	PO or IV	2 × weekly
	(b) $30-50$ mg/m^2	PO or IV	weekly
	(c) 15 mg/m^2/d × 5	IV or IM	Q 2–3 wks
II.	Moderate dose		
	(a) $50-150$ mg/m^2	IV push	Q 2–3 wks
	(†b) 240 mg/m^2	IV 24-h infusion	Q 4–7 wks
	(†c) $0.5-1.0$ g/m^2	IV 36–42-h infusion	Q 2–3 wks
III.	High dose		
	†$1-12$ g/m^2	IV 1–6h	Q 1–3 wks

* Based on Refs 44, 195, 196.
† With leucovorin rescue.

causes single- and double-strand DNA breaks that may be dose-related.

BLM is rapidly absorbed after intra-muscular (IM) injection, with a half-life similar to that seen with rapid intravenous (IV) injection or prolonged IV infusion. Peak plasma concentrations after IM injection are approximately one-third to one-half of those observed after rapid IV administration.[54]

Absorption after subcutaneous (SC) injection seems less predictable than with the other routes. BLM is excreted primarily by the kidneys and in patients with creatinine clearances below 25–35 ml/min the plasma half-life of the drug increases exponentially as the creatinine clearance decreases.[54] Evidence obtained in experimental animals[55] suggests increased therapeutic efficacy with continuous

TABLE 14.3   PROSPECTIVE TRIALS COMPARING DOSES AND SCHEDULES OF MTX

Investigators and MTX dose schedule	Evaluable patients*	Response CR + PR	Response Rate (%)	Median response duration	Median survival duration	Toxicity
Levitt *et al.*[46]						
(a) 80–230 mg/m^2 × 30 h infusion, Q 2 wks	16	7	44	12 wks	NA	Mainly haematological, with less leukopenia but not less thrombo-cytopenia in Group (b).
(b) 140–1080 mg/m^2 × 36–42 h infusion, Q 2 wks, with LR 36–42 h after MTX	25	15	60	11 wks	NA	
Woods *et al*[47]						
(a) 50 mg/m^2 IV bolus + LR 24 h after MTX	23	6	26	6 wks	32 wks overall	Group (c) – severe GI, renal and myelo-toxicity. Relatively mild in (a) and (b).
(b) 500 mg/m$_2$ IV bolus + LR 24 h after MTX	27	7	26	7 wks		
(c) 5 g/m^2 bolus + LR 24 h after MTX	22	10	45	12 wks		
DeConti and Schoenfeld[48]						
(a) 40 mg/m^2 IV bolus weekly	81	21	26	105 d	154 days	(a) Significantly more skin and mucosal toxicity.
(b) 240 mg/m^2 IV bolus + LR 42 h later, Q 2 wks	80	19	24	42 d	133 days	
(c) MTX + LR as in (b) CTX 0.5 g/m^2 rapid IV infusion just before MTX ARA-C 300 mg/m^2 IV in 15 min., after MTX	76	14	18	49 d	98 days	(c) Gave more haemato-logical toxicity than others.
Kirkwood *et al.*[49]						
(a) 40–200 mg/m^2 IV bolus, d 1 and 4 weekly, LR d 2 and 5	19	12	63	12 wks	NA	Moderate renal and mild GI/mucosal toxicity in both arms; myelotoxicity rare in (a) and more frequent in (b)
(b) 1–7.5 g/m^2 IV bolus weekly; LR 24 h after MTX	30	9	30	11 wks	NA	
Tejada *et al.*[50]						
(a) 50 mg/m^2 PO, weekly	21	5	24	NA	NA	Minimal to moderate reversible and tolerable
(b) 25 mg/m^2 PO, d 1 and 2 weekly	20	13	65	NA	NA	
(c) 50 mg/m^2 PO d 1 + *CP* 20 mg/m^2 IV d 1, weekly	21	13	62	NA	NA	
Vogler *et al.*[51]						
(a) 125 mg/m^2 PO Q 6 h × 4, weekly + LR	49	11	22	6.3 months	NA	Haematological toxicity less on regimen (c) and similar on (a) and (b). Regimen (b) in general more toxic.
(b) 60 mg/m^2 IV push weekly	61	19	31	5.4 months	NA	
(c) 15 mg/m^2 Q 6 h × 4 weekly	44	12	27	5.8 months	NA	

* All patients had prior surgery and/or radiotherapy.

(7-day) IV infusion compared to intermittent schedules. Direct comparative trials in the clinic, however, are lacking.

The chief major organ toxicity of BLM is progressive pulmonary fibrosis, which may be fatal in up to 6% of cases. Other toxic effects include characteristic skin changes, fever and chills in as many as 50% of patients, rare instances of severe and potentially fatal anaphylatic reactions, nausea and vomiting, stomatitis, and occasionally myelo-suppression.[54]

Table 14.4 illustrates the experience with BLM in head and neck cancer. The response rates range from 6% to 45%; response durations have generally not exceeded 2–3

months.[63] Because of the initial clinical activity and relative lack of myelotoxicity, BLM was rapidly incorporated into combination regimens despite the need for further clarification of dose and schedule dependency.

Cisplatin

This platinum coordination complex (*cis*-diammine dichloroplatinum(II)) (DDP) is one of a series shown by Rosenberg *et al.*[64] to have significant activity against experimental tumours. Subsequent clinical trials have revealed a very broad spectrum of effectiveness in human malignancies.[65]

DDP inhibits DNA synthesis, with the formation of intrastrand crosslinks in DNA.[66]

TABLE 14.4   PHASE II TRIALS OF BLEOMYCIN

Investigators, and BLM dose schedule	Evaluable patients*	Response CR + PR	Response Rate (%)	Response duration	Survival duration	Toxicity
Bonadonna *et al.*[56]						
(a) 10, 15 or 30 mg/m^2 IV, 2 × weekly	24	7	29			High incidence of pulmonary toxicity at the high doses (above 10 mg/m^2, 2 × weekly)
(b) 15 mg/m^2/d × 5–8 IV	32	17	53			
(c) 30 mg/m^2/d × 8 IV	6	4	67			
Totals	62	28	45	2–5 months	NA	
Halnan *et al.*[57]						
30 mg IV *or* IM, 2 × weekly	55	24	44	NA	NA	Erythema and mucosal ulcerations; stomatitis, fever and mild pulmonary toxicity
Haas *et al*[58]						
10 mg/m^2 IV *or* IM, 2 × weekly	64	12	19	NA	NA	Mild to moderate fever, chills and skin toxicity; pulmonary toxicity; nausea and vomiting
Yagoda *et al.*[59]						
0.25 mg/kg IV daily until skin or mucosal toxicity	46	6	13	Range: 1–11 months	NA	Skin and mucosal toxicity; fever, chills, nausea and vomiting
Durkin *et al.*[60]						
10 mg/m^2 IV *or* IM, 2 × weekly	81	5	6	2–3 months	NA	Minor skin and GI; fever, six patients with pulmonary toxicity (one severe)
EORTC[61]						
10–20 mg/m^2/d × 10–38 days IV *or* IM (total 150–820 mg) *or* 20 mg/m^2 IV 2 × weekly	54	9	17	NA	NA	Fever, nausea and vomiting, rashes, mucosal lesions, pulmonary lesions
Wasserman *et al.*[62]						
A review and analysis of various dose schedules	158	24	15	NA	NA	NA

* Patients previously treated with surgery and/or radiotherapy; some also had chemotherapy.

Zwelling *et al.*[67] have demonstrated the presence of interstrand crosslinks after reaction with either the *cis*- or *trans*-isomer, as well as protein–DNA crosslinks after DDP treatment. The biological significance of these reactions is not known. The drug binds to plasma proteins, and is >90% bound within 24 hours. Plasma clearance is biphasic, with rapid early disappearance but a long terminal half-life of up to 3 days.[66] The dose-limiting toxicity is renal, but vigorous hydration with concomitant diuresis is protective.[65] Other clinically important side-effects are nausea and vomiting, mild myelosuppression, ototoxicity, hypomagnesaemia, neurotoxicity, and alopecia.

Experience with DDP in head and neck cancer (Table 14.5) has shown responses in about one-third of patients; as with other drugs, durations have been very short. When DDP administration is accompanied by careful hydration and forced osmotic diuresis, nephrotoxicity can be largely prevented. Debilitating nausea and vomiting were very

TABLE 14.5   PHASE II TRIALS OF CISPLATIN

Investigators, and DDP dose schedule	Evaluable patients*	Response		Response duration	Survival duration	Toxicity
		CR + PR	Rate (%)			
Wittes *et al.*[68] 2.5–4.5 mg/kg in 20–30 min. infusion Q 3 wks; with hydration and mannitol diuresis	26[a]	8	31	Median 4 months	NA	Consistent nausea and vomiting; mild myelo-suppression, transient tinnitus; renal well controlled by hydration and diuresis
Jacobs[69] 80 mg/m² 24 h infusion, Q 3–4 wks	29[a]	9	31	7 PR–mean 5.8 months 2 CR–7 and 8 months	NA	Mild myelosuppression; mild ototoxicity and peripheral sensory changes
Panettiere *et al.*[70] 50 mg/m² d 1 and 8, Q 4 wks	65[b]	16	25	median 3.5 months	NA	Moderate nausea and vomiting, mild myelo-suppression; moderate reversible renal toxicity
Creagan *et al.*[71] 90 mg/m² CIVI over 24 h with hydration and mannitol	23[c]	4	17	median time to progression: 7 weeks	Median 29 wks	Moderate to severe nausea and vomiting. Mild renal and haematological toxicity
Sako *et al.*[72] (a) 120 mg/m² rapid IV infusion	15[c]	5	33	1, 4, 6, 6, 8 months	NA	Significant GI and renal toxicity, and ototoxicity in both arms
(b) 20 mg/m² rapid IV infusion Both arms with hydration and mannitol diuresis; courses Q 3 wks	15[c]	4	27	1, 5, 5, 8 months		
Randolph and Wittes[73] 50 mg/m²/wk; *no* prehydration or diuresis	13[c]	4	30	1+ to 3+ months	NA	Dose-limiting nephro-toxicity in 50%; significant myelosuppression and GI. More nephrotoxic than with higher doses and hydration

* Prior treatment with (a) radiotherapy and some chemotherapy, (b) surgery and/or radiotherapy, or (c) surgery and/or radiotherapy, and some chemotherapy.

TABLE 14.6   RANDOMIZED COMPARISONS OF MTX AND CISPLATIN

Investigators and treatment	Evaluable patients*	Response		Median response duration	Median survival duration	Toxicity
		CR + PR	Rate (%)			
Hong et al.[74]						
DDP 50 mg/m² IV push d 1 and 8 Q 4 wks	21	6	29	92 days	6.3 months	More nephrotoxicity, nausea and vomiting
vs.						
MTX 40−60 mg/m² IV push weekly	17	4	23	84 days	6.1 months	More mucositis and myelosuppression
Grose et al.[75]						
DDP 50 mg/m² IV d 1 and 8 Q 4 wks	48	4	8.5	8 wks	18 wks	More renal toxicity
vs.						
MTX 15 mg/m² IM d 1−3 Q 3 wks	44	8	18	18 wks ($P = 0.12$)	20 wks ($P = 0.99$)	More myelosuppression

* All with prior surgery and/or radiotherapy.

significant side-effects in the past but are now largely preventable with metoclopramide administration in appropriate doses.

Randomized Comparisons of Single Agents

Clinical trials comparing directly the activity of single agents in recurrent head and neck cancer are very sparse (Table 14.6). In a small study, Hong et al.[74] compared DDP and MTX prospectively and found no obvious differences in response rate, duration of response, or survival; MTX appeared to be better tolerated. In a similar trial performed in the Southwest Oncology Group (SWOG) MTX had a higher response rate (30% vs. 9%), but the apparent differences in response rates, durations, and survival were not significant.[75]

INVESTIGATIONAL AGENTS

The relatively limited efficacy of standard agents serves to emphasize the need for new active drugs in the treatment of head and neck cancer. Recently a number of investigational agents[76−92] have been tested in advanced disease; unfortunately, only a handful have shown signs of activity (Table 14.7).

Methyl G

Methylglyoxal-bis (guanylhydrazone) (Methyl G, Methyl GAG, mitoguazone) has been in

TABLE 14.7   INVESTIGATIONAL DRUGS EVALUATED IN ADVANCED HEAD AND NECK CANCER

Agent	No. of responders/ no. of evaluable patients	Response rate (%)	Reference
Ftorafur	1/14	7	76
Pyrazofurin	2/22	9	77
Vindesine	9/57	16	78−80
Maytansine	1/31	3	81
m-AMSA	3/43	7	82, 83
Methyl G	12/47	25	84, 85
Dianhydrogalactitol	7/37	19	86, 86a
Thioproline	0/16	0	87
ICRF 159	2/23	9	88
Dibromodulcitol	3/12	25	89
VP-16	1/24	4	90
AZQ	0/18	0	91

clinical trials for over 20 years.[93] In the early 1960's the drug was administered on a daily schedule producing substantial anti-tumour activity, but at the cost of severe toxicity.[94] Subsequently, Knight *et al.*[95] designed a weekly infusion schedule that was associated with acceptable toxicity and good anti-tumour activity in a variety of solid tumours.

In head and neck cancer the extent of activity of methyl G by this schedule is not clear. Studies at the Walter Reed Army Medical Center showed significant activity in relapsed disease.[84] Nine of 22 patients (40%) responded, including two complete responses; all of the patients had failed conventional radiotherapy and surgery, and 15 had failed prior chemotherapy. On the other hand, a trial at the Memorial Sloan–Kettering Cancer Center yielded only three partial responses in 25 adequately treated patients.[85] The agent is particularly appealing for incorporation into combinations since its toxic effects do not overlap significantly with those of other agents.

M-AMSA

The drug, 4′-(9-acridinylamine)-methane-sulfon-m-anisidide (AMSA), is an acridine derivative synthesized by Cain and Atwell[96] with activity in a wide spectrum of murine tumours. In humans it has clear activity in the treatment of relapsed acute leukaemia.[97] Two studies[82,83] in head and neck cancer have shown a combined response rate of only 6% (three PR in 43 patients). Further evaluation of this compound in previously untreated patients is probably not worthwhile.

Vindesine

Vindesine has recently undergone evaluation at several centres. Among 57 patients with advanced epidermoid carcinoma of the head and neck,[78–80] only seven brief partial responses were seen. The low level of activity was particularly disappointing since most of the patients had good performance status, including 14 with no prior chemotherapy.

Dianhydrogalactitol (DAG)

Investigators at the Mayo Clinic have evaluated this compound in 28 patients with inoperable advanced carcinomas of the head and neck.[86] All but one of the patients had failed prior surgery and/or radiation therapy and 12 had prior chemotherapy. In 11 cases the disease remained stable during three courses of therapy, but there were no objective responses.

In another trial conducted by the SWOG[86a] one partial response was observed in nine evaluable patients with squamous cell carcinomas.

Diaziquone (AZQ)

AZQ is one of a series of lipophilic aziridinylbenzoquinones synthesized by Chou *et al.*[98] and known to cross-link DNA. The drug has been evaluated in Phase I and in preliminary Phase II trials, where it has shown activity in primary brain tumours.[99] A single Phase II trial in 18 heavily pretreated patients with epidermoid head and neck cancer produced no objective responses.[91]

Dibromodulcitol (DBD)

In a Phase I study of DBD in 96 patients, there were 20 objective remissions, including one of 13 cases of head and neck cancer (100). A Phase II trial[89] produced 51 objective responses (28%) among 181 patients. There were two partial and one complete remissions among 12 patients with head and neck cancer; the complete responder was still in remission 48 months from start of therapy at the time of the report.

DBD + BLM

Based on the modest activity seen with DBD[89,100] in head and neck cancer, BLM was added to DBD[101] and activity of the two drugs was compared to BLM alone. Forty-four patients were treated with BLM + DBD and 12 (27%) achieved a partial regression. BLM alone produced 4/18 responses (22%). Within the limitations imposed by the small number of

TABLE 14.8   PHASE II TRIALS OF 2-DRUG COMBINATIONS OF BLEOMYCIN, CISPLATIN AND MTX

Investigators and treatment	Evaluable patients*	Response CR + PR	Rate (%)	Response duration	Survival duration	Toxicity
Yagoda et al.[102] BLM (15 u IV) MTX (15 mg/m² IV) at 4 – 14 d intervals	15[a]	8	53	3 + months (mean)	NA	Mild, reversible mucositis and/or myelosuppression
Broquet et al.[103] BLM (30 mg IV 2 × weekly) MTX (0.4 mg/kg IV 2 × weekly)	15[a]	9	60	9 weeks (average)	NA	Severe haematological and pulmonary toxicity
Medenica et al.[104] BLM (15 mg IV weekly) MTX (0.6 mg/kg IV weekly)	26[a]	13	50	35 weeks (average)	NA	Mild haematological only
Mosher et al.[105] BLM (20 mg/d × 5 IM) alternating weekly with MTX (240 mg/m² × 2 IV in 36 h) + LR	4[b]	2	—	NA	NA	Severe skin and mucosal toxicity, fever and myelosuppression.
Wittes et al.[106] DDP (2 mg/kg IV, Q 3 wks) BLM (0.25 mg/kg IV daily until toxicity; then 1 – 2 mg daily maintenance)	24[c]	3	13	4 months (median)	NA	Severe nephrotoxicity
Bianco et al.[107] DDP (30 mg/m² IV d 1 – 3 Q 3 wks) with diuresis BLM (15 mg/m² IM, d3, 10, and 17, Q 3 wks)	7[a]	2	—	2 + weeks and 2 months	NA	One fatal septicaemia in a leukopenic patient; otherwise, only moderate myelosuppression
Pitman et al.[108] DDP (80 mg/m² 24 h infusion, Q 2 wks × 2) with hydration, followed by MTX (3 gm/m² IV/1 h weekly × 4) with LR	9[a]	6	66	NA	NA	First regimen caused more nephrotoxicity, myelosuppression and mucositis − CP compromised ability to give subsequent MTX−LR
vs. MTX followed by DDP (same dose schedules)	11[a]	6	54	NA	NA	
Moran et al.[109] MTX (30 mg/m² IV) d 1 DDP (50 – 60 mg/m² IV) d 2 courses Q 22 d	23[a]	8	35	4 months (median)	6 months (median)	Mild stomatitis and leukopenia; transient creatinine rise

* Prior treatment with (a) surgery and/or radiotherapy, (b) radiotherapy, or (c) surgery and/or radiotherapy, some chemotherapy.

patients, the addition of DBD appeared to add little to BLM.

DRUG COMBINATIONS

Armed with several drugs having reproducible activity and motivated by evidence in other tumour types that multi-drug combinations may possess substantially more activity than single agents do, investigators have been actively exploring the potential of combination chemotherapy. The rationale behind these exploratory studies has varied from empirically combining two or more active agents to more complex considerations of cell kinetics or pharmacology.

Phase II Trials with Combinations of BLM, DDP, and MTX

The combination of MTX and BLM has been the two-drug regimen most frequently studied (Table 14.8), mostly in broad Phase II trials.[102–105] Response rates in head and neck cancer of 50 – 60% were reported in individual studies of 15 or more evaluable patients.[102–104] In one trial at the University Hospital in Geneva,[103] partial remission was obtained in 60% of the cases, but at the price of serious haematological and pulmonary toxicity. A subsequent re-evaluation of the combination at lower doses achieved a similar response rate and more prolonged response duration, with only mild and reversible myelosuppression.

With the introduction of DDP into the clinic, evidence for its activity in head and neck cancer emerged directly from Phase I trials.[71] Wittes et al.[106] studied the new agent combined with BLM in a group of heavily pretreated patients. This trial, performed before the protective effect of virorous osmotic diuresis was appreciated, yielded a low response rate and unacceptable degrees of nephrotoxicity. Other investigators,[107] using hydration, obtained somewhat better results with less toxicity, but results did not suggest that the combination was superior to either single agent.

The combination of DDP and MTX[108] produced severe toxicity, especially when MTX was given after DDP. In the same trial with a limited number of patients, this drug combination given in the reverse order produced similar response rates at the cost of substantially less toxicity.[108] Other investigators[109] using lower doses obtained a 35% partial response rate with mild toxicity.

Because these three drugs were among the most frequently tested and active single agents, and exhibited a relative lack of overlapping toxicities (especially with low-dose MTX), studies of three-drug regimens proceeded rapidly (Table 14.9). In seven of these studies,[110-116] 52% of 149 patients obtained complete or partial responses with a variety of dose schedules. Disappointingly, the durations of response and survival were as short as with single-agent treatment.

Trials of Other Combinations (Table 14.10)

Livingston et al.[117] obtained a 34% response rate in a broad Phase II trial using a combination of BLM, CTX, Vincristine (VCR), and MeCCNU, but the duration of response and median survival times were not reported. In an attempt to delay development of clinically evident drug resistance and to decrease toxicity, the same group[118] used several agents sequentially. This regimen, which was designed for administration in five cycles over 36 weeks,

produced a 43% response rate in the first three treatment cycles with a median duration of 25 weeks. The authors concluded that the results with the regimen would most probably not exceed those achievable by MTX alone.

Wheeler and Baker[119] observed impressive activity with high-dose BLM given in a 4-day continuous infusion with VCR and mitomycin-C (MMC), with or without MTX depending on prior treatment history. The high overall response rate of 73% (19/26) was obtained at the cost of severe pulmonary toxicity in 19% of patients; median reponse duration was not reported. In a subsequent small pilot trial in 26 patients the same group observed no obvious improvement in response rate when these drugs were incorporated into two putatively non-cross resistant combinations used sequentially.[119a]

Price and Hill,[120] have constructed a multi-drug regimen based on cytokinetic considerations and have achieved a 50% overall response rate with median survival duration of about 10 months in responders. Other investigators,[121] using a very similar regimen, have not been able to reproduce these results and have seen moderately severe toxicity. Creagan et al.[122-124] demonstrated response rates varying from 0% to 64% with three different dose schedules of CTX, adriamycin (ADM), and DDP (CAP). It is unclear to what extent treatment-related or patient-related factors are responsible for the variability in these results.[143]

In 1979 Cadman et al.[143] reported that exposure of L1210 leukaemia cells *in vitro* to MTX at concentrations of 0.1–100 M, followed by 10 M 5FU, produced a synergistic effect on cell killing. These experimental findings have been applied by the Yale group to a number of tumour types, including head and neck cancer, for which moderate doses of MTX have been followed 1 hour later by 5FU administration, and subsequently LR.[125] Of 23 evaluable patients with recurrent disease, 12 (52%) achieved partial and three (13%) complete responses. In Ringborg's[125a] series of 16 evaluable previously treated patients, six

TABLE 14.9   PHASE II TRIALS OF THREE-DRUG COMBINATIONS OF BLEOMYCIN, CISPLATIN, AND MTX

Investigators and treatment	Evaluable patients	Response		Median Response Duration	Median Survival Duration	Toxicity
		CR + PR	Rate (%)			
Ervin et al.[110] Two 4-wk courses: *DDP* (20 mg/m²) d 1–5 as 2 h infusion after hydration *BLM* (10 u/m²) d 3–7 as continuous infusion *MTX* (200 mg/m²) d 15 and 22 + LR	11[a]	11	100	>4 months	NA	Moderate nausea and vomiting; mild nephrotoxicity; severe granulocytopenia in 28% and thrombocytopenia in 20%
Vogl and Kaplan[111] Q 3 wk courses: *MTX* (40 mg/m² IM) d 1 and 15 *BLM* (10 u IM) d 1, 8 and 15 *DDP* (50 mg/m²) IV d 4 with hydration and diuresis	31[c]	19	61	PR–3 months CR–7+ months	PR–3 months CR–not reached at time of report	Mild myelosuppression and azotaemia; nausea and vomiting from cisplatin severe in some cases
Leone and Ohnuma[112] Unspecified dose schedule of high-dose *MTX–LR, BLM* and *DDP*	24[a]	6	25	2 months	NA	Stomatitis and moderate myelosuppression; nausea and vomiting; slight creatinine rise in 5 patients
Caradonna et al.[113] *BLM* (15 mg/m² IV) d 1 *MTX* (20 mg/m² IV) d 1 *DDP* (120 mg/m² IV/30 min) d 2 with hydration and diuresis *BLM* and *MTX* at 15 and 40 mg/m² IV respectively Q 2 wks × 4 doses, and entire 3-drug regimen repeated at 10 wks. No one got more than 2 courses	19[d]	14	74	4 months	6 months (responders) 2 months (non-responders)	Moderate to severe pulmonary, renal, myelosuppression, nausea and vomiting, and mucositis

Investigators and treatment	Evaluable patients	Response CR + PR	Response Rate (%)	Median Response Duration	Median Survival Duration	Toxicity
Murphy et al.[114] DDP (100 mg/m² d 2 with hydration and diuresis MTX (30 mg/m² IV) d 1 and 15 BLM (30 mg) d 1; then weekly × 6 (180 mg)	24[a]	11	46	5 months	NA	Moderate to severe nephrotoxicity, nausea and vomiting, stomatitis, neuropathy, pulmonary fibrosis, and myelosuppression
Von Hoff et al.[115] Q 4 wk courses: DDP (50 mg/m²) d 1 after hydration BLM (6 u/m² SC, Q 8 h × 12) d 1–4 MTX (7.5 mg/m² IM) d 4–6	26[e]	9	35	3 months	4 months (responders) 3 months (non-responders)	Substantial renal toxicity and myelosuppression, mucositis, nausea and vomiting. Two cases of pulmonary toxicity (BLM)
Belt et al.[116] 2 courses at 21-day interval BLM (25 u/d × 4) d 1–4 MTX (30 mg/m²) d 6 and 7 DDP (100 mg/m²) d 15	12[a]	7	58	36 wks	NA	Mucositis; mild myelosuppression, nausea and vomiting, nephrotoxicity

[a] Prior surgery and/or radiotherapy
[b] No prior treatment
[c] 26 prior surgery and/or RT, including 1 with prior chemotherapy; 5 no prior therapy
[d] 15 prior surgery and/or RT; 2 with prior chemotherapy; 2 no prior therapy
[e] 22 prior surgery and/or RT; 4 no prior therapy

TABLE 14.10   OTHER MULTIDRUG COMBINATIONS IN UNCONTROLLED TRIALS

Investigators and treatment	Evaluable patients	Response		Duration response	Duration survival	Toxicity
		CR + PR	Rate (%)			
Livingston *et al.*[117]						
CTX (800–1000 mg/m² IV) d 1 Q 4–6 wks						Severe myelosuppression in 20%; bleomycin lung damage (4%); dose-limiting VCR neuropathy (11%)
VCR (0.5–1 mg IV) d 2, then twice weekly × 12–48 doses						
MeCCNU (100 mg/m² PO) d 1 and Q 4–6 wks	32[a]	11	34	NA	NA	
BLM (7.5–30 mg IV) d 2 (6 h after VCR), then twice weekly × 12–48 doses						
Livingston *et al.*[118]						
Sequential therapy:	28[a]	12	43	25 wks median	24 wks median	Moderate myelosuppression, mucositis, stomatitis
(A) 1st 6 wks:						
CTX (18 mg/m² IV) d 1 and 22						
VCR (0.75–1 mg IV) d 2; then weekly × 6		(9 responses were after 1st cycle of therapy; 2 after 2nd and 1 after 3rd)				
BLM (30 u IV) d 2 (6 h after VCR); then weekly × 6						
(B) Next 12 wks:						
MTX (30 mg/m² IM weekly × 12) (escalate dose 10 mg/m² weekly until toxicity)						
(C) Next 6 wks:						
ADM (60 mg/m² IV) d 1; 45 mg/m² IV) d 22						
MeCCNU (100 mg/m² PO) d 1						
(D) Next 6 wks:						
MTX (weekly × 6 at dose tolerated in (B))						
(E) Next 6 wks:						
ADM and MeCCNU as in (C)						

Investigators and treatment	Evaluable patients	Response CR + PR	Response Rate (%)	Duration response	Duration survival	Toxicity
Wheeler and Baker[119] (BOMI) VCR (2 mg IV d 1 and 29) MMC (15 mg/m² IV d 1) BLM (20 u/d × 4 continuous infusion starting d 1 and 29) or	7ª	4	73 overall	4 months median	NA	Severe pulmonary toxicity due to cumulative BLM and MMC. Nausea and vomiting, fever, and stomatitis
(BOMIM) VCR, MMC, and BLM, as above plus MTX 30 mg/m² IV weekly beginning d 6	19ª	15				
Wheeler et al.[119a] BOMI as above plus, MTX (30 mg/m² twice weekly followed by LCV 24 h later a single dose given 36–42 h or 60–72 h after BLM) ADM (40 mg/m²) CTX (400 mg/m²) DDP (80 mg/m² in 24 h infusion (above started at 10 wks for responders to BOMIM or immediately for non-responders))	26ᵏ	17	65	Median NA	NA	Moderately severe pulmonary, renal, gastrointestinal and bone marrow toxicities
Price and Hill[120] In a 24-h period, Q 2–3 wks.: VCR (2 mg IV at 0h) BLM (60 mg/6 h infusion from 12 to 18 h) MTX (100 mg IV at 12, 15 and 18 h) Hydrocortisone (500 mg IV at 12 and 18 h) 5FU (500 mg IV at 18 h) Leucovorin (15 mg PO or IM Q 6 h × 4 starting at 26 h)	40ª	20	50	NA	320 days median for responders	Very minimal toxicity
Raafat and Oster[121] Same regimen as Price and Hill,[120] Q 3–4 wks	15ª	2	13	5 wks and 28 wks	NA	Moderate haematological; 3 cases severe stomatitis, but mostly mild or no stomatitis

TABLE 14.10 Cont.

Investigators and treatment	Evaluable patients	Response CR + PR	Response Rate (%)	Duration response	Duration survival	Toxicity
Creagan et al.[122] CTX (400 mg/m² and ADM (40 mg/m² and DDP (40 mg/m²) with no hydration or diuresis). Regimen repeated on 1 day.	25^c	16	64	7 months median	11 months median	Moderately severe myelosuppression, nausea and vomiting, stomatitis, malaise
Creagan et al.[123] ADM (40 mg/m²) d 1 CTX (400 mg/m²) d 3 DDP (20 mg/m²/1 h) d 1–3 with hydration Repeated Q 4 wks	12^a	0	—	NA	5 months median all patients	Moderate to severe nausea and vomiting; moderate myelo-suppression
Creagan et al.[124] CTX (200 mg/m² IV) Q 4 wks ADM (30 mg/m²) DDP (90 mg/m²/24 h) with hydration and diuresis	17^d	7	41	4.6 months median time to progession	NA	Moderate to severe nausea and vomiting; mild myelosuppresion
Pitman et al.[125] MTX (125–250 mg/m² IV + LR) 5FU (600 mg/m² IV 1h) after MTX repeat Q 2 wks	23^h 12^b	15 10	65 83	3.6 months NA	11.5 months 12 months	Mild to moderate diarrhoea, mucositis, nausea and vomiting, myelosuppression
Ringborg et al.[125a] As above	16^j 20^b	9 14	52 70	NA NA	NA NA	Mild gastrointestinal and haematological toxicities
Jacobs[126] MTX + LR as above[124] followed by 5FU as above	30^e	5	17	19+, 4 +, 5, 5 and 7 + months	8 months (mean)	More severe neutropenia and diarrhoea
Thatcher et al.[127] ADM (30 mg/m² IV) Q 3 wks × 6 5FU (500 mg/m² IV) d 1 and PO d 3–6, Q 3 wks × 3 BLM (10 mg/m² IM 2 × weekly) total dose 100 mg/m² Retinol palmitate (vitamin A) (400,000 U/m² IM weekly × 6) MTX (after completing vit. A course, 30 mg/m²/wk × 4 IV)	25^a	10	40	14 wks median	38.5 wks median	No marked myelosuppression; GI toxicities, vomiting and mucositis, not severe

Investigators and treatment	Evaluable patients	Response CR + PR	Response Rate (%)	Duration response	Duration survival	Toxicity
Woods et al.[128] VCR (2 mg IV) d 1 MTX (200 mg/m² IV 24 h infusion) d 1, with LR BLM (15 mg/d in 48 h IV infusion) d 2 repeated Q 3 wks	33[i]	8	24	16 wks median	28 wks median	Minimal myelosuppression
Brown et al.[129] VLB (4 mg/m² IV) d 1 BLM (15 mg/d IM) d 1–7	23[b]	17	74	NA	NA	Relatively minor nephrotoxicity; moderate myelosuppressions; nausea and vomiting; some BLM skin toxicity
DDP (60 mg/m² IV 6 h infusion) Repeat Q 3 wks	22[a]	10	45	4 months median	NA	
Huang et al.[130] BLM (100 u SC) d 1 and 4 MTX (20 mg PO) d 1 and 4 VLB (8 mg/m² IV) d 1 CCNU (175 mg/m² PO) d 1 Repeat Q 4–6 wks; in 2nd–6th courses, BLM dose is 20 units Hydroxyurea (2 g PO) d 1 and 4 substituted for BLM after reaching total dose of 220 units	38[a]	19	50	NA	34 wks median all patients	Mild to moderate nausea and vomiting, and myelosuppression
Presant et al.[131] BCNU (100 mg/m² IV/30 min) CTX (400 mg/m² IV bolus) ADM (40 mg/m² IV bolus) 18–24 h after BCNU and CTX Repeated Q 28 d	29[f]	9	31	Mean time to progression 5.4 months (PRs) 6 + months (CR)	Mean 8.8 months (PRs) 7 + months (CRs)	Moderate myelosuppression; nausea and vomiting
Amer et al.[132] VCR (0.5 mg/m² IV) d 1 and 4 BLM (30 u/d – continuous IV infusion over d 1 and 4) DDP (120 mg/m² IV) d 6 with hydration and diuresis	27[a]	13	48	NA	median 7 months (responders) 1.5 months (non-responders)	Mild haematological; one fatality with nephrotoxicity

TABLE 14.10 Cont.

Investigators and treatment	Evaluable patients	Response CR + PR	Response Rate (%)	Duration response	Duration survival	Toxicity
Lester et al.[133] CTX (600 mg/m² IV) d 1 and 8 VCR (1 mg IV) and MTX (120 mg/m² IV) d 2 and 9, followed 6h later by BLM (15 mg/m² IV) and Adriamycin (25 mg/m² IV) on d2 and 9 LR d 3 and 10 Repeated Q 28 d	39ᵃ	14	36	NA	7–30 + months (CRs) 2 + –19 + months (PRs)	Severe myelosuppression and mucositis
Kish et al.[134] DDP (100 mg/m² IV) with hydration and diuresis 5FU (1000 mg/m²/d) in 96 h infusion 2nd course in 3 weeks	26ᵃ	23	88	NA	13 alive (NED) at 60 + wks	Mild to moderate myelosuppression, nausea and vomiting
Forastiere et al.[135] CP (60 mg/m² IV) Q 21 d CTX (600 mg/m² IV) Q 21 d	23ᵃ	9	39	Median 7 + months	NA	Mild myelosuppression, nausea and vomiting
Spaulding et al.[136] VLB (1.25 mg/m²/d) d 1–5 continuous infusion	21ᵍ	6	28	4–9 months	NA	Primarily nausea and vomiting; no myelosuppression or mucositis
5FU (2 mg/kg/d) d 2–5 continuous infusion Repeated Q 4 wks	7ᵇ	7	100			
Eisenberger et al.[138] BLM (15 u/m² IV) d 1 Hydroxyurea (1000 mg/m² d 8–15, Q 2 wks) After BLM, total dose 300 u, hydroxyurea continued alone	19ᵃ	9	47	Median 130 days to progression	Median 250 days	Mild to moderate myelosuppression; one patient with pulmonary fibrosis
Medenica et al.[139] BLM (15 mg IV) weekly MTX (0.6 mg/kg) weekly Hydroxyurea (1000 mg/m²) 3 oral doses weekly Maintenance with MTX and BLM at same dosage 2 × monthly, and 2500 mg/m² 4 HU Q 2 wks	32ᵇ	21	66	Mean 43 wks (CRs) 355 wks (PRs)	NA	Mild to moderate myelosuppression, mucositis, nausea and vomiting, one patient with reversible lung toxicity

Investigators and treatment	Evaluable patients	Response CR + PR	Response Rate (%)	Duration response	Duration survival	Toxicity
Cortes et al.[140] BLM (15 u/24 h) d 1–3 continuous infusion CTX (500 mg IV(d 5 MTX (50 mg IV) d 5 5FU (500 mg IV) d 5 Repeated Q 3 wks for 8 courses	39[d]	21	54	Median 11 months (CRs) 7 months (PRs)	Median 15 months (CRs) 10 months (PRs)	Mild myelosuppression
Costanzi et al[141] BLM (7.5 mg/m^2 in 48 h continuous infusion) MTX (30 mg/m^2 IV push) d 3 alternating Q 10–14 days with BLM as above Hydroxyurea (2 g/m^2 PO) d 3	17[a]	10	59	1–8 months	NA	Mild to moderate myelosuppression and GI toxicity
Plasse et al.[142] BLM (7.5 u/m^2/d) continuous infusion × 3 days (d 1–4, 8–11) followed on days 5 and 12 with CTX (300 mg/m^2), MTX (30 mg/m^2) and 5FU (300 mg/m^2) Repeated Q 28 d	24[c]	5	21	Median 3.9 months	Median 4.4 months (responders) 3.5 months (non-responders)	Severe pulmonary toxicity in 2 patients; 1 died. Mild stomatitis, GI, hepatic and renal effects

* Abbreviations: VCR – vincristine; VLB – vinblastine; 5FU – 5-Fluorouracil; BCNU – carmustine; CCNU – lomustine.
a Prior surgery and/or RT.
b No prior therapy.
c Prior surgery and/or RT – 10 also had CT.
d Prior surgery and/or RT – 2 also had CT.
e Prior surgery and/or RT – 16 also had CT.
f Prior surgery and/or RT – 24 also had CT.
g Prior surgery and/or RT – some had CT.
h 2–3 surgery and/or RT – 5 also had CT.
i Prior surgery and/or RT – 4 no prior therapy.
j Prior radiation – some had CT.
k 21 – Prior surgery and/or radiotherapy; 11 no prior therapy.
l Prior surgery and/or RT; 9 had prior CT.
m Prior RT – 33; no prior therapy – 6.

(37%) achieved partial and three (19%) complete responders. Jacobs[126] has been unable to confirm these results and has seen substantial toxicity as well. Again here, patient selection may have had much to do with apparent differences in effectiveness in these two trials, inasmuch as the latter series of patients had had a heavier history of chemotherapy pretreatment.

In a small prospective randomized trial by Browman *et al.*[125b] sequential MTX and 5FU was compared to the simultaneous use of both agents at the same dose. In patients with recurrent disease the simultaneous administration produced responses (CR + PR) in 11 of 16 patients (68%) as opposed to five of 13 (38%) receiving the sequential schedule (Table 14.11). The median duration of response was 5.5 months for all responders and differences between arms were not significant. Although no definitive conclusions can be made about the relative value of sequential and simultaneous use of these drugs it seems unlikely that sequenced administration will result in a significant therapeutic advance for patients with recurrent or metastatic disease.

The partial cell-synchronizing effect of BLM[137] in tumour models *in vivo* has been the basis for at least five trials (Table 14.10). After BLM administration, various drug schedules were employed and response rate ranged from 21% to 59%.[138–142] As in other studies, these responses were relatively brief and survival data, where available, failed to show any significant advantage for the responders over the entire treated group.

Not surprisingly, randomized trials are much fewer in number than uncontrolled Phase II studies of drug combinations. Most of the randomized trials (Tables 14.6, 14.8, and 14.9) were primarily designed to compare the efficacy of the most active combination regimens with single drugs. Only five of the studies, which were conducted as multi-centre cooperative trials, included enough patients for appropriate statistical analysis (Table 14.11). Lehane *et al.*[144] compared MTX to a combination of MTX, MeCCNU, and BLM.

The results failed to demonstrate the superiority of the combination over MTX alone (Table 14.12). The authors' inclination to attribute the rather long median survival time of the complete responders (84 weeks) to an effect of therapy is not justified since there is no way to exclude the influence of tumour and/or host factors. As noted previously, the Eastern Cooperative Oncology Group (ECOG) study,[48] comparing standard dose MTX, moderately high-dose MTX + LR, or combined high-dose MTX + CTX + Ara-C, based on biochemical and pharmacological studies showing evidence of therapeutic synergism among these drugs,[150] produced no statistically significant differences in response rates or survival. The duration of response differed somewhat between treatments, with $P < 0.04$ (three-way analysis) favouring standard dose MTX.

Williams *et al.*[145] randomized 220 patients in the Southeastern Cancer Study Group (SECSG) to either MTX or DDP + vinblastine (VLB) + BLM. Analysis of 136 evaluable cases showed no significant differences in response rates, duration of responses, or survival. Interestingly, a statistically significant difference in response rates favouring the combination (43%) over MTX alone (9%) did occur in patients with distant metastases (almost one-third of patients in each treatment arm).

In another ECOG study, Vogl and Schoenfeld[146] compared standard MTX versus MTX + DDP + BLM given on an ambulatory basis. In earlier Phase II trials this combination had produced impressive response rates suggesting superiority over the historical experience with MTX. The randomized trial, however, showed some improvement in response rate with the combination but no superiority in response duration or survival.

Jacobs *et al.*[147] compared DDP alone versus a combination of DDP and moderate-dose MTX + LR in 80 evaluable patients. The combination showed no significant superiority over the single agent and was significantly more toxic.

TABLE 14.11   RANDOMIZED TRIALS

Investigators and treatment	Evaluable patients*	Response CR + PR	Response Rate (%)	Duration response	Duration survival	Toxicity
Lehane et al.[144]						
(a) MTX (15 mg/m²/dx3 IM, Q 3 wks) vs	106[a]	35	33	17 wks median	30 wks median	Slightly more myelotoxicity with arm (b)
(b) MTX (15 mg/m²/dx3 IM) MeCCNU (200 mg/m² PO) d 1 BLM (12.5 u/m² IM on wks 3, 4, 5, and 6 Repeated Q 6 wks	90[a]	21	24	14 wks median	26 wks median	
Williams et al.[145]						
(a) MTX (45–60 mg/m² IV) weekly vs.	68[a]	11	16	21 wks	29 wks	Toxicity roughly comparable. Arm (a) slightly more myelosuppression and mucositis; arm (b) more renal and GI effects.
(b) DDP (60 mg/m²) d 1 VLB (0.1 mg/kg) d 1 and 15 BLM (15 u IV weekly)	66[a]	13	20	16 wks	23 wks	
Vogl and Schoenfeld[146]						
(a) MTX (40–60 mg/m²/wk) vs.	83[a]	29	35	5 months median time to progression	Both (a) and (b) – 5.6 months	Arm (b) slightly more toxic
(b) MTX (40 mg/m²) d 1 and 15 BLM (10 u IM) d 1, 8, and 15 DDP (50 mg/m² IV) d 4	81[a]	39	48	5.8 months median time to progression		
Jacobs et al.[147]						
(a) DDP (80 mg/m²) Q 3 wks vs.	41[a]	7	18	Median time to progression 210 days	Median 370 days	Arm (b) more toxic; myelosuppression and mucositis
(b) DDP (80 mg/m²) Q 3 wks MTX (250 mg/m² + LR) Q wk	39[a]	13	33	140 days	267 days	

TABLE 14.11 Cont.

Investigators and treatment	Evaluable patients*	Response CR + PR	Response Rate (%)	Duration response	Duration survival	Toxicity
Drelichman et al.[148] (a) MTX (40 mg/m² IV) weekly	24[a]	8	33	NA	24 wks median	No severe toxicity with either arm. More nausea and vomiting with (b); more stomatitis and diarrhoea with (a)
vs. (b) DDP (100 mg/m² IV) d 1 with hydration and diuresis VCR (1 mg d 2 and 5) BLM (30 u as 96 h continuous infusion) d 2–5 Repeated Q 21 d × 3 Allopurinol (300 mg PO) daily	27[a]	11	41		17 wks median	
Davis and Kessler[149] (a) DDP (3 mg/kg IV over 4–6 h) with diuresis	30[a]	4	13	mean 4.2 months	NA	Arm (a) major toxicity was renal; renal and myelosuppression in arm (b); nausea and vomiting in both arms
vs. (b) DDP (as above) MTX (50 mg/m² IV) d 1 and 15 BLM (15 mg/m² IV) 2 × weekly. Repeated Q 4 wks	27[a]	3	11	mean 5.2 months	NA	
DeConti and Schoenfeld[48] (a) MTX (40 mg/m² IV bolus) weekly	81[a]	21	26	105 days median	154 days median	(a) Significantly more skin and mucosal toxicity; (c) more haematological toxicity than other
(b) MTX (240 mg/m² IV bolus + LR) Q 2 wks	80[a]	19	24	42 days median	133 days median	
(c) MTX + LR, as in (b) CTX (0.5 g/m² rapid IV infusion just before MTX) ARA-C (300 mg/m² IV/15 min., after MTX)	76[a]	14	18	49 days median	98 days median	

Investigators and treatment	Evaluable patients*	Response		Duration response	Duration survival	Toxicity
		CR + PR	Rate (%)			
Clavel *et al.* (EORTC)[149a]						
(a) *DDP* (50 mg/m² IV) d 4 *MTX* (40 mg/m² IV) d 1 and 15 *VCR* (2 mg IV) d 1, 8 and 15 *BLM* (10 u IV) d 1, 8 and 15	17[a]	8	47	NA	NA	Mild overall toxicities; (b) less nausea and vomiting
(b) As above without DDP						
Browman *et al.*[125b]						
(a) *MTX* (200 mg/m² IV)	13[a]	5	38	Median duration for all responders in both (a) and (b) 5.5 months	NA	Moderate diarrhoea, conjunctivitis and leucopenia in both arms
5FU (600 mg/m² IV 1h after MTX) *LCV* (at 24 h courses given on d 1 and 8, Q 3 wks) (sequential)	21[b]	6	29		NA	
(b) *5FU* just before *MTX* at the same doses with *LCV*	16[a]	11	68		NA	
(simultaneous)	23[b]	13	57		NA	
Tejada *et al.*[50]						
(a) *MTX* (50 mg/m² PO) weekly	21[a]	5	24	NA	NA	Minimal to moderate reversible to tolerable
(b) *MTX* (25 mg/m² PO) d 1 and 2 weekly	20[a]	13	65	NA	NA	
(c) *MTX* (50 mg/m² PO) d 1 *DDP* (20 mg/m² IV) d 1	21[a]	13	62	NA	NA	

* Prior therapy: [a] surgery and/or RT as primary treatment — no prior chemotherapy;
                  [b] previously untreated

TABLE 14.12   UNCONTROLLED ADJUVANT CHEMOTHERAPY TRIALS*

Investigators and induction chemotherapy	Patients†	Response to induction	Comment
Randolph et al.[158] Wittes et al.[159]			
(a) DDP (120 mg/m² IV) d 1, with diuresis BLM (10 mg/m² IVP) d 3 BLM (10 mg/m² CIVI) d 3–10 Repeat DDP on d 22	21 (Stage IV, unresectable)	Overall 71% 4 CR (19%) 11 PR (52%)	See text
(b) MTX (40 mg/m²) VLB – (7 mg/m²), and BLM (20 mg/m² IV) d 1 BLM (20 mg/m² CIVI) d 1–4 DDP (100 mg/m²) d 5	21 (Stage III and IV)	10 PR (48%)	Severely myelotoxic; follow-up too brief for analysis of survival and time to progression
(c) DDP (120 mg/m² IV) max. 3 doses	22 (Stage III and IV)	Overall 40% 1 CR (4%) 8 PR (36%)	Maximal responses observed by 3rd course; follow-up too brief for survival analysis
Elias et al[160] DDP (100 mg/m² IV) with hydration and diuresis BLM (15 mg/m² IVP; then 15 mg/m² /d x 5 CIVI) MTX (1.5 g/m² over 36 h + LR) 1 course	(A) 22 (Stage III and IV) (B) 11 (Prior surgery and/or RT)	Overall 73% 4 CR (18%) 12 PR (54%) 6 PR (55%)	See text
Pennachio et al.[161] DDP (120 mg/m²) (d 1' and 22, with hydration and diuresis BLM (15 mg/m² IVP followed by 15 mg/m²/d CIVI) d 3–9	41 (2 prior surgery or RT) (Stage IV, unresectable)	Overall 70% 7 CR (17%) 22 PR (53%)	Nineteen patients became resectable after induction. See text
Spaulding et al.[162] DDP (80 mg/m²) d 1, with hydration and diuresis VCR (1.4 mg/m² IVP) d 2, followed in 6 h by BLM (15 mg/m²/d x 5 CIVI) Repeat course d 22	47 (49 primaries) (Stage III and IV resectable)	Overall 89% 11 CR (22%) 33 PR (67%)	See text
Amrein et al.[162a] DDP (80 mg/m² 24 h. CIVI) with hydration and diuresis d 1 VCR (1 mg/m² IV) d 3 BLM (15 u/m² IV Bolus and 15 u/m² CIVI) d 2–5	37 (Stage III and IV) 18 resectable (19 unresectable)	Overall 67% 2 CR (5%) 23 PR (62%)	Median survival for the entire group not reached at the time of the report. Estimated median survival for patients with resectable disease was 16 months.

Investigators and induction chemotherapy	Patients†	Response to induction	Comment
Price and Hill[120,163] In a 24 h period on d 1 and d 14: VCR (2 mg IV) at 0 h BLM (60 mg/6 h CIVI) from 12–18 h MTX (100 mg IV) at 12, 15 and 18 h Hydrocortisone (500 mg IVP at 12 and 18 h) 5FU (500 mg IV) at 18 h LR (15 mg PO or IM Q 6 h × 4) Starting at 26 h	195 (Stage III and IV)	Overall 67% (8 CR and 123 PR)	Most responsive sites were nasopharynx and oral cavity. *See text*
Weaver et al.[164] DDP (100 mg/m² IV) d 1, with hydration and diuresis BLM (30 mg/d CIVI) d 2–5 VCR (1 mg IV) d 2 and 5 Repeat course in 3 wks	75 (Stage III and IV)	Overall 80% 21 CR (28%) 39 PR (52%)	Median survival for Stage III 91.3 wks vs. 67.1 wks for Stage IV. *See text*
Kish et al.[134] DDP (100 mg/m² IVP) with hydration and diuresis 5FU (1 g/m²/d CIVI × 4 days) Allopurinol 300 mg daily 2 courses, at 3 wk intervals	26 (2 prior RT) (Stage IV unresectable)	Overall 88% 5 CR (19%) 18 PR (69%)	*See text*
Weaver et al.[165] DDP (100 mg/m² IVP) with hydration and diuresis 5FU (1 g/m²/d CIVI + 5 days) Allopurinol, 300 mg daily 3 courses, at 3 wk intervals	61 (Stage III and IV)	Overall 93% 33 CR (54%) 24 PR (39%)	*See text*
Perry et al.[166] VLB (4 mg/m² IV) d 1 BLM (15 mg IM) d 1–7 DDP (60 mg/m² IV) d 8 2–4 courses	64 (Stage III and IV)	Overall 66% 14 CR (22%) 28 PR (44%)	Median survival of entire group was 15.6 months. After surgery and/or RT, no clear survival advantage due to induction CT at 36 months follow-up compared to historical controls
Feldmann et al.[167] BLM (30 mg) CTX (300 mg/m²) ADM (30 mg/m²) DDP (30 mg/m²) 2 courses	18 (Stage III and IV)	Overall 100% 6 CR (33%) 12 PR (66%)	10 (55%) disease-free after 2–24 months follow-up

TABLE 14.12 Cont.

Investigators and induction chemotherapy	Patients†	Response to induction	Comment
Schaefer *et al.*[168] DDP (100 mg/m² CIVI 16 h on d 1 and d 21)	28 (Stage IV inoperable and incurable by RT alone)	Overall 36% 1 PR (3.5%) 9 improved (32%)	11 (39%) had a CR after RT. 19 patients had their disease controlled after treatment (16 CT + RT + S, 3 CR + RT) with a median survival of 15 months.
Popkin *et al.*[169] BLM (15 mg/m² IVP) followed by: BLM (15 mg/m²/d × 7 CIVI)	20	Overall 30% 1 CR 5 PR	7-day CIVI appeared to yield a response rate similar to intermittent IV bolus.
Israel *et al.*[170] (a) DDP (20 mg/m²/d × 5) BLM (5 mg/m²/d × 5 CIVI)	57 (12 inoperable)	Overall 78% 10 CR (17%) (8 CRs in resectable patients)	Projected 2-year survival 53% for operable patients and 38% for inoperable patients
(b) DDP + BLM (as above) Mitomycin C (6 mg/m²) d 1, Q 3 wks	53 (9 inoperable)	Overall 90% 13 CR (24%) (12 CRs in resectable patients)	Projected 12 months survival 92% for operable patients and 51% for inoperable patients
Ervin *et al.*[171] MTX (3–7 g/m²/wk × 4 + LR) Responders given added 4 weekly courses after local therapy	21 (Stage IV unresectable)	11 PR (52%)	6 PRs (55%) disease-free at 3 years; 8 PRs were resectable after induction CT
Schuller *et al.*[172] DDP (50 mg/m² IV) d 1 MTX (40 mg/m²) d 1 BLM (15 mg/m² IV or IM) d 1 and 8 VCR (2 mg IVP) d 1 Q 3 wks × 3	58 (Stage III and IV)	Overall 66% 15 CR (26%)	Primary goal was to obtain pilot data for a prospective randomized trial. Principal interest was response rate to induction CT and acute toxicity

Investigators and induction chemotherapy	Patients†	Response to induction	Comment
Glick et al.[173] DDP (80–100 mg/m² 24 h CIVI) d 1 BLM (15 mg/m² IVP) d 3; then CIVI (15 mg/m²/d × 5) d 3–7 Repeat CP on d 22	29 (Stage III and IV unresectable)	14 PR (48%)	Median follow-up of 13 months (4–19 months) 12 alive NED and 8 alive with disease
Marcial et al.[174] VCR (1.5 mg/m² IVP) followed in 6 h by BLM (15 mg/d 48 h CIVI) followed in 24 h by MTX IV, IM, or IA (200 mg/m²) Q 6 h × 4 + LR	39 (33 evaluated after CT) (37 evaluated after RT and surgery)	Overall 61% 2 CR (6%) 18 PR (54%)	After CT, RT yielded 17 CR (46%); this was increased to 24 CR (65%) with surgery on 7 post-RT failures. Median survival was 11 months
Vogl et al.[175] (a) MTX (40 mg/m² IM) d 1 and 15 BLM (10 mg IM) d 1, 8 and 15 DDP (50 mg/m² IV) d 4 Q 3 wks × 2	9	6 PR	Median survival for all patients and median time to progression for CRs (after total therapy) were both 10 months. All but 2 patients were dead by 30 months
(b) MTX, BLM and DDP (as above) Mitomycin-C (10 mg/m² IV) d 1 Q 3 wks × 2	13	Overall 77% (17/22) 2 CR 9 PR	
Ervin et al.[197] Two 4-wk courses: DDP (20 mg/m²) d 1–5 as 2 h infusion after hydration BLM (10 u/m²) d 3–7 as continuous infusion MTX (200 mg/m²) d 15 and 22 + LR)	93 (mostly Stage IV)	88% overall 24% CR	Median follow-up 14.5 months. Disease-free survival appeared to correlate with response. 89% of the responders became disease-free after local therapy versus 20% of non-responders. Dose-limiting toxicity in 15%.

* Abbreviations: IVP – IV push; CIVI – continuous IV infusion; CT – chemotherapy; RT – radiotherapy
† Only evaluable patients, previously untreated, unless otherwise stated.

Among the remaining three smaller trials one[50,148,149] suggested an advantage for the combination over the single agent. Tejada *et al.*[50] reported significant differences in response rates favouring MTX + DDP or split-dose MTX over standard MTX. Because of the small patient population in each treatment arm, however, definite conclusions are impossible.

An ongoing randomized trial by the European Organization for Research on the Treatment of Cancer (EORTC)[149a] is comparing the combination of MTX, VCR, and BLM with the same drugs plus DDP; interim results indicate slightly higher response rates for the platinum-containing combinations.

ADJUVANT CHEMOTHERAPY

Although surgery and radiotherapy are relatively effective in controlling early disease, approximately 40–50% of the more advanced cases can be expected to recur locoregionally, and 20–25% will develop distant metastases.[151] As demonstrated in the previous section, chemotherapy is of very limited value in patients with reccurent and/or metastatic disease but appears to have greater activity in previously untreated patients. Accordingly chemotherapy has been applied as the initial treatment of patients with advanced head and neck cancer in the hope that such treatment may:

(1) significantly reduce tumour bulk and improve chances for local control and perhaps cure;
(2) eradicate small foci of subclinical disease elsewhere and thus reduce the chances of systemic relapse.

In addition, if it can be shown clearly that the addition of chemotherapy to standard local therapy improves local control rates, one can easily imagine the possibility that the need for extensive and radical surgical operations could be revised in favour of more anatomically conservative procedures.

Extensive preclinical investigations support the use of adjuvant chemotherapy administered after treatment of the primary tumour. The fundamental background for the clinical application is found in the basic principles of the cell-kill hypothesis of Skipper *et al.*[152] A single cancer cell is capable of proliferating to massive and lethal numbers; a relationship exists between drug dose and schedule and cytotoxicity; a given dose level of a drug or drug combination kills a constant fraction of tumour cells, rather than a fixed cell number. Several cytokinetic studies[153–155] on the effect of the size of the tumour burden have found a higher percentage of dividing cells in smaller tumours, which theoretically should be more sensitive to cytotoxic drugs. On the other hand there are no good animal models for the use of chemotherapy as initial treatment, in the manner most commonly employed in the clinic for advanced head and neck cancer. Theoretically one might worry about the likelihood of having efficient selection of a resistant cell population if chemotherapy is used when body burden of tumour is maximal, instead of after initial cytoreduction.

The first large-scale trial in the United States was performed by the Radiation Therapy Oncology Group (RTOG) in largely unresectable Stage IV patients randomized to pre-irradiation MTX versus the same radiation doses and schedules alone.[156] This trial failed to demonstrate any advantage for the MTX-treated group over the controls. Tarpley *et al.*[157] at the National Cancer Institute treated patients with resectable disease with high-dose MTX plus LR repeated twice before surgery performed between days 12 and 15. When the disease-free interval of the MTX-treated patients was compared to that of matched historical controls from the same institution, there was a statistically significant difference (10.13 months for MTX *vs* 6.78 months for controls). However, the two groups showed no significant differences in survival and incidence of recurrence.

These two early studies showed the feasibility of giving chemotherapy prior to local treatment. After 1975 the identification of DDP as an active agent and the proliferation of active combinations with tolerable toxicity and higher response rates prompted the design of new studies.

Uncontrolled Trials

The group at the Memorial Sloan–Kettering Cancer Center[158] initially reported high response rates in unresectable Stage IV patients treated with combined DDP and BLM ('a', Table 14.12). There were four CR and 11 PR for an overall response rate of 71%. Nineteen of the 21 patients subsequently received radiotherapy; at 2-year follow-up all but one had recurred with a median time to progression of 12 months for those who had CRs and 8 months for PRs. Long-term benefits were not apparent in this group, but the study did show that DDP-based therapy was feasible in the context of multimodality treatment. The same group of investigators[159] subsequently tested DDP alone and combined with MTX, VLB, and BLM without apparent improvement in response rates compared to DDP and BLM, and, in the case of the combinations with MTX, with much-increased toxicity.

These results with DDP and BLM were confirmed in trials at the Boston Veterans Administration Hospital,[161] where similar remission induction rates were achieved. At the completion of subsequent local therapy the CR rate was 73%. After 20 months follow-up 53% of the patients were alive; the median survival had not been reached, but was projected at 29 months. The overall disease-free survival was 41% (17/41). In patients who received chemotherapy, surgery, and radiotherapy the overall median survival and disease-free survival were 21.7 and 17 months respectively; for chemotherapy and radiotherapy these were 20 and 18 months. All seven patients who were CRs after chemotherapy were alive at 20 months and six were disease-free. The survivorship of the study population was superior to that of 41 historical controls treated with radiotherapy only.

Elias *et al.*[160] evaluated DDP + BLM +

HD–MTX–LR induction therapy in 22 untreated patients (Group A) and in 11 who had previous local therapy (Group B). The overall response rate was 66% (22/33), including 73% for the Group A patients and 55% in Group B. Eighteen of the 22 patients in Group A received all three drugs, while four could tolerate only DDP and BLM. Of the 22 Group A patients, 12 underwent surgery and six received radiotherapy; at 6–18 months follow-up, 17 were still alive (10 disease-free).

Using DDP, BLM, and VCR as induction, Spaulding *et al.*[162] reported a response rate of 89% (22% CR, 67% PR) in 47 patients. A significant increase in the probability of disease-free and overall survival was reported when the resectable patients were compared to a multi-institution historical control group. However, the extent of disease was not specified for patients in the study population or for the historical controls, and this alone could account for the difference observed.

Amrein *et al.*[162a] with a similar combination incorporating DDP by 24-hour continuous intravenous infusion, reported somewhat lower response rates (67%) in 37 previously untreated patients. Estimated median survival for all patients was 16 months; among 18 patients with resectable disease 51% remained disease-free at 12 months and median survival was 16 months.

Price and Hill[120,163] used kinetic considerations in designing a multi-drug regimen that yielded an overall response rate of 67% (131/195), including eight CR and 123 PR. Following radiotherapy, the CR rate was 63% (124/195); among the responders to chemotherapy the rate was 72% (94/131) versus 47% (30/64) among non-responders. The median survival after attainment of CR therapy was 52.4 months vs. 7.8 months in patients who still had residual disease; 46% of the former group were alive at 5 years in contrast to 9% of the latter patients. Median survival for induction chemotherapy responders was superior to non-responding patients (33 months vs. 20 months). It seems quite clear from these data that attainment of CR is a good prognostic sign. Because of the lack of a randomized control group, however, the ultimate efficacy of the regimen is still unproved.

Al-Sarraf and his associates investigated two different drug combinations in three sequential studies in patients with resectable and unresectable Stage III and IV disease.[134,164,165] In the first trial[164] DDP + BLM + VCR produced significant response rates (28% CR; 52% PR) among 75 patients; 68 subsequently underwent surgery and/or radiotherapy. Overall median survival was significantly better for responders to chemotherapy than for non-responders (CRs, 80 weeks; PRs, 79 weeks; less than PR, 35 weeks).

The second combination,[134] DDP + 5FU + allopurinol, was given in two courses to 26 inoperable Stage IV patients. An overall response rate of 88% (23/26) was observed (19% CR, 69% PR), and 21 of the responders underwent radiotherapy and/or surgery. After at least 1 year of follow-up, 13 patients were still alive without evidence of disease.

These encouraging results led to the third trial,[165] which increased the period of 5FU infusion to 5 days and the number of chemotherapy courses to three. The overall response rate among 61 patients was 93%, including a particularly impressive CR rate of 54% (33/61). Thirteen of the complete responders underwent surgery, with nine showing no histological evidence of tumour at the primary site or in the neck dissection specimen; eight other CRs also showed no tumour in biopsies before radiotherapy. Thus, more than 50% of the clinical CRs had no histological evidence of residual tumour after chemotherapy. Paradoxically, the very efficacy of this drug regimen brought with it its own problems in patient management. Subsequent local therapy was intended in all – but 17 patients, 13 of them with CRs, refused surgery after chemotherapy. Although 11 eventually received radiotherapy, six refused all additional treatment; three of these suffered recurrence in 4–7 months. Efforts to confirm the activity of this regimen are presently in progress at several centres. One important

additional observation is that the failure to achieve response (at least 25% tumour reduction) to induction chemotherapy was almost invariably associated with a low likelihood of obtaining tumour clearance with subsequent local treatment. This might not be due specifically to an absence of tumour sensitivity to chemotherapy, but rather to other tumour and/or host factors associated with generally poor prognosis and unresponsiveness to any form of therapy.

Response to chemotherapy or other modalities is usually defined by reduction in bulk of primary tumour and neck nodes. Data from these pilot trials suggest that response to chemotherapy, particularly complete response, may be more probable with decreasing initial bulk of disease (Table 14.13), though this relationship, if real, certainly is not a striking one quantitatively. It is not clear whether probability of response in these trials has any relationship to degree of differentiation in head and neck carcinomas. Such relationships, if they exist, will probably only be convincingly demonstrated in the context of large clinical trials showing relatively high CR rates.

In summary the uncontrolled trials performed to date suggest that response rates to chemotherapy in previously untreated patients are indeed higher than in those who have already failed local therapy. Furthermore, the use of chemotherapy initially does not appear

TABLE 14.13 COMPLETE RESPONSE RATE TO CHEMOTHERAPY ACCORDING TO PRIMARY TUMOUR SIZE AND NODAL STATUS[158,161,165]

Tumour size and nodal status	Number of CRs	Total patients	CR rate (%)
T3 or less	29	62	47
T4	17	57	30
Total	46	119	39
N0 & N1	10	26	39
N2 & N3	25	80	31
Total	35	106	33

to interfere with subsequent surgery or radiotherapy, provided that the patients consent to local treatment; the experience at Wayne State University, however, indicates that this may be a significant problem in precisely those patients for whom the stakes are highest (the CRs).

Controlled Trials

The encouraging preliminary results in many of the pilot studies discussed previously have motivated a few controlled clinical trials of adjuvant chemotherapy. The vast majority of the pilot studies have explored the feasibility of using chemotherapy as initial treatment, rather than as a post-surgical or post-radiation adjuvant. This is sharp contrast to the preferred strategy in other epithelial cancers such as breast in which chemotherapy has usually followed local therapy. The apparent preference of head and neck oncologists for initial chemotherapy is probably a result of the preoccupation with local control that has been such a persistently difficult problem in advanced stages; the striking tumour regressions that chemotherapy produces in previously untreated patients have made it reasonable to anticipate improved locoregional control rates if chemotherapy is given when tumour is maximally responsive.

In addition, the use of chemotherapy as an adjuvant *after* completion of local treatment has certain problems when applied to head and neck cancers. Local therapy in these diseases, unlike breast cancer for example, is often protracted, involving combinations of one or more surgical resections, reconstructive procedures, and radiotherapy. The post-operative period is frequently marked by major or minor problems with wound infections, graft or flap viability, and nutrition. All these features of local therapy impose inevitable delays on the start of any planned chemotherapy regimen, delays which might well prejudice chances of success. Moreover, patients who have been through the rigors of combined local therapy may be disinclined to subject themselves to the inconveniences and potential toxicity of

systemic chemotherapy. There are currently no hard data on whether patients with head and neck tumours are less likely to agree to such an approach than other patients. For whatever reasons, however, no such trials have been completed and reported in the literature.

Of all the controlled studies, only one has been reported in final form. As previously discussed, the RTOG randomized 712 patients with Stage III and IV disease to receive either MTX (25 mg IV Q 3 days for a total of five doses) prior to irradiation or the same dose of irradiation alone.[156] No differences between the two groups emerged in time to progression or survival. A multivariate analysis failed to demonstrate any advantage of either treatment for various sub-groups according to primary site and initial stage of disease.

Tejada and Chandler[176] have treated Stage III and IV patients with a timed sequence of MTX and DDP; treatment design was based on experimentally determined head and neck cancer kinetic perturbations.[50] Patients were subsequently randomized to receive either maintenance chemotherapy, as given for induction, or no further treatment. A preliminary analysis has shown no differences in time to progression or survival.

The Head and Neck Contracts Program, a multi-institutional consortium supported by the NCI, has completed accrual on a three-arm adjuvant trial for patients with Stage III and IV resectable epidermoid cancer from six sites in the oral cavity and larynx. In this trial the following treatment policies are compared in prospective randomized fashion: (1) standard local therapy (surgery and postoperative irradiation); (2) initial chemotherapy with DDP + BLM, followed by standard local therapy; (3) same as arm (2), followed by six treatments at monthly intervals with 24-hour infusions of DDP. Preliminary results[177] indicate an overall response rate of approximately 49% (7% CR) to the single course of induction chemotherapy. Analysis of treatment effects on time to relapse, patterns of relapse, and survival is in progress. Results from this trial will be very important as a point of departure for future multimodality studies, since it represents the only large-scale controlled study of the efficacy of a cisplatin-based regimen. Table 14.14 illustrates the design of the above studies and some of the currently open randomized trials of combined modality treatment in this disease.

INTRA-ARTERIAL CHEMOTHERAPY

Intra-arterial chemotherapy (IAC) has been used for over 20 years in the treatment of localized tumours; the rationale is that delivery of high drug concentrations to such tumours will yield better tumour cell kill and minimize systemic toxicity.[178,179] With a natural history characterized by local recurrence, and the presence of a well-defined vascular supply, many head and neck cancers are suitable for regional drug delivery. Use of this approach also has been prompted by encouraging results obtained with various drugs administered IA in different organs.[180,181]

Nevertheless, these factors alone do not provide sufficient grounds for widespread use of IAC. Certain pharmacokinetic considerations must be observed in choosing a target organ and drug(s), i.e. the total body clearance of a given drug, the perfusion rate of the target organ, and the extraction ratio of the drug by the target region.[182-184] Areas with low perfusion rates and drugs that are rapidly eliminated from the body (high total body clearance) offer ideal settings for IAC. Similarly, use of a drug with a high ratio of extraction by the target organ decreases systemic toxicity by limiting the total amount of drug available to the circulation. Other factors of concern in the use of IAC include the mechanism(s) of drug action, the duration of exposure and the tumour doubling time. Theoretically, tumours with short doubling times are more sensitive to cell-cycle-specific agents such as MTX and may be killed more efficiently as infusion is prolonged. On the other hand, tumours with longer doubling times may be more effectively treated by the alkylating agents or

anthracycline antibiotics, where the length of infusion may be less crucial to cytotoxicity.[184,185] Unfortunately, these principles have been applied infrequently in clinical studies.

Techniques

The most common approach for IA infusion is by retrograde placement of a catheter through the superficial temporal artery,[186,187] a technique successful in 75% of the cases. Occasionally the catheter is positioned in the common carotid artery through an incision in the neck. More recently, with the introduction of totally implantable infusion pumps, many of the complications of IA infusion have been overcome.[188] The pump is placed in a subcutaneous pocket superficial to the fascia of the pectoral major muscle and a branch of the external carotid that does not infuse the region of the neoplasm is selected to receive the catheter. The catheter tip is advanced until it is located at the origin of the vessel from the external carotid, and then it is securely tied.

Clinical Studies

The early trials of IAC in head and neck cancer were prompted by the activity of intravenous MTX. In summarizing 19 studies of MTX by intra-arterial infusion, Carter[45] noted that the overall response rate of 53% in 340 evaluable patients did not suggest clearcut superiority over that obtained by systemic administration.

Combination regimens have also been studied by this route. In a 10-year series (1961–71) comprising 94 patients with advanced head and neck cancer at the Lahey Clinic Foundation, Oberfield *et al.*[186] employed prolonged IA infusion of 5FU, FUdR and MTX-leucovorin. Most patients had failed previous surgery and radiotherapy. Of the 94 patients, 47 achieved at least a 30% objective tumour regression, including 19 with at least 50% and 24 with 100% regression. Among the 24 complete responders, regression persisted for more than 6 months in 10, and for more than 1 year in nine. Nineteen of the 24 complete

TABLE 14.14   RANDOMIZED TRIALS OF COMBINED MODALITY TREATMENT IN THE UNITED STATES

Investigators	Study	Design	
Tejada *et al.*[176]	*MTX* (50 mg/m² PO) d 1 *DDP* (20 mg/m² IV) d 2 *wkly × 4* → Surgery and/or RT →		*MTX + CP* for 1 year
HNCP[177]	(A) No therapy →	→	No therapy
	(B) *DDP* (100 mg/m²) d 1 *BLM* (15 mg/m² IV) d 3; then 15/mg² CIVI, d 3–7 *1 course* →	S U R G E R Y [box]	No therapy G + RT
	(C) *DDP + BLM* as above →		*CP* (80 mg/m²) 24 hr CIVI monthly × 6
SEG Protocol 356	(A) *MTX* (70 mg/m² IV) Q 6 h × 4 + LR *BLM* (30 mg IV) weekly × 6 *DDP* (2 mg/kg) Q 3 wks × 2 → Surgery ± RT		
	(B) No therapy		
SWOG Protocol 8006	(A) *DDP* (50 mg/m² IV) d 1 *MTX* (40 mg/m² IV) d 1 *BLM* (15 mg/m² IV) d 1, 8 *VCR* (2 mg IV) Q 3 wks Repeat Q 3 wks × 3 → Surgery ± RT		
	(B) No therapy		

responders survived longer than 6 months and 13 (54%) survived over 1 year. As usual, objective regression was associated with increased duration of response and survival.

Toxicity in this series was common, with 45% of the patients experiencing systemic effects, including two deaths, and 30% having local side-effects. Technical complications, such as inadequate catheter placement, premature displacement or leakage, occurred in 44%. Objective regression was related to systemic toxicity, i.e. better responses were seen in patients with severe toxicity, but survival was markedly decreased in comparison to patients without toxicity. On the other hand, mild to moderate toxicity correlated with better response-survival.

In a smaller trial,[189] a combination of 5FU, MTX, and BLM was administered IA in 15 patients whose tumours were refractory to radiotherapy or radiotherapy plus surgical resection. Thirteen (87%) of the cancers regressed to some extent, but only six of these were greater than 50% regressions. The median duration of response was only 2.5 months; actuarial 1-year survival was 32%.

A more recent study[190] employed IAC with BLM and MTX (plus leucovorin) prior to high-dose radiotherapy and, where possible, surgery. This prospective trial conducted between 1973 and 1978 included 20 patients, of whom 18 were evaluable for response and toxicity. Catheters were placed in the external carotid artery via the superficial temporal artery and placement was confirmed by injection of fluorescein. The 9-day drug regimen consisted of 24-hour infusion of BLM (0.75 mg/kg; maximum daily dose, 60 mg) alternating every other day with MTX (0.5 mg/kg daily; maximum daily dose, 25 mg); leucovorin was given each day after MTX administration. The mean interval between IAC and radiation therapy was 2 weeks (range 1–4 weeks); between radiation and surgery it was 6 weeks (range 4–8 weeks).

After IAC, five (28%) of the 18 patients had a partial response while seven had minimal responses; six tumours did not change. There

was no complete tumour regression after IAC alone. The combination of IAC and radiation therapy was used in all 18 patients and produced six complete and seven partial responses, as well as three minor responses. Surgery was performed in 11 patients. At the end of all therapy, 10 (56%) of the 18 patients were judged free of disease; nine of them had undergone surgery, and one was operable but refused hemiglossectomy. Two patients had persistent disease after surgery and six suffered from persistent, unresectable tumours after IAC and radiotherapy. The best results were obtained in patients with tumours of the maxillary antrum; here, four of five patients were alive and free of disease 29, 24, 18, and 12 months after beginning treatment.

Toxicity in this study was moderate. Four patients suffered complications due to catheterization. In two of them the catheters had to be removed between the sixth and eighth days because of extravasation. Another patient had a mild paralysis of the forehead after the incision and thrombosis occurred in one patient's catheter.

Many other studies in the United States and abroad have been conducted using combinations of MTX with mitomycin C, ADM, 5FU, VLB, and BLM.[191–194] All have reported response rates between 50% and 70% in patients previously unexposed to chemotherapy. However, few have reported duration of response; in those that have, the median duration has always been less than 8 months.

Future Directions

After two decades of use the role of IAC in head and neck cancer remains to be clearly defined. The lack of controlled trials comparing IAC *versus* conventional IV regimens prevents any reasonable conclusions about its relative efficacy in the palliation of advanced disease or in reducing tumour burden prior to radiotherapy or surgery. Although response rates in some studies appear to be higher with IAC[186,189,190,192] than with systemic treatment, this has not been translated into meaningful survival advantage.

CONCLUSIONS

As we have seen, chemotherapy has very limited utility in patients who have already failed local therapy or who have distant metastases on presentation. A minority of such patients may be expected to respond to treatment, and responses, even when achieved, only last a few months in the majority of cases. Long-term disease-free survival is not therefore a realistic goal of therapy for this subset of patients with the drugs currently available.

This state of affairs has important implications for the testing of experimental drugs. Since patients without prior chemotherapy are in better general condition than their counterparts who have already failed one or more drug regimens and are less likely to exhibit drug resistance, such patients should be the focus of new drug testing in the future. Once a patient has failed primary local therapy and is not likely to be cured by further local measures, he should be given the opportunity of participating in trials of new therapies, if such studies are available in his community or within reasonable referral range.

Provided that a meaningful informed consent is obtained, the policy of suggesting experimental chemotherapy before standard drugs poses no ethical problem at all, since the efficacy of conventional chemotherapy is so limited. A judgement about the effectiveness of a new drug can usually be made 4 – 6 weeks after start of treatment, and the patient can quickly be switched to standard therapy if the new drug is not helping. By restricting trials of new agents to patients with no prior chemotherapy, the chance of missing an active agent is minimized, and patients who are unlikely to benefit are spared exposure to potentially toxic therapy. If the new drug turns out to be active in patients previously untreated with chemotherapy, those who have failed other drugs might then be entered in a second stage.

The short response durations of head and neck cancer have been one of its most frustrating features. Even trials which have documented a modest increase in response rate with the use of drug combinations[146] have failed to show a significant increase in time to progression. Why the emergence of clinically significant drug resistance should be such a striking problem with these tumours is, of course, unknown, but the clinical observation suggests that cells derived from these tumours might be an interesting and productive system for laboratory studies on mechanisms of drug resistance in human tumours.

The use of chemotherapy as an adjuvant to local treatment is now common practice, at least in centres which are devoted to cancer clinical trials. The literature is full of small pilot studies which have documented over and over again that the approach is feasible. Single-institution studies, however, cannot muster the sample sizes necessary for properly controlled trials of large numbers of patients; such trials will be necessary not only to answer questions of efficacy but also to approach the issues of primary site specificity and patterns of relapses, which are of great importance in designing new therapeutic strategies. In general the multimodality approach to head and neck cancer has not fared well in the cooperative groups; except for RTOG and more recently the Northern California Oncology Group, studies have suffered from lack of physician interest and poor patient accrual. Since most of the clinical cooperative groups in the US are based on medical oncology, the failure to accrue adequate numbers of previously untreated head and neck cancer patients is not surprising. It seems clear that a surgically based group such as the recent Head and Neck Contracts Group offers a much better chance of success.

REFERENCES

1. Silverberg, E. (1975). *CA-A Cancer Journal for Clinicians,* Jan./Feb., p.6.
2. Harrison, D., Espiner, H., and Glazebrook, G. (1963). In G. Fairley, and J. Simister, (Eds), *Cyclophosphamide,* Williams & Wilkins, Baltimore, p.48.

3. Foye, L.V., Chapman, C.G., Willett, F.M., and Adams, W.S. (1960). *Arch. Intern. Med.*, **106**, 365.

4. Solomon, J., Alexander, M.D., and Steinfeld, J.L. (1963). *JAMA*, **183**, 165.

5. Bergsagel, D., and Levin, W. (1968). *Cancer Chemother. Rep.*, **52**, 120.

6. Moore, G., Bross, I., Ausman, R., Nadler, S., Jones, R., Slack, N., and Rimm, A. (1968). *Cancer Chemother. Rep.*, **52**, 661.

7. Karnofsky, D., Abelman, W., Craver, L., and Burchenal, J. (1948). *Cancer*, **1**, 634.

8. Hurley, J., Ellison, E., Riesch, J., Schulte, W. (1960). *JAMA*, **174**, 1696.

9. Olson, K., and Greene, J. (1960). *J. Nat. Cancer Inst.*, **25**, 133.

10. Weiss, A., Jackson, L., and Carabasi, R. (1961). *Ann. Intern. Med.*, **55**, 731.

11. Staley, C., Kerth, J., Cortes, N., and Preston, F. (1961). *Surg. Gynecol. Obstet.*, **112**, 185.

12. Ansfield, F., Schroeder, J., and Curreri, A. (1962). *JAMA*, **181**, 295.

13. Moore, G., Bross, I., Ausman, R., Nadler, S., Jones, R., Slack, N., and Rimm, A. (1968). *Cancer Chemother. Rep.*, **52**, 641.

14. White, J., Ricketts, W., and Strudwick, W. (1962). *J. Nat. Med. Assoc.*, **54**, 315.

15. Gold, G., Hall, R., Shnider, B., Selawry, O., Colsky, J., Owens, A., Dederick, M., Holland, J., Brindley, C., and Jones, R. (1959). *Cancer Res.*, **19**, 935.

16. Young, C.W., Ellison, R., Sullivan, R., Levick, S., Kaufman, R., Miller, E., Woldow, I., Escher, G., Li, M., Karnofsky, D., and Burchenal, J. (1960). *Cancer Chemother. Rep.*, **6**, 17.

17. Jacobs, E., Luce, J., and Wood. D. (1968). *Cancer*, **22**, 1233.

18. Lerner, H., and Beckloff, G. (1968). *JAMA*, **192**, 1168.

19. Bloedow, C. (1964). *Cancer Chemother. Rep.*, **40**, 39.

20. Smart, C., Rochlin, D., Nahum, A., Silva, A., and Wagner, D. (1964). *Cancer Chemother. Rep.*, **34**, 31.

21. Kenis, Y., De Smedt, J., and Tagnon, H.J. (1966). *Eur. J. Cancer*, **2**, 51.

22. Krakoff, I.H. (1975). *Cancer Chemother. Rep.*, **6**, 253.

23. Blum, R.H., (1975). *Cancer Chemother. Rep.*, **6**, 247.

24. Humphrey, E., Hymes, A., Ausman, R., and Ferguson, D. (1961). *Surgery*, **50**, 881.

25. Papac, R.J., and Fisher, J.J. (1971). *Cancer Chemother. Rep.*, **55**, 193.

26. Marsh, J.C., DeConti, R.C., and Hubbard, S.P. (1971). *Cancer Chemother. Rep.*, **55**, 599.

27. Ramirez, G., Wilson, W., Grage, T., and Hill, G. (1972). *Cancer Chemother. Rep.*, **56**, 787.

28. Hoogstraten, B., Gottlieb, J., Caoili, E., Tucker, W.G., Talley, R.W., and Haut, A. (1973). *Cancer*, **32**, 38.

29. Broder, L.E., and Hansen, H.H. (1973). *Eur. J. Cancer*, **9**, 147.

30. DeConti, R.C., Hubbard, S.P., Pinch, P., and Bertino, J. (1973). *Cancer Chemother. Rep.*, **57**, 201.

31. Dowell, K.E., Armstrong, D.M., Aust, J.B., and Cruz A.B. Jr. (1975). *Cancer*, **35**, 1116.

32. Tranun, B.M., Haut, A., Rivkin, S., Weber, E., Quagliana, J.M., Shaw, M., Tucker, W.G., Smith, F.E., Samson, M., and Gottlieb, J. (1975). *Cancer*, **35**, 1148.

33. Firat, D., and Tekuzman, G. (1975). *Cancer Chemother. Rep.*, **59**, 1021.

34. Jackson, R.C., and Niethammer, D. (1977). *Eur. J. Cancer*, **13**, 567.

35. Zaharko, D.C., Fung, W., and Yang, K.H. (1977). *Cancer Res.*, **37**, 1602.

36. White, J.C. (1981). *Cancer Treat. Rep.*, **65**, (Suppl. 1), 3.

37. Goldin, A., Venditti, J.M., Kline, I., and Mantel, N. (1966). *Nature*, **212**, 1548.

38. Ensminger, W.D., and Frei, E. (1977). *Cancer Res.*, **37**, 1857.

39. Leyva, A., Nederbrogt, H., Lankelma, J., and Pinedo, H.M. (1981). *Cancer Treat. Rep.*, **65**, (Suppl. 1), 45.

40. Henderson, E.S., Adamson, R.H., and Oliverio, V.T. (1965). *Cancer Res.*, **25**, 1018.

41. Chabner, B.A., Donehower, R.C., and Schilsky, R.L. (1981). *Cancer Treat. Rep.*, **65**, (Suppl. 1), 51.

42. Jacobs, S.A., Stoller, R.G., Chabner, B.A., and Johns, D.G. (1976). *J. Clin. Invest.*, **57**, 534.

43. Solter, R.G., Hande, K.R., Jacobs, S.A., Rosenberg, S.A., and Chabner, B.A. (1977). *New Engl. J. Med.*, **297**, 630.

44. Bertino, J.R. (1981). *Cancer Treat. Rep.*, **65**, (Suppl. 1), 131.

45. Carter, S.K. (1977). *Sem. Oncol.*, **4**, 413.

46. Levitt, M., Mosher, M., DeConti, R., Farber, L., Skeel, R., Marsh, J., Mitchell, M., Papac, R., Thomas, E., and Bertino, J. (1973). *Cancer Res.*, **33**, 1729.

47. Woods, R.L., Fox, R.M., and Tattersall, M.H.N. (1981). *Br. Med. J.*, **282**, 600.

48. DeConti, R., and Schoenfeld, D. (1981). *Cancer*, **48**, 1061.

49. Kirkwood, J., Canellos, G., Ervin, T., Pitman, S., Weichselbaum, R., and Miller, D. (1981). *Cancer*, **47**, 2414.

50. Tejada, F., Murphy, E., and Zubrod, C.G.

(1980). *Proc. Int. Head and Neck Oncol. Conf.*, Abst. 2.14, National Cancer Institute.

51. Vogler, W., Jacobs, J., Moffitt, S., Velez-Garcia, E., Goldsmith, A., Johnson, L., and Mackay, S. (1979). *Cancer Clin. Trials*, **2**, 227.

52. Barranco, S.C., and Humphrey, R.M. (1971). *Cancer Res.*, **31**, 1218.

53. Saunders, G.F., Haidle, C.W., Saunders, P.P., and Kuo, M.T. (1975). In *Pharmacological Basis of Cancer Chemotherapy*, Williams & Wilkins, Baltimore, p.507.

54. Crooke, S.T. (1978). In S.K. Carter, *et al.* (Eds), *Bleomycin: Current Status and New Developments*, Academic Press, Baltimore, p.1.

55. Sikic, B.I., Collins, J., Mimnaugh, E., and Gram, T. (1978). *Cancer Treat. Rep.*, **62**, 2011.

56. Bonadonna, G., Tancini, G., and Bajetta, E. (1976). *Prog. Biochem. Pharmacol.*, **11**, 172.

57. Halnan, K.E., Bleehen, N.M., Berwin, T., Deelay, T., Harrison, D., Howland, C., Kunkles, P., Ritchie, G., Wiltshaw, E., and Todd, I. (1972). *Br. Med. J.*, **4**, 635.

58. Haas, C., Coltman, C., Gottlieb, J., Haut, A., Luce, J., Talley, R., Samol, B., Wilson, H., and Hoogstraten, B. (1976). *Cancer*, **38**, 8.

59. Yagoda, A., Mukherji, B., Young, C., Etcubanas, E., Lamonte, C., Smith, J., Tan, C., and Krakoff, I. (1972). *Ann. Intern. Med.*, **77**, 861.

60. Durkin, W.J., Pugh, R.P., Jacobs, E., Sadoff, L., Pajak, T., and Bateman, J. (1976). *Oncology*, **33**, 260.

61. EORTC Clinical Screening Group (1970). *Br. Med. J.*, **2**, 643.

62. Wasserman, T., Comis, R., Goldsmith, M., Handelsman, H., Penta, J., Slavik, M., Soper, W., and Carter, S.K. (1975). *Cancer Chemother. Rep.*, **6**, 399.

63. Turrisi, A., Rozencweig, M., Von Hoff, D., and Muggia, F. (1978). In S. Carter *et al.*, (Eds), *Bleomycin: Current Status and New Developments*, Academic Press, Baltimore, p.151.

64. Rosenberg, B., Van Camp, L., and Krigas, T. (1965). *Nature*, 205, 698.

65. Durant, J. (1980). In A. Prestayko *et al.* (Eds), *Cisplatin: Current Status and Future Developments*, Academic Press, p.317.

66. Prestayko, A. (1980). In A. Prestayko *et al.* (Eds), *Cisplatin: Current Status and Future Developments*, Academic Press, p.1.

67. Zwelling, L.A., Kohn, K.W., Ross, W.E., Ewig, R.A.G., and Anderson, T. (1978). *Cancer Res.*, **38**, 1762.

68. Wittes, R., Cvitkovic, E., Shah, J., Gerold, F., and Strong, E. (1977). *Cancer Treat. Rep.*, **61**, 359.

69. Jacobs, C. (1980). In A. Prestayko *et al.* (Eds), *Cisplatin: Current Status and Future Developments*, Academic Press, p.423.

70. Panettiere, F., Lehane, D., Fletcher, W.S., Stephens, R., Rivkin, S., McCracken, J.D. (1980). *Med. Ped. Oncol.*, **8**, 221.

71. Creagan, E.T., O'Fallon, J.R., Woods, J.E., Ingle, J.N., Schutt, A.J., Nichols, W.C. (1983). *Cancer*, **51**, 2020.

72. Sako, K., Razack, M., and Kalnins, I. (1978). *Am. J. Surg.*, **136**, 529.

73. Randolph, V., and Wittes, R. (1978). *Eur. J. Cancer*, **14**, 753.

74. Hong, W.K., Schaefer, S., Issell, B., Cummings, S., Luedke, D., Bromer, R., Fofonoff, S., D'Aoust, J., Shapshay, S., Welch, J., Levin, E., Vincent, M., Vaughan, C. and Strong, S. (1983). *Cancer*, **52**, 206.

75. Grose, E.W., Lehane, D., Dixon, D.O., Fletcher, W.S., Stuckey, W.J. (1983). Submitted *Cancer Treat. Rep.*

76. Campbell, M., and Al-Sarraf, M. (1980). *Cancer Treat. Rep.*, **64**, 713.

77. Cheng, E., Currie, V., and Wittes, R.E. (1979). *Cancer Treat. Rep.*, **63**, 2047.

78. Cheng, E., Young, C.W., and Wittes, R.E. (1980). *Cancer Treat Rep.*, **64**, 1141.

79. Sledge, G.W., Von Hoff, D.D., Clark, G.M., Griffin, C., and Oines, D.W. (1982). *Proc. Am. Soc. Clin. Oncol.*, **1**, C-788, 203.

80. Kaplan, B.H., Vogl, S.E., Cinberg, J., Berenzweig, M., and O'Donell, M. (1982). *Proc. Am. Soc. Clin. Oncol.*, **1**, C-775, 199.

81. Creagan, E.T., Fleming, T.R., Edmonson, J.H., and Ingle, J.N. (1979). *Cancer Treat. Rep.*, **63**, 2061.

82. Ratanatharathorn, V., Drelichman, A., Sexon-Porte, M., and Al-Sarraf, M. (1982). *Am. J. Clin. Oncol.*, **5**, 29.

83. Forastiere, A.A., Young, C.W., and Wittes, R.E. (1981). *Cnacer Chemother. Pharmacol.*, **6**, 145.

84. Perry, D.J., Crain, S., Weltz, M., Wilson, J., Davis, R.K., Woolley, P., Forastiere, A., Taylor, H.G., and Weiss, R. (1983). *Cancer Treat. Rep.*, **67**, 91.

85. Thongprasert, S., Bosl, G.J., Geller, N.L., Wittes, R.E. Submitted for publication.

86. Edmonson, J.H., Frytak, S., Letendre, L., Kvols, L.K., and Eagan, R.T. (1979). *Cancer Treat. Rep.*, **63**, 2081.

86a. Haas, C.D., Lehane, D., Bottomly, R. (1983). *Medical and Pediatric Oncology*, **11**, 281.

87. Boccardo, R., Barbieri, A., Canobio, L., Guarneri, D., Merlano, M., and Rosso, R. (1982). *Cancer Treat. Rep.*, **66**, 585.

88. Sah, M.K., Engstrom, P.R., Catalano, R.B.,

Paul, A.R., Bellet, R.E., and Creech, R.H. (1982). *Cancer Treat. Rep.*, **66**, 557.

89. Andrews, N.C., Weiss, A.J., Wilson, W., and Nealon, T. (1974). *Cancer Chemother. Rep.*, **58**, 653.

90. Nissen, N.I., Pajak, T.F., Leone, L., Bloomfield, C.D., Kennedy, B.J., Ellison, R.R., Silver, R.T., Weiss, R.B., Cuttner, J., Falkson, G., Kung, F., Bergevin, P.R., and Holland, J.F. (1980). *Cancer*, **45**, 232.

91. Forastiere, A.A., Crain, S.M., Callahan, K., Van Echo, D., Mattox, D., Thant, M., Von Hoff, D.D., and Wiernik, P.H. (1982). *Cancer Treat. Rep.*, **66**, 2097.

92. Creagan, E.T., Nichols, W.C., and O'Fallon, J.R. (1981). *Cancer Treat. Rep.*, **65**, 827.

93. Mihich, E. (1963). *Cancer Res.*, **23**, 1375.

94. Freireich, E.J., Frei, E., III, and Karon, M. (1962). *Cancer Chemother. Rep.*, **16**, 183.

95. Knight, W., Livingston, R.B., Fabian, C., and Costanzi, J. (1979). *Proc. Am. Assoc. Cancer Res.*, **20**, C-115, 319.

96. Cain, B.F., and Atwell, G.J. (1974). *Eur. J. Cancer*, **10**, 539.

97. Legha, S.S., Keating, M.J., McCredie, K.B., Bodey, G.P., and Freireich, E.J. (1982). *Blood*, **60**, 484.

98. Chou, F., Kahn, A.H., and Driscoll, J.S. (1976). *J. Med. Chem.*, **19**, 1302.

99. Bender, J.F., Grillo-Lopez, A.J., and Posada, J.G., Jr. (1983). *Investigational New Drugs*, **1**, 71.

100. Andrews, N.C., Weiss, A.J., Andsfield, F.J., Rochlin, D.B., and Mason, J.H. (1971). *Cancer Chemother. Rep.*, **55**, 61.

101. Issell, B.F., Borsos, G., Aoust, J.C.D., Banhidy, F., Crooke, S.T., and Eckhardt, S. (1982). *Cancer Chemother. Pharmacol.*, **8**, 171.

102. Yagoda, A., Lipman, A.J., Winn, R., Schulman, P., and Cohen, F. (1975). *Proc. Am. Assoc. Cancer Res.*, **16**, C-1105, 247.

103. Broquet, M.A., Jacot-Descombe, E., Montandon, A., and Alberto, P. (1974). *Schweiz. Med. Wochenschr.*, **104**, 18.

104. Medenica, R., Alberto, P., and Lehman, W. (1976). *Schweiz. Med. Wochenschr.*, **106**, 799.

105. Mosher, M., DeConti, R., and Bertino, J. (1972). *Cancer*, **30**, 56.

106. Wittes, R., Brescia, F., Young, C., Magill, G., Golbey, R., and Krakoff, I. (1975). *Oncology*, **32**, 202.

107. Bianco, A., Taylor, S.G., Reich, S., Merrill, J., and DeWys, W. (1979). *Cancer Treat. Rep.*, **63**, 158.

108. Pitman, S., Minor, D., Papac, R., Knopf, T., Lowenthal, I., Nystrom, S., and Bertino, J. (1979). *Proc. Am. Assoc. Cancer Res.*, **20**, C-529, 419.

109. Moran, M., Goepfort, H., Byers, R., Guillamondagui, O., Larson, D., and Medina, J. (1982). *Proc. Am. Soc. Clin. Oncol.*, **1**, C-756, 195.

110. Ervin, T., Weichelbaum, R., Miller, D., Meshal, M., Posner, M., and Fabian, R. (1981). *Cancer Treat. Rep.*, **65**, 787.

111. Vogl, S., and Kaplan, B. (1979). *Cancer*, **44**, 26.

112. Leone, L., and Ohnuma, T. (1979). *Proc. Am. Assoc. Cancer Res.*, **20**, C-342, 374.

113. Caradonna, R., Paladine, W., Ruckdeschel, J., Goldstein, S., Olson, J., Jask, J., Silvers, S., Hillinger, S., and Horton, J. (1979). *Cancer Treat. Rep.*, **63**, 489.

114. Murphy, W., Valdivieso, M., Bodey, G., and Freireich, E. (1980). *Proc. Am. Assoc. Cancer Res.*, **21**, 666, 166.

115. Von Hoff, D., Alberts, D., Mattox, D., Coulthard, S., Dana, B., Manning, M., Myers, J., and Griffin, C. (1981). *Cancer Clin. Trials*, **4**, 215.

116. Belt, R., Davidner, M., and Mundis, R. (1982). *Proc. Am. Soc. Clin. Oncol.*, **1**, C-773, 199.

117. Livingston, R., Einhorn, L., Bodey, G., Burgess, M., Freireich, E., and Gottlieb, J. (1975). *Cancer*, **36**, 327.

118. Livingston, R., Einhorn, L., Burgess, M., and Gottlieb, J. (1976). *Cancer Treat. Rep.*, **60**, 103.

119. Wheeler, R.H., Liepman, M.K., Baker, S.R., Earhart, R.H., Bull, F.E., Ensminger, W.D. (1980). *Cancer Treat. Rep.*, **64**, No. 8–9, 943.

119a. Wheeler, R., Baker, S.R., Liepman, M.K., and Ensminger, W.D. (1983). *Medical and Pediatric Oncology*, **11**, 12.

120. Price, L.A., and Hill, B. (1981). *Cancer Treat. Rep.*, **65**, (Suppl. 1), 149.

121. Raafat, J., and Oster, M. (1980). *Cancer Treat. Rep.*, **64**, 187.

122. Creagan, E.T., Flemming, T.R., Edmonson, J., Ingle, J., and Woods, J.E. (1981). *Cancer*, **47**, 240.

123. Creagan, E.T., Flemming, T.R., Edmonson, J., Ingle, J., and Woods, J.E. (1981). *Cancer*, **47**, 2549.

124. Creagan, E.T., O'Fallon, J.R., Schutt, A.J., Rubin, J., Richardson, R., and Woods, J.E. (1982). *Proc. Am. Soc. Clin. Oncol.*, **1**, C-770, 198.

125. Pitman, S., Kowal, C., and Bertino, J. (1983). *Seminars in Oncology*, Vol. 10, No. 2, Suppl. 2 (June).

125a. Ringborg, V., Gosta, E., Kinnman, J., Lundqvist, P., and Strander, H. (1983). *Cancer*, **52**, 971.

125b. Browman, G.P., Young, J.E.M., Archibald,

S.D., Khiel, K., Russell, R., and Levine, M.N. (1983). *Proc. Am. Assoc. Clin. Oncol.*, C-616, 158.

126. Jacobs, C. (1982). *Cancer Treat. Rep.*, **66**, 1925.

127. Thatcher, N., Blackledge, G., and Crowther, D. (1980). *Cancer*, **46**, 1324.

128. Woods, R.L., Stewart, J., Fox, R., and Tattersall, M.H. (1979). *Cancer Treat Rep.*, **63**, 1997.

129. Brown, A., Blom, J., Butler, W., Garcia-Guerrero, G., Richardson, M., and Henderson, R. (1980). *Cancer*, **45**, 2830.

130. Huang, A., Lucas, V., Baughn, S., and Cole, T. (1980). *Cancer*, **45**, 2038.

131. Presant, C., Ratkin, G., Klahr, C., and Brown, C. (1979). *Cancer*, **44**, 1571.

132. Amer, M., Izbicki, R., Vaitkevicius, V., and Al-Sarraf, M. (1980). *Cancer*, **45**, 217.

133. Lester, E., Johnson, C.M., Kaplan, A., and Matz, G. (1982). *Proc. Am. Soc. Clin. Oncol.*, **1**, C-782, 201.

134. Kish, A., Drelichman, A., Jacobs, J., Hoschner, J., Kinzie, J., Loh, J., Weaver, A., and Al-Sarraf, M. (1982). *Cancer Treat. Rep.*, **66**, 471.

135. Forastiere, A., Crain, S.M., Coker, D., Elias, E., Amornmarn, R., and Wiernik, P. (1982). *Proc. Am. Soc. Clin. Oncol.*, **1**, C-762, 196.

136. Spaulding, M.B., De Los Santos, R., Sanani, S., Canty, R., and Sundquist, N. (1982). *Proc. Am. Soc. Clin. Oncol.*, **1**, C-772, 199.

137. Barranco, S.C., Luce, J., Romsdahl, M.M., and Humphrey, R. (1973). *Cancer Res.*, **33**, 882.

138. Eisenberger, M., Denefrio, J., Silverman, M., and Lessner, H.E. (1982). *Cancer Treat. Rep.*, **60**, 1439.

139. Medenica, R., Alberto, P., and Lehman, N.W. (1981). *Cancer Chemother. Pharmacol.*, **5**, 145.

140. Cortes, E.P., Kalra, J., Amin, V.C., Attic, J., Eisenloud, L., Khafif, R., Wolk, D., Asal, I., Sciubba, J., Akbiyik, M., and Heller, K. (1981). *Cancer*, **47**, 1966.

141. Costanzi, J., Loukas, D., Gagliano, R., Griffiths, C., and Barranco, S. (1976). *Cancer*, **38**, 1503.

142. Plasse, T., Ohnuma, T., Goldsmith, M., Brooks, S., Holland, S.F., and Biller, H. (1982). *Proc. Am. Soc. Clin. Oncol.*, **1**, C-755, 194.

143. Cadman, E., Heimer, R., and Davis, L. (1979). *Science*, **205**, 1135.

144. Lehane, D., Lane, M., Gad-el-Mawla, N., Thomas, L.C., O'Bryon, R.N., Fletcher, W.S., Dixon, D.O. Submitted *Cancer Treat. Rep.*, 1983.

145. Williams, S., Einhorn, L., Velez-Garcia, E., Essessee, I., Ratkin, C., Birch, R., and Garrard, J. (1982). *Proc. Am. Soc. Clin. Oncol.*, **1**, C-784, 202.

146. Vogl, S., and Schoenfeld, D. (1983). *Cancer*, in press.

147. Jacobs, C., Meyers, F., Hendrickson, C., Kohler, M., Carter, S.K. (1983). *Cancer*, in press.

148. Drelichman, A., Cummings, G., Al-Sarraf, M. (1983). *Cancer*, **52**, 399.

149. Davis, S., and Kessler, W. (1979). *Cancer Chemother. Pharmacol.*, **3**, 57.

149a. Clavel, M., Wildiers, J., Von Rijmenant, M., Bruntsch, V., Kirkpatrick, A., Rozencweig, M. (1983). *Proc. Am. Assoc. Clin. Oncol.*, C-618, 158.

150. Avery, T.L., and Roberts, D. (1974). *Eur. J. Cancer*, **10**, 425.

151. Kramer, S., Gelber, R., Snow, J., Davis, L., Marcial, V., and Lowry, J. (1980). *Proc. Int. Head and Neck Oncol. Res. Conf.*, Abst. 1.1, National Cancer Institute.

152. Skipper, H.E., Schabel, F.M., and Wilcox, W.S. (1964). *Cancer Chemother. Rep.*, **35**, 1.

153. Griswold, D.P. (1975). *Cancer Chemother. Rep.*, **5**, 187.

154. Skipper, H.E. (1978). *Cancer*, **41**, 936.

155. Schabel, F.M. (1976). *Am. J. Roentgenol.*, **126**, 500.

156. Fazecas, J., Sommer, C., and Kramer, S. (1980). *Int. J. Radiat. Oncol. Biol. Phys.*, **6**, 533.

157. Tarpley, J., Chretien, P., Alexander, J., Hoye, R., Block, J., and Ketcham, A. (1975). *Am. J. Surg.*, **130**, 481.

158. Randolph, V., Vallejo, A., Spiro, R., Shah, J., Strong, E., Huvos, A., and Wittes, R. (1978). *Cancer*, **41**, 460.

159. Wittes, R., Heller, K., Randolph, V., Howard, J., Vellejo, A., Farr, H., Harrold, C., Gerold, F., Shah, J., Spiro, R., and Strong, E. (1979). *Cancer Treat. Rep.*, **63**, 1533.

160. Elias, E.G., Chretien, P.B., Monnard, E., Kahn, T., Bouchelle, W., Wiernik, P., Lipson, S., Hande, K., and Zentai, T. (1979). *Cancer*, **43**, 1025.

161. Pennacchio, J., Hong, W.K., Shapshay, S., Gillis, T., Vaughn, E., Bhutani, R., Uemakli, A., Katz, A., Bromer, R., Willet, B., and Strong, S. (1982). *Cancer*, **50**, 2795.

162. Spaulding, M., Kahn, A., De Los Santos, R., Klotch, D., and Lore, T. (1982). *Am. J. Surg.*, **144**, 432.

162a. Amrein, P.C., Fingert, H., Weiszman, S.A. (1983). *Am. J. Clin. Oncol.*, **1**, (7), 421 (July).

163. Price, L.A., and Hill, B.T. (1982). *Proc. Am. Soc. Clin. Oncol.*, **1**, C-786, 202.

164. Weaver, A., Loh, J., Vandenberg, H., Powers, W., Fleming, S., Mathog, R., and Al-Sarraf, M. (1980). *Am. J. Surg.*, **140**, 549.

165. Weaver, A., Flemming, S., Kish, J., Vandenberg, H., Jacob, J., Crissman, J., and Al-Sarraf, M. (1982). *Am. J. Surg.*, **144**, 445.

166. Perry, D.J., Davis, R.K., and Weiss, R.B. (1982). *Proc. Am. Soc. Clin. Onocol.*, **1**, C-749, 193.

167. Feldman, J., Ellingwood, K., and Clarkson, D. (1982). *Proc. Am. Soc. Clin. Onocol.*, **1**, C-751, 193.

168. Schaefer, S., Middleton, R., Carder, H., Sudderth, J., Graham, M., Anderson, R., and Frenkel, E. (1981). *Proc. Am. Assoc. Cancer Res.*, **22**, C-374, 428.

169. Popkin, J., Bromer, R., Byrne, R., Licciardello, J., Gehr, G., Amick, R., and Hong, W. (1982). *Proc. Am. Soc. Clin. Oncol.*, **1**, C-777, 200.

170. Israel, L., Aguilera, J., Soudant, J., Penot, J.C., and Breau, J.L. (1982). *Proc. Am. Soc. Clin. Oncol.*, **1**, C-779, 200.

171. Ervin, T.J., Karp, D.D., Weishelbaum, R.R., and Frei, E., III (1982). In S. Salmon, and S. Jones (Eds), *Therapy of Cancer, III*, Grune & Stratton, p.183.

172. Schuller, D., Wilson, H., Smith, R., Bately, F., and James, A. (1983). *Cancer*, **51**, 15.

173. Glick, J.H., Marcial, V., Richter, M., and Velez-Garcia, E. (1980). *Cancer*, **46**, 1919.

174. Marcial, V.A., Velez-Garcia, E., Figueroa-Valles, N.R., Cintron, J., and Vallecillo, L. (1980). *Int. J. Radiat. Oncol. Biol. Phys.*, **6**, 717.

175. Vogl, S.E., Lerner, H., Kaplan, B.H., Coughlin, C., McCormick, B., Camacho, F., and Cinberg, J. (1982). *Cancer*, **50**, 840.

176. Tejada, F., and Chandler, J.R. (1982). *Proc. Am. Soc. Clin. Oncol.*, **1**, C-774, 199.

177. Baker, S.R., Makuch, R.W., and Wolf, G.T. (1980). *Proc. Int. Head and Neck Oncol. Conf.*, Abst. 5.12, National Cancer Institute.

178. Klopp, C.T., Alford, T.E., Bateman, J., Berry, G.N., and Winship, T. (1950). *Ann. Surg.*, **132**, 811.

179. Sullivan, R.D., Jones, R. Jr., Schonobel, T.G. Jr., and MacShorey, J. (1953). *Cancer*, **6**, 121.

180. Shah, P., Baker, L.H., and Vaitkevicius, V.K. (1977). *Cancer Treat. Rep.*, **61**, 1565.

181. Ansfield, F.J., Ramirez, G., Davis, H.L., Wirtanen, G., Johnson, R., Bryan, G., Manalo, F., Borden, E., Davis, T., and Esmaili, M. (1975). *Cancer*, **36**, 2413.

182. Hsiao-Sheng, G.C., and Gross, J.F. (1980). *Cancer Treat. Rep.*, **64**, 31.

183. Eckman, W.W., Patlak, C.S., and Fenstermacher, J.D. (1974). *J. Pharmacokinet. Biopharm.*, **2**, 257.

184. Collins, J.M., and Dedrick, R.L. (1982). In *Pharmacologic Principles in Cancer Treatment*, Saunders, Philadelphia, p.77.

185. Skipper, H.E., Schabel, F.M. Jr., Mellet, L., Montgomery, J., Wilkoff, L., Lloyd, H., and Brockman, R.W. (1970). *Cancer Chemother. Rep.*, **54**, 431.

186. Oberfield, R.A., Cady, B., and Booth, J.C. (1973). *Cancer*, **32**, 82.

187. Cruz, A.B., McInnis, W.D., and Aust, J.B. (1974). *Am. J. Surg.*, **128**, 573.

188. Baker, S.R., Wheeler, R.H., Ensminger, W.D., and Niederhuber, J.E. (1981). *Head and Neck Surg.*, **4**, 118.

189. Donegan, W.L., and Harris, P. (1976). *Cancer*, **38**, 1479.

190. Zielke-Tenme, B.C., Stevens, K.R., Everts, E.C., Moseley, H.S., and Ireland, K. (1980). *Cancer*, **45**, 1527.

191. Misra, N.C., Jaiswal, M.S., and Singh, R.V. (1974). *Indian J. Surg.*, **35**, 441.

192. Molinari, R., de Palo, G.M., Preda, F., Gennari, L., and Di Pietro, S. (1971). *Tumori*, **57**, 111.

193. Krisch, A., and Muska, K. (1977). *Cesk. Otolaryngol.*, **26**, 345.

194. Freckman, H.A. (1972). *Am. J. Surg.*, **124**, 501.

195. Wittes, R.E. (1981). Recent Results in *Cancer Res.*, **76**, 276.

196. Million, R., Cassizzi, N., Wittes, R.E. (1982). In V. DeVita *et al.* (Eds), *Principles and Practice of Oncology*, J.B. Lippencott Company, Philadelphia, pp. 301–386.

197. Ervin, T.J., Weichselbaum, R.R., Miller, D., Posner, M.R., Fabian, R.L., Tuttle, S.A., Frei, E., III. *Proc. Am. Soc. Clin. Oncol.*, **2**, C-640, 164.

Chapter 15

Concurrent Radiotherapy and Chemotherapy

Karen K. Fu
Dept. of Radiation Oncology, University of California Hospital, San Francisco, CA, USA.

INTRODUCTION

The principal objective of combining chemotherapy with radiotherapy (XRT) for the treatment of advanced head and neck cancer is to improve the therapeutic ratio through the enhancement of local control and reduction of distant metastases without excessively enhancing normal tissue effects. Improved tumour control can result from sole additivity of either therapy or direct interactions between drug and radiation leading to increased tumour cell kill.[57] Chemotherapy may sensitize the cells to radiation, interfere with repair of sublethal or potentially lethal radiation damage, induce cell synchrony, and reduce tumour mass leading to reoxygenation and decreased fraction of resistant hypoxic cells. Radiation may improve drug accessibility to tumour cells and reduce tumour volume leading to increased cell proliferation and chemosensitivity. If the enhanced effects of combined therapy are purely additive, then the two modalities can be administered either sequentially or concurrently with the same results. However, if the enhanced effects result from the direct interaction between drug and radiation, it is necessary that the two modalities be administered concurrently and in close temporal proximity. This review summarizes the results of clinical studies in which chemotherapy was administered concurrently during the course of radiotherapy for patients with previously untreated advanced squamous cell carcinoma in the head and neck.

BLEOMYCIN AND RADIOTHERAPY

Bleomycin has been shown to enhance radiation lethality in mammalian cells *in vitro*[36,60] and enhance tumour effect of radiation in murine squamous carcinoma *in vivo*.[25,45]

Bleomycin administered as a single agent has an overall response rate of 31% for advanced squamous cell carcinoma of the head and neck.[18] It has been the chemotherapeutic agent most frequently used concurrently with radiotherapy for head and neck cancer. Of the 13 studies combining bleomycin and radiotherapy reviewed (Table 15.1), only five of these were randomized[7,13,27,37,51] and in one study[27] the combined bleomycin and radio-

TABLE 15.1 CONCURRENT BLEOMYCIN AND RADIOTHERAPY (XRT) FOR ADVANCED HEAD AND NECK CANCER

Reference	Primary site	No. of patients	XRT dose schedule	Bleomycin dose schedule	Response rate CR	Response rate PR	Survival
Berdal (1976)[4]	Various sites	>300 210 patients observed 1–3.5 yrs	350 R/d Mon.– Sat., rest 1 week, 350 R/d Mon.–Sat. Total dose 4200 R to skin, 2500 R to tumour	15 mg/d IM 1 h before XRT Mon.–Sat. first wk, then 15 mg/ d IM on Mon., Wed., Fri. for 2 wks. Total dose 180 mg (Nov. 1971–May 1973). Bleo. dose subse-quently lowered to 45–80 mg given before and during the early part of XRT at 15–30 mg b.i.w. until Dec. 1973 changed to total dose of 0.7 mg/kg/wk in 3 weekly injec-tions	115/212 (54%)	68/212 (32%)	Patients surviving 1–3.5 yrs: Larynx: 75/90 (83%) Hypopharynx: 9/21 (43%) Oral cavity: 9/21 (43%) Tongue: 8/13 (62%)
De la Garza et al. (1976)[10]	Various sites	20	4000–6000 rad ? fractionation	15 mg IV b.i.w. total dose 150–300 mg	CR + PR: 14/20 (70%)		5 alive NED 9–16 months 5 alive with disease 6–16 months
Tanaka et al. (1976)[59]	Oral cavity	39	2500–3000 rad/ 2.5–3 wks + further treatment with surgery in 15, XRT in 17 and chemotherapy in 4 patients	7.5 mg IM t.i.w. in 4 patients. 10 mg IV b.i.w. in 2 patients. 15 mg IV b.i.w. in 33 patients.	11/29 (38%)		2-y survival rate 30/39 (76.9%)

Reference	Primary site	No. of patients	XRT dose schedule	Bleomycin dose schedule	Response rate CR	Response rate PR	Survival
Cachin et al. (1977)[7]	Oropharynx	220 (186 evaluable) XRT – 87 XRT + bleo. 99	Prescribed dose: 7000 rad to the primary in 7–8.5 wks. 5000–5500 rad in 5–6 wks to the regional lymph nodes. Actual dose: XRT alone group: 6403 ± 204 rad/47 ± 2 d. XRT + bleo. group: 6288 ± 168 rad/52 ± 2 d.	15 mg IM or IV 2 h before XRT b.i.w. × 5 wks to a total dose of 150 mg.	Primary site: XRT: 67.9% XRT + bleo: 67.0% Regional nodes: XRT: 49% XRT + bleo: 62%	13.1% 17.0% 26% 14%	Median survival: 15 months in both groups. 2 yr actuarial survival: XRT ~45%; XRT + bleo. ~42%.
Kapstad et al. (1978)[27]	Various sites	32 (29 evaluable) XRT pre-op 14. XRT + bleo. 15	3000 rad/5 wks at 150 rad × 5/ wk during wks 1,2,4 and 5, no XRT during wk 3. Surgery during wk 8.	15 mg IM 1 h before XRT t.i.w. to a total dose of 180 mg.	XRT + bleo: 5 (27%) XRT alone: 1 (7%) Evaluated at 2 wks after treatment	5 (33%) 3 (21%)	N/A.
Kapstad (1978)[26]	Various sites	30 (17 initial and 13 recurrent disease)	Initial disease: Total dose: 4000–5000 rad at 150 rad × 5/ wk during wk 1, 2, 4, 5, 6 and 7. Recurrent disease: Total dose: 0–4000 rad.	15 mg IM 1 h before XRT t.i.w. to a total dose of 60–300 mg in initial disease and 30–225 mg in recurrent disease.	Initial: 7/17 (41%) Recurrent: 0	5/17 (29%) 2/13 (15%)	N/A.

TABLE 15.1 Cont.

Reference	Primary site	No. of patients	XRT dose schedule	Bleomycin dose schedule	Response rate CR	PR	Survival
Rygard and Hansen (1979)[44]	Primarily larynx and oral cavity	33	1630 ±85 – 1720 ±75 CRE r.e.u. at 160–200 rad/d.	Variable: 1970 – 1972: 10 – 15 mg IM $\frac{1}{2}$–1 h before XRT 2–3 ×/wk. 1972 on: 0.7 mg/kg/wk IM $\frac{1}{2}$–1 h before XRT. Total dose 103–124 mg	15 (45%)		Median survival: 15 months
Seagren et al. (1979)[48]	Various sites	19	5040 rad/28 fractions/5.5 wks + surgery (2 patients) or ^{192}Ir implant (7 patients) or further XRT (6 patients)	15 u IM b.i.w. to a total dose of 165–180 u	11 (58%) after 5040 rad	7 (37%)	1-yr crude survival = 68%. Disease-free survival = 57%
Shanta and Krishnamurthi (1980)[51]	Oral cavity, primarily buccal mucosa	157	5500–6000 rad/ 6.5–7 wks. 3 treatments/wk in the XRT + bleo. group and 6500 rad/6.5–7 wks. 5 treatments/wk in the control group	10 – 15 mg IA or IV b.i.w. or t.i.w. on non-irradiation days, i.e., Tue., Thur. and occ. Sat. to a total dose of 150–250 mg, or 30 mg IM b.i.w. × 2 wks before XRT and 30 mg IM × 1 during XRT to a total dose of 150 mg	XRT + bleo: 78.6% XRT alone: 19.1% Recurrence-free rate at 5 yrs: XRT + bleo: 71.8% XRT alone: 17.0%		5-yr disease-free survival: XRT + bleo: 65.5% XRT alone: 23.5%

Reference	Primary site	No. of patients	XRT dose schedule	Bleomycin dose schedule	Response rate		Survival
					CR	PR	
Morita (1980)[37]	Oral tongue	45	XRT alone: 4000 rad/4 wks + 4000−6000 rad/5−7 d with radium implant. XRT + bleo: 2000−4000 rad in 2 wks + 4000−6000 rad/5−7 d with radium needle implant	5 mg/d IM 5 × /wk to a total dose of 50−60 mg	2-year local control rate: XRT alone: 15/23 (65%) XRT + bleo: 17/22 (73%)		N/A
Shah *et al.* (1981)[50]	Oral cavity	59	4000−6000 rad at 200 rad/d, 6 d/wk	15 mg IV $\frac{1}{2}$ h before XRT t.i.w.	XRT alone: 18 (50%) XRT + bleo: 11 (47.8%)	3 (8.3%) 4 (17.4%)	Median Survival R NR XRT 6M 6M XRT + bleo: 7M12D 5M22D R = Responder NR = Non responder

TABLE 15.1 Cont.

Reference	Primary site	No. of patients	XRT dose schedule	Bleomycin dose schedule	Response rate CR	Response rate PR	Survival
Silverberg et al. (1981)[53]	Various sites	42	Prescribed dose: 6500 rad at 180 rad/d, 5 d/wk. Actual dose: 4997 – 7546 rad. Median: 6649 rad in complete responders, 4620 – 7360 rad (median 6480 rad) in partial responders	15 u IV b.i.w. in 19 patients. 5 u IV b.i.w. in 18 patients. 2 u IV t.i.w. in 2 patients. 15 u IV weekly in 1 patient. 10 u IV b.i.w. in 1 patient. Total dose: 20 – 255 u (mean 93 u) in complete responders, 36 – 180 u (mean 91 u) in partial responders	23 (52%)	18 (43%)	Median survival: 392 d (85 – 1076 + d) in complete responders. 212 d (59 – 581 d) in partial responders
Fu et al. (1982)[13]	Various sites	79	7000 rad at 180 rad/d 5 d/wk	5 u IV b.i.w. during XRT. Bleo. 15 u/wk + MTX 25 mg/m²/ wk × 16 wk after completion of XRT	47% with XRT + bleo. treatment vs. 38% with XRT alone in the primary site; 60% vs. 37% in the regional lymph nodes at 90 d after randomization	35% vs. 19% in the primary site; 27% for both groups at 90 d after randomization	Median survival 432 days with XRT + bleo. vs. 369 d with XRT alone. 2-yr survival 48% with XRT + bleo. vs. 28% with XRT alone

therapy treatments were followed by planned surgery. The randomized study by Shanta and Krishnamurthi reported the most significant difference in tumour response and survival between the combined treatment and XRT alone groups.[51] Favourable response, defined as total healing within the irradiated volume at 8 weeks after the completion of radiotherapy, was 78.6% in the study group and 19.1% in the control group. The 5-year recurrence free rate was 71.8% and 17% in the study and control groups respectively. The 5-year actuarial disease-free survival was 65.5% in the study group and 23.5% in the control group. The difference was statistically significant in the patients who received intra-arterial or intravenous bleomycin ($P = 0.05$), but not significant in the patients who received intramuscular bleomycin. There was also a significant difference in survival rates with respect to site and T stage, being greater for buccal mucosa as compared to gingiva, and for T_3 as compared to T_4 disease. It should be noted that the total doses of bleomycin were different for the different routes of administration and the XRT dose fractionation was also different for the study and control groups.

Morita reported similar results for tongue cancer treated with XRT alone or in combination with bleomycin.[37] Two-year local control rates of 65% and 73% were achieved for the XRT alone group and the combined treatment group respectively, although the combined treatment group received a lower external beam dose. Both groups received radium needle implant following the external beam irradiation. The incidence of osteonecrosis was 20% in the XRT alone group but 0% in the combined treatment group. Thus, it would appear that the therapeutic ratio is greater in the combined treatment group.

The clinical trial of the Northern California Oncology Group (NCOG) differs for most of the other studies in that the bleomycin dose during XRT is 5 u IV b.i.w. instead of 10–15 u IV or IM b.i.w. to t.i.w., used in most other studies.[13] In contrast to most studies which showed marked enhancement of radiation

mucositis in the combined treatment group necessitating interruption of XRT and decrease of total XRT dose, there has been no significant difference in XRT dose or treatment days between the XRT alone group and the combined treatment group in this study. The degree of mucositis has been more severe by one grade point in the combined treatment group. Although patients randomized to the combined treatment group should receive maintenance chemotherapy with bleomycin 15 u IV and methotrexate (MTX) 25 mg/m^2 IV weekly for 16 weeks after XRT, only one-third of the patients in the combined treatement group have received greater than 50% of the prescribed maintenance chemotherapy dose. Thus, the observed difference in the locoregional tumour response is probably primarily due to the bleomycin administered during XRT. Although preliminary results suggest a greater locoregional tumour response in the combined treatment group, the difference in survival has not yet reached statistical significance.

In contrast to the above three studies, the European Organization for Research on Treatment of Cancer (EORTC) study on carcinoma of the oropharynx[7] showed no significant difference in either the tumour regression rate evaluated 6 weeks after the completion of XRT, or in survival at 15 months follow-up between the XRT control group and XRT + bleomycin group. However, the incidence of severe mucositis and epidermatitis was significantly greater in the combined treatment group, which necessitated delay of XRT in 22% and the interruption of treatment in 5% of the patients.

In the randomized study reported by Kapstad *et al.*,[27] in which bleomycin was administered during preoperative XRT, 4/15 (27%) of the patients in the combined treatment group, compared to 2/14 (14%) in the XRT alone group, had no tumour in the surgical specimen. However, this difference was not statistically significant.

Thus far, although three randomized studies have shown enhanced locoregional tumour response,[13,37,51] only the study from India[51] has demonstrated a statistically significant improvement in survival. Most of the non-randomized studies showed no, or equivocal, enhancement of tumour response by bleomycin.

5-FLUOROURACIL (5FU) AND RADIOTHERAPY

5FU, a halogenated pyrimidine which inhibits the synthesis of thymidine by blocking the enzyme thymidylate synthetase is toxic to mammalian cells. When combined with XRT it has been shown to enhance anti-tumour effects in transplanted murine solid tumours and leukaemic cells *in vivo*.[21,61,62]

As a single agent, 5FU has an overall response rate of 15% in advanced head and neck cancer.[18] 5FU has been used concurrently with XRT in at least six studies (Table 15.2). Four of these studies[17,24,47,52] involved intra-arterial infusion of 5FU during the course of XRT. The 5FU dose schedule was variable among the different series. The only randomized study, which also had the longest follow-up, was conducted at the University of Wisconsin and reported by Lo *et al.*[31] As shown in Table 15.2, although the 2-year NED rate was significantly better in the combined treatment group, 49% with XRT + 5FU vs. 18% with XRT alone ($P < 0.05$); the difference in 5-year survival was statistically significant only in the patients with oral cavity cancer, 40% vs. 13% ($P < 0.05$). There was no difference in the incidence of distant metastasis between the combined treatment and control groups. This study suggests the importance of primary site in the evaluation of response to combined chemotherapy and radiotherapy.

Two non-randomized studies from Japan[28,47] also suggest an enhanced tumour response by 5FU. Sato *et al.*[47] observed the complete disappearance of tumour in 38 of 57 patients with carcinoma of the paranasal sinuses after completion of XRT and intra-arterial 5FU infusion. However, 16 of the 38 patients had further treatment consisting of

total resection in one, partial resection in 12, and intracavitary irradiation with ^{137}Cs in three patients. Toxicity was also significant in that 66% of the patients developed severe reaction and 50% required interruption of treatment. Furthermore, in patients followed for 48 months or longer, five patients became blind and four patients had decreased vision. It is noteworthy that blindness, retinal and optic nerve injury, and injury to the anterior eye were also reported by Goepfert *et al.*[17] in patients with carcinoma of the paranasal sinuses treated with XRT and intra-arterial 5FU.

The other non-randomized study suggesting enhanced tumour response was reported by Komiyama *et al.*,[28] in which vitamin A was administered in addition to 5FU during XRT (Table 15.2). This series consisted of 33 patients with laryngeal cancer (12 supraglottic and 23 glottic primaries) and 15 patients with hypopharyngeal cancer or cervical oesophageal cancer, and included patients with Stage I and II disease as well as more advanced disease. The XRT dose was variable. Fifteen patients with laryngeal cancer and four with hypopharyngeal cancer had additional surgery. The 3-year survival was 17/18 (94%) in those receiving 5FU, vitamin A, and XRT and 10/15 (67%) in those who had further surgery, with an overall 3-year survival of 82%.

Jesse *et al.*[24] observed a local control rate of 40% in 25 patients with advanced head and neck cancer who received intra-arterial 5FU during the initial part of a course of XRT. However, 33% of the patients without local recurrence later developed distant metastasis.

In the study reported by Shigematsu,[52] in which treatment was allocated by odd or even case numbers on admission, a number of agents including 5FU, cyclohexanol succinate and amethohepazone were used during XRT in patients with maxillary sinus cancer. In 25 patients who received 5FU the recurrence-free rate was significantly different from the XRT control group at 1 year, but not at 2 years (Table 15.2). There was no difference in the

TABLE 15.2   CONCURRENT 5FU AND RADIOTHERAPY (XRT) FOR ADVANCED HEAD AND NECK CANCER

Reference	Primary site	No. of patients	Radiation dose schedule	5-FU dose schedule	Response rate CR	PR	Survival
Jesse et al. (1969)[24]	Various head and neck sites	25	200 rad/d, d 2–6 and d 8–13 and continued to a total dose of 6000–7000 rad	5FU 4–8 mg/kg/d IA on d 1–5 and 7–12. Total dose 2500–12000 mg with an average dose of 5000 mg	10/25 (40%) NED with no local recurrence		10/25 (40%) surviving 10–60 months
Sato et al. (1970)[47]	Paranasal sinuses	57	7000 rad/44 d at 200 rad/d + total resection in 6. partial resection in 20 and intracavitary ^{137}Cs in in 6 patients	250 mg/d IA beginning d 10 after XRT started to a total dose of 5000 mg or until toxicity	38/57 (67%) including 16 patients with further surgery or XRT		57% 2-yr survival
Shigematsu et al. (1971)[52]	Maxillary sinuses	XRT + 5FU 25. XRT alone 38.	Planned dose: 8000 rad/8 wks	5FU: 5–10 mg/kg/d IA to total dose of 5 g/4–7 wks	Recurrence-free rate at 1 yr: XRT + 5FU: 8/17 (47%) XRT alone: 7/30 (23%) $P<0.05$ At 2 yrs: XRT + 5FU: 3/8 (38%) XRT alone: 5/17 (29%)		2-yr crude survival: XRT + 5FU: 5/9 (56%) XRT alone: 10/17 (59%)
Goepfert et al. (1973)[17]	Nasal cavity and paranasal sinuses	26	6000–7000 rad/ 6–7 wks starting on d 2 of infusion	5FU 6 mg/kg/24 h IA in 21 patients. MTX 50 mg/d IA until systemic toxicity developed and then 5FU in 3 patients. 2 patients received MTX+leucovorin × 15 d	11/23 (48%) who completed treatment had no local recurrence 28–84 months (median – 44 months)		Determinate survival: 2-yr 47.8% 5-yr 26.6%

TABLE 15.2 Cont.

Reference	Primary site	No. of patients	Radiation dose schedule	5-FU dose schedule	Response rate CR	PR	Survival
Lo et al. (1976)[31]	Oral cavity and oropharynx	XRT 68 XRT + 5FU 68	6000–7000 rad/ 6–10 wks	5FU 10 mg/kg/d IV × 3 d then 5FU 5 mg/kg d 4 and Q Mon., Wed., and Fri. until end of treatment	Oral cavity: Initial: XRT 8/33 (24%) XRT + 5FU 16/33 (48%) After salvage: XRT 9/33 (27%) XRT + 5FU 20/33 (61%) Oropharynx: Initial: XRT 10/23 (43%) XRT + 5FU 13/33 (57%) After salvage: XRT 11/23 (48%) XRT + 5FU 13/23 (57%) 2 yr NED (all sites): XRT 12/68 (18%) XRT + 5FU 33/68 (49%) $P < 0.05$		5-yr survival 13% with XRT vs. 32% with XRT + 5FU for the entire group, 13% vs. 40% for oral cavity ($P < 0.05$).
Komiyama et al. (1978)[28]	Larynx, hypopharynx	48	6000–7000 rad/ 6–7 wks or 3000–4000 rad/ 3–4 wks with a 3 wk split followed by surgery or additional 3000–4000 rad	FAR: vitamin A 50 000 iu IM 6–10 h before and 5FU 250 mg IV 1 h before XRT. Total 5FU dose 1500– 11 000 mg. Vitamin A 60–220 × 10⁴ iu	Larynx: FAR: 15/18 (83%) FAR + surgery: 9/15 (60%) Hypopharynx: FAR: 1/4 (25%) FAR + surgery: 7/11 (64%)		>3-yr survival: FAR: 17/18 (94%) FAR + surgery: 10/15 (67%) Overall: 27/33 (82%)

2-year crude survival between the study and control groups. Furthermore, severe mucositis in the combined treatment group made it impossible to deliver the planned XRT dose of 8000 rad/8 weeks.

Thus, it appears that 5FU when used concurrently with XRT improved local control as well as survival in patients with oral cavity cancer. Patients with tumours of other primary sites had no significant improvement in survival, although there is a suggestion of improved local control. 5FU enhanced radiation mucositis, and intra-arterial 5FU during XRT of paranasal sinus cancer can be associated with an increase in incidence of late injury to the eye resulting in blindness or impaired vision.

METHOTREXATE (MTX) AND RADIOTHERAPY

MTX can potentially enhance radiation effects by producing partial synchronization of tumour cells. MTX has been one of the chemotherapeutic agents most frequently used in combination with XRT for advanced head and neck cancer. However, most of the studies are non-randomized, and MTX and XRT were usually administered sequentially rather than concurrently.[18] Results of concurrent MTX and XRT are shown in Table 15.3. In a randomized study by Condit,[8] 40 patients with advanced head and neck cancer received split course XRT alone vs. split XRT + intravenous MTX every 2 weeks for four doses (Table 15.3). Five patients in each treatment group failed to complete the planned treatment because of complications of advanced disease. An additional five patients randomized to receive combined treatment developed severe MTX toxicity after partial therapy. Thus, only 10/20 (50%) in the combined treatment group and 15/20 (75%) of the XRT alone group completed treatment. There was no significant difference in the remission rate.

Other non-randomized studies[2,29,32,35] also suggest no significant improvement in tumour response or survival. Enhanced toxicity,

primarily radiation mucositis, varied with the timing of drug and radiation administration. A higher incidence of moderate and severe mucositis was observed when MTX was administered concurrently with XRT than when it was administered sequentially with XRT. Late normal tissue complications were also more common with concurrent XRT and MTX. Lustig *et al.*[32] noted a 25% incidence of late soft tissue complications, 25% incidence of severe oedema, 4% radionecrosis, and 6% severe fibrosis with concurrent MTX and XRT, but decreased incidence of soft tissue complications and sever oedema (14% and 22% respectively). No radionecrosis or severe fibrosis occurred with intravenous MTX administered prior to XRT. For the XRT alone group the incidence of soft tissue necrosis was 8%, severe oedema was 10%, and no radionecrosis or severe fibrosis was observed. Thus, MTX administered concurrently with XRT appeared to increase the incidence of acute and late normal tissue toxicity without improvement of tumour response or patient survival.

HYDROXYUREA (HU) AND RADIOTHERAPY

HU has been shown to selectively kill cells in the S phase, inhibit DNA synthesis, block cells at the G_1–S border,[54,55,65] and inhibit the repair of potentially lethal radiation damage.[40] These experimental results suggest that HU when combined with XRT may have enhanced effects on proliferating tumour cells.

There have been a number of randomized, as well as non-randomized, studies combining HU and XRT for advanced squamous cell carcinoma of the head and neck (Table 15.4). In an early randomized study by Richards and Chambers,[41] 40 patients were randomized to receive XRT alone or XRT combined with HU. Twelve patients from the XRT alone group and 11 patients from the combined treatment group subsequently underwent resection of the primary tumour. An additional patient from the XRT alone group

TABLE 15.3   CONCURRENT METHOTREXATE (MTX) AND RADIOTHERAPY (XRT) FOR ADVANCED HEAD AND NECK CANCER

Reference	Primary site	No. of patients	Radiation dose schedule	MTX dose schedule	Response rate CR	Response rate PR	Survival
Condit (1968)[8]	Various sites	40	1800–2500 rad/ 3 d × 2 courses with a 4 wk break in between. Total dose 3600–5000 rad/31 d	1–4 mg/kg IV Q 2 wks × 4 during XRT	XRT alone: 12/15 (80%) of patients who completed treatment or 12/20 (60%) of patients entered. XRT + MTX: 9/10 (90%) of patients who completed treatment or 9/20 (45%) of patients entered.		N/A
Bagshaw and Doggett (1969)[2]	Various sites	22	Average total dose 6310 rad/ 46 d at 225 rad/d	25 mg/8h/d IA + Citrovorum 6 mg IM q.i.d. Total dose: 700 mg/ 18 d–2160 mg/ 44 d	XRT alone: 6/16 (38%) XRT + MTX: 7/22 (32%)		XRT alone: 5/16 (31%) alive NED XRT + MTX: 5/22 (23%) alive NED
Kramer (1969)[29]	Various sites	57	1st series: 6500 rad/6.5–8 wks starting d 6 after first dose MTX	2.5 mg PO t.i.d.	35/57 (61.4%)		3-yr disease-free survival 18/57 (31.6%)
		41	2nd series: XRT started d 5–8 after first dose of MTX XRT started the day after last dose of MTX	25 mg PO Q 3 d to toxicity or 25 mg IV Q 3 d to toxicity or 25 mg IV Q 3 d × 5	28/41 (68%)	7/41 (17%)	
Mason and Ediger (1970)[35]	Various sites	30	Total dose of 6000 rad in 6 wks	50 mg/d IA + 6 mg Citrovorum IM Q 6 h × 6–10 d	6/30 (20%)	10/30 (33%)	N/A
Lustig (1976)[32]	Various sites	48	Average XRT dose: 6579 rad/ 6.5 wks starting on 5 after MTX	2.5 mg PO t.i.d. to toxicity average total dose 99.8 mg (50–215 mg)	CT + PR = 24/48 (50%)		3-yr survival 33% (median 20 months)

TABLE 15.4   CONCURRENT HYDROXYUREA (HU) AND RADIOTHERAPY (XRT) FOR ADVANCED HEAD AND NECK CANCER

Reference	Primary site	No. of patients	Radiation dose schedule	HU dose schedule	Response rate		Survival
					CR	PR	
Richards and Chambers (1969)[41]	Various sites	40	Various dose schedules ranging from 4000 to 9000 rad in 21–84 d	80 mg/kg PO Q 3 d to 20–350 g total dose in 15–206 d	XRT alone: 1/7 XRT + surgery: 3/13 XRT + HU: 7/9 XRT + HU + surgery: 6/11	4/7 2/9	5-yr survival: XRT: 1/7 (14%) XRT + surgery: 6/13 (46%) XRT + HU–3/9 (33%) XRT + HU + Surgery: 7/11 (64%)
Stefani et al. (1971)[58]	Various sites	126	6000–10,000 rad/8–12 wks orthovoltage XRT ± intraoral cone, interstitial or intravacitary application	80 mg/kg PO b.i.w.	Primary tumour: XRT + HU: 20/48 (42%) XRT + placebo: 22/47 (47%) Node: XRT + HU 14/41 (34%) XRT + placebo: 13/30 (43%)	23/48 (48%) 16/47 (34%) 18/41 (44%) 14/30 (47%)	XRT + HU: 13/59 (22%) alive without disease 4/59 (7%) alive with disease XRT + placebo: 17/55 (31%) alive without disease 11/55 (20%) alive with disease. At 6–33 months follow-up
Rominger (1971)[43]	Various sites	10 previously untreated, 16 recurrent	2000–7000 rad/ 2–7 wks	80 mg/kg PO Q 3 d	—		Average survival 6.4 months with 3 patients alive NED 4–14 months, in previously untreated patients. Average survival 3 months in recurrent cases
Richards and Chambers (1973)[42]	Various sites	610	No details given	1500 mg daily	—		5-yr tumour-free survival: XRT ± surgery: 48/187 (25%) XRT + HU ± surgery: 258/423 (61%) XRT alone 38/101 (37%) XRT + HU 83/168 (49%) XRT + surgery + HU: 118/185 (63%) Surgery + XRT + HU: 57/70 (81%)

TABLE 15.4 Cont.

Reference	Primary site	No. of patients	Radiation dose schedule	HU dose schedule	Response rate CR	Response rate PR	Survival
Hussey and Abrams (1975)[23]	Various sites	40 randomized (4 recurrent) 32 Pilot non-randomized (16 recurrent)	No previous RX: 4500–7500 rad/ 4.5–9 wks at 850 rad/wk. Recurrent tumours: Most patients received 5000–6000 rad given dose in 5–6 wks	30 mg/kg 4 h prior to XRT and 30 mg/kg immediately after XRT on Mon., Wed., Fri.	Pilot study: No previous RX: 9/16 (56%) Recurrent: 11/16 (69%) Randomized study: XRT only: No previous RX: 6/12 (50%) Recurrent: 3/4 (75%) XRT + HU: No previous RX: 13/18 (72%) 3/6 (50%)	Local control: 8/16 (50%) 6/16 (38%) 5/12 (42%) 1/4 (25%) 7/18 (39%) 2/6 (33%)	NED at 24 months: Pilot study: No previous RX: 7/15 (47%) Recurrent: 1/16 (6%) Randomized study: XRT only: No previous RX: 3/11 (27%) Recurrent: 1/4 (25%) XRT + HU: No previous RX: 6/17 (35%) Recurrent: 1/6 (17%)
Lerner (1977)[30]	Various sites	100	Dose not specified. 3–5 treatments/wk for 10 wks or shorter time (+ surgery in 44 patients)	80 mg/kg PO Q 3 d beginning 1 wk prior to start of XRT, continued during XRT and indefinitely thereafter	73%	27%	42% alive NED.

underwent radical neck dissection. The incidence of tumour in the surgical specimen was greater in the XRT alone group than in the combined treatment group (10/12 vs. 5/11). The main effect of HU was seen on lymph nodes; none of the 11 patients in the combined treatment group had positive lymph nodes in the surgical specimen, whereas 7/13 patients in the XRT alone group had nodal disease remaining. No enhancement of radiation mucositis was observed.

In contrast to the report by Richards and Chambers,[41] the randomized study reported by Stefani et al.[58] showed no significant difference in primary tumour regression, cervical node response, or survival between the placebo group and the HU group. HU-enhanced radiation mucositis necessitated modification of radiation dose schedule in some patients. The incidence of distant metastasis was greater in the HU group than the placebo group (22.8% vs. 7.5%).

Although a pilot study at the M. D. Anderson Hospital suggested promising results in patients with advanced or recurrent squamous cell carcinoma of the head and neck treated with combined HU and XRT, their subsequent randomized study failed to demonstrate better local control with this combined treatment.[23] HU enhanced radiation mucositis to a greater degree than radiation dermatitis. This study illustrated the importance of randomized trials in clinical studies.

Available evidence in the literature suggests no significant therapeutic gain by combining HU with XRT in advanced squamous cell carcinoma of the head and neck.

CISPLATIN (DDP) AND RADIOTHERAPY

Recently DDP has been used with increasing frequency in the treatment of advanced or recurrent squamous cell carcinoma of the head and neck. Laboratory studies have shown that DDP may act as a hypoxic cell radiosensitizer, interfere with repair of sublethal and potentially lethal radiation damage, and enhance radiation lethality of mammalian cells.[11] As an adju-

vant to XRT it is usually given in combination with a number of other chemotherapeutic agents and administered sequentially with XRT.[1,16,63,64] Two recent reports suggest that DDP may be used concurrently with XRT with acceptable toxicity. (Table 15.5). In the study reported by Coughlin et al.[9] DDP was administered along with bleomycin prior to XRT and then three times a week during the course of XRT. After 4800 rad the patients were given 2-week rest periods and then reevaluated for surgical resection or further XRT to 7000 rad. Complete regression was achieved in 7/8 patients treated with XRT and 4/4 patients who underwent surgery. Three patients required a 1–2-week rest after 3000 rad due to mucositis.

In a pilot study of the Eastern Cooperative Oncology Group (ECOG), in which DDP at 10–30 mg/m^2/week was administered with conventional XRT, early results demonstrated a high rate of complete regression, 15/18 (83%) with a low incidence of early regional relapse (7%).[20] The incidence of severe mucositis was related to the dose used, being 1/12 with 10–20 mg/m^2/week and 6/13 with 30 mg/m^2/week. Based on these results ECOG has embarked on a randomized trial comparing XRT + DDP at 20 mg/m^2/week to XRT alone.

The value of DDP used as a single agent concurrently with XRT awaits results of further clinical trials.

MISCELLANEOUS SINGLE AGENT CHEMOTHERAPY AND RADIOTHERAPY (XRT)

A number of other single chemotherapeutic agents, including 6 MP, BUdR, and razoxane (ICRF159), have been combined with XRT for advanced squamous cell carcinoma of the head and neck (Table 15.6). In a double-blind controlled clinical trial of XRT and razoxane versus XRT + placebo, 14/18 pairs of patients matched by sex, tumour site, and tumour stage were evaluable for tumour response.[3] More favourable tumour response

TABLE 15.5   CONCURRENT (*CIS*—PLATINUM (*DDP*) AND RADIOTHERAPY (XRT) FOR ADVANCED HEAD AND NECK CANCER

Reference	Primary site	No. of patients	Radiation dose schedule	CP dose schedule	Response rate		Survival
					CR	PR	
Coughlin et al. (1982)[9]	Various sites	12	4800 rad at 200 rad/d, starting d 22, followed by surgery or further XRT to 7000 rad after a 2-wk rest	120 mg/m²/1½ h on d 1 + bleo. 15 u/m²/d IV on d 2–5. + DDP 120 mg/m²/1½ h IV on d 21. DDP 20 mg/m² IV 1 h before XRT t.i.w. beginning on d 28.	DDP + XRT: 7/8 (88%) DDP + XRT + surgery: 4/4 (100%)		—
Haselow et al. (1982)[20]	Various sites	23 18 evaluable	180 rad/d/5 d/wk to 6800–7600 rad	DDP: 10 mg/m²/wk: 4 patients 20 mg/m²/wk: 6 patients 30 mg/m²/wk: 13 patients	15/18 (83%) NED at 2–16 months (median 5 months)		

TABLE 15.6   CONCURRENT MISCELLANEOUS SINGLE AGENT CHEMOTHERAPY AND RADIOTHERAPY (XRT) FOR ADVANCED HEAD AND NECK CANCER

Reference	Primary site	No. of patients	Radiation dose schedule	Drug dose schedule	Response rate CR	PR	Survival
Bagshaw and Doggett (1969)[2]	Various sites	XRT alone 16 XRT + 6MP 9	XRT alone: average total dose 6360 rad/45 d at 225 rad/d XRT+6MP: average total dose 6513 rad/43 d at 225 rad/d	6 Mercapto-purine 0.3–1 mg/kg 24 h IA. Total dose: 380 mg/20 d to 190 mg/37 d	Local control: XRT alone: 6/16 (38%) XRT+6MP: 2/9 (22%)		XRT alone: 5/16 (31%) alive NED XRT + 6MP: 0/9 alive NED
Bagshaw and Doggett (1969)[2]	Various sites	15	XRT alone: average total dose 6360 rad/45 d XRT + BUdR: average total dose 5900–6340 rad/47–57 d	BUdR 500 mg/d IA with or without methotrexate before BUdR to an average total BUdR dose of 17 g	Local control: XRT + BUdR: 5/15 (33%) XRT alone: 6/16 (38%)		XRT + BUdR: 4/15 alive NED XRT alone: 5/16 (31%)
Bakowski et al. (1978)[3]	Various sites	90 patients entered (1975–76) 18 pairs or 36 matched for evaluation	5800–6800 rad in 38–61 d at 200 rad/fraction	ICRF 159 (Razoxane) 125 mg in the morning. 62.5 mg in the evening of each day of irradiation	Razoxane + XRT: 7/18 (39%), 3 recurrent at 3 and 5 months. Placebo + XRT: 10/18 (56%), 3 recurrent at 7 and 9 months	Razoxane + 2/36	—
Morita (1980)[37]	Paranasal sinuses	23	4000–5000 rad/ 4–5 wks	Methotrexate 0.2 mg/d + BUdR 200 mg/d IA to a total BUdR dose of 4000–5000 mg/20–25 d	2-yr local control: 3/21 (14.3%) vs. historical XRT alone: 19/47 (40.4%)		—
		22	4000 rad/4 wks + surgical removal of residual tumour	Methotrexate 0.2 mg/d + BUdR 200 mg/d IA to a total BUdR dose of 4000 mg/20 d	2-yr local control: 14/22 (63.6%)		

was obtained in the XRT + placebo group than the XRT + razoxane group (10/18 or 56% vs. 7/18 or 39%). The incidence of mucositis was similar in both groups. Similarly, 6 MP when combined with XRT appeared to have a less favourable tumour response, but enhanced radiation mucositis more than XRT alone.[2] BUdR, a radiosensitizer, infused intra-arterially during XRT with or without preceding MTX markedly enhanced the radiation mucositis without improvement of local control or survival.[2,37]

MULTI-DRUG CHEMOTHERAPY AND RADIOTHERAPY (XRT)

In the past, combined treatment for advanced inoperable head and neck cancer consisted of a XRT and a single chemotherapeutic agent. More recently, multi-drug combination chemotherapy concurrent with XRT has been tried by a number of institutions (Table 15.7).

One of the earliest studies employing multi-drug XRT concurrent with XRT was reported by O'Connor *et al.* in 1979.[38] Ninety-two patients, treated with a multi-drug regimen of vincristine, bleomycin, and MTX with leucovorin rescue combined with a synchronous course of XRT were compared with a historical group of 92 patients treated with XRT alone. There was statistically significant improvement in 4-year crude survival rate, 56.1% vs. 24.5% ($P < 0.001$); and disease-free survival, 56.5% vs. 21.8% ($P < 0.000001$), in the combined treatment group. In a recent update of the study,[39] of 198 patients treated since 1974 the crude actuarial survival was 41% and the probability of recurrence-free was 52% at 60 months (Table 15.7). Local control above the clavicle was maintained in 62% of the patients. The incidence of treatment-related deaths was 7.5%. However, in the combined treatment group severe and premature mucositis necessitated interruption of treatment up to 1-2 weeks in many patients, and dysphagia

and consequent dehydration necessitated tube feeding in one-third of the patients.

Stimulated by the early reported results of this study, the Radiation Therapy Oncology Group (RTOG) conducted a pilot study in which two cycles of vincristine, bleomycin, and MTX, similar to the regimen used in the above study, were administered prior to XRT and three cycles were planned concurrently with XRT.[15] Ten of 11 patients completed XRT and 8/11 (73%) had complete local clearance. The chemotherapy programme did not appear to decrease the risk of distant metastases, as 5/11 (45%) patients developed distant metastases. Only 2/11 (8%) were in continuous complete remission for a follow-up period of 1-18 months (median 8 months). Toxicity was substantial, necessitating interruption of XRT in eight cases and only 7/11 tolerated their full chemotherapy cycles during XRT. Two patients developed osteonecrosis and one patient had carotid rupture. Performance status and weight uniformly decreased during XRT. It was felt that, although the combined treatment led to improved tumour response, the morbidity of the treatment regimen was prohibitive for continued study.

A similar experience was reported in another RTOG pilot study employing a different multi-drug regimen consisting of cyclophosphamide, vincristine, and bleomycin during XRT followed by cyclophosphamide, MTX, and bleomycin after completion of XRT.[12] A planned 2-week break was instituted after 1800 rad. At the time of death or last follow-up (2-24 + months with a median of 7 months), the disease was controlled at the primary site in eight patients (53%) and in the neck in 12 patients (80%) and in all sites in seven patients (47%), but only 6/15 (40%) survived more than 1 year. Toxicities, primarily mucositis and infection, were severe, and three patients had fatal complications. In addition, two patients developed late osteonecrosis. Only seven of the 15 patients received maintenance chemotherapy after XRT and only one of the seven completed the

TABLE 15.7   CONCURRENT MULTI-DRUG CHEMOTHERAPY AND RADIOTHERAPY (XRT) FOR ADVANCED HEAD AND NECK CANCER

Reference	Primary site	No. of patients	Radiation dose schedule	Drug dose schedule	Response rate CR	PR	Survival
Bitter (1977)[6]	Oral cavity	20	200 rad/d × 4 wks to 6000 rad	Bleomycin 30 mg/h IA Q 4 d × 4, then 5 mg IA Q 4 d to a total dose of 180–200 mg. MTX 240 mg/m²/20 h IA immediately after bleomycin Q 4 d × 4, plus Leucovorin rescue.	10/20 (50%) 14/20 (70%) 4 after surgical salvage		83.8% at 1 yr.
O'Connor et al. (1982)[39]	Various sites	198	Total dose amount at 6000–6600 rad at 180–200 rad/d	VBM: 0 h VCR 2 mg IV 6 h bleo 30 mg IM 24 h MTX 200 mg/1000 cc saline 24 h infusion 48 h Leucovorin 50 mg IV followed by 9 mg Leucovorin IM Q 6 h × 5 doses for 4 courses, i.e., before XRT at 2000 rad, at 4000 rad and after completion of XRT. XRT interupted during drug administration	Local control above the clavicle – 62%		5-yr actuarial crude survival: 41%

TABLE 15.7 Cont.

Reference	Primary site	No. of patients	Radiation dose schedule	Drug dose schedule	Response rate CR	Response rate PR	Survival
Glick et al. (1979)[15]	Various sites	11	6600–7400 rad/ 7–8 wks, 175–200 rad/d, 5 fractions per wk	VBM: VCR 1.4 mg/m^2 IV (Max. 2.0 mg) + bleo. 30 units IV followed 6 h later by (5 patients); MTX 60 mg/m^2 IV–200 mg/m^2 IV with leukovorin rescue. 2 cycles VBM alone followed by 3 cycles VBM + XRT. MTX maintenance: MTX 30 mg/m^2 IV/wk × 2 courses. Escalate to 35 mg/m^2 IV/wk × 2 then 40 mg/m^2 IV/wk × 6 months followed by 40 mg/m^2 IV Q 2 wks × 6 months	8/11 (73%)	2/11 (18%)	2 patients alive NED at 16 and 18 months. 1 patient alive with local control but distant metastases at 12 months.

Reference	Primary site	No. of patients	Radiation dose schedule	Drug dose schedule	Response rate CR	Response rate PR	Survival
Bezwoda et al. (1979)[5]	Various sites	58	XRT alone: Day 0 start XRT at 250 rad/d × 13, to 3250 rad t.d. Nodes to 2600 rad at 1 cm, beginning d 17 split 3 wks then d 39 resume XRT to total tumour dose of 6500 rad and 5200 rad at 1 cm to lymph nodes. Total duration 55 d	XRT + chemotherapy: Day 0: start with 1 24 h cycle of 2 mg VCR + 40 mg adria. IV at time 0. 60 mg bleo. infusion in 6 h at 6 h and MTX 30 mg PO at 6, 9, 12 h and 500 mg 5FU IV at 12 h HU 2000 mg PO at 18 h and 6 MP 200 mg at 24 h. Day 7: XRT starts 250 rad/d × 13 to 3250 rad, nodes to 2600 rad at 1 cm. Day 24: Split 3 wks Day 28: Chemotherapy. Day 39: XRT resumes to total tumour dose of 6500 rad and 5200 rad at 1 cm. Day 63: Chemotherapy Total duration 63 d.	XRT: 1/28 (3.1%) XRT + chemotherapy: 1/30 (3.3%)	13/28 (46.4%) 16/30 (53.3%)	Mean survival: XRT 18 wks XRT + chemotherapy: 36 wks ($P < 0.05$)

TABLE 15.7 Cont.

Reference	Primary site	No. of patients	Radiation dose schedule	Drug dose schedule	Response rate CR	Response rate PR	Survival
Fu *et al.* (1979)[12]	Various sites	15	6500–7500 rad in 9–11 wks with planned 2-wk break at 1800 rad	CTX 750 mg/m² IV d 1. VCR 1.4 mg/m² IV d 2. Bleo. 15 u IV d 3, 4, and 5, and 5 u IV d 8 and 10 then 5 u IV b.i.w. during XRT. Remission consolidation: CTX 500 mg/m² IV d 1 MTX 25 mg/m² IV d 1, 8, 15 and 22. Bleo. 15 u IV/wk on d 1 Q 4 wks × 6 cycles	Primary 53% Nodes 80%		6/15 (40%) survived ⩾ 1 yr
Hollmann *et al.* (1979)[22]	Various sites	69	5 rad – 6680 rad, average 4430 rad, with betatron (39 patients); 4004 rad with gammatron (20 patients) 2480 rad with X-ray (10 patients)	MTX 25 mg/2 h/d (a.m.) IA. Bleo. 15 mg/2 h/d (p.m.) IA. Leucovorin 12.5 mg/d IM. Mean total dose: MTX 507 (50–1200) Bleo. 286 (45–450) Great variation of drug doses	N/A		15/53 (28.3%) alive > 1 yr

Reference	Primary site	No. of patients	Radiation dose schedule	Drug dose schedule	Response rate CR	Response rate PR	Survival
Smith et al. (1980)[56]	Various sites	36	5500–6500 rad in 5.5–6.5 wks to the primary and 4000–5000 rad in 5–6 wks to the nodes	5FU: 110 mg/m² IV 3x/wk 1 h before XRT. Adria. 7 mg/wk IV on d 1. Bleo.: 4.5 u/m²/a.l.k. IV or IM on d 1 and 4	20/30 (67%)	10/30 (33%)	19/30 (63 %) alive 3–27 months
Malaker et al. (1980)[33]	Various sites	29	6000–6600 rad in 61–64 d. 3 split courses: 2000 rad/10 fractions d 5–17 and d 27–39 and 2600 rad/13 fractions d 49–64	VBM (same as O'Connor et al.) on d 1, 22, 44 and 3 courses after XRT during 4, 5 and 6 months	Primary: 23/29 (79%) Nodes: 6/17 (35%)	7/17 (41%)	N/A
Seagren et al. (1982)[49]	Various sites	24	180 rad/fraction d 1–5 and 8–12 to total dose of 5400 rad in 10 wks No treatment d 13–28. 3 cycles of 28 d Additional RX: 1. 7000 rad T.D. 4 patients 2. Implant 11 patients 3. Radical neck 4 patients 4. No further treatment 5 patients	CTX: 1 g/m² IV d 2, 4, 9 and 11 each. Total: CTX 3 g/m² Bleo. 180 u	16/24 (67%) 11/16 subsequently recurred loco-regionally		4/24 (17%) alive NED with minimum follow-up of 29 months

prescribed treatment. It was concluded that treatment morbidity and complications were too prohibitive for this treatment programme to progress to a randomized trial.

The only randomized trial comparing multi-drug chemotherapy + XRT to XRT alone was reported by Bezwoda et al., from South Africa.[5] A seven-drug (vincristine, adriamycin, bleomycin, MTX, 5FU, HU, and 6 MP) combination chemotherapy regimen was administered before, during, and after a split course of XRT (Table 15.7). Although a significant difference in survival was found between the two groups (median survival 18 weeks for XRT alone vs. 56 weeks for XRT + chemotherapy ($P < 0.05$), only 1/28 (3.6%) in the XRT alone group and 1/30 (3.3%) in the combined treatment group had a complete response. Both the survival and the tumour response rates were lower than most reported series of advanced head and neck cancer treated with XRT with or without chemotherapy. The degree and incidence of toxicity were greater in the combined treatment group, and one patient died of infection.

Smith et al.[55] reported a complete response rate of 66% and a partial response rate of 33% in 36 patients treated with 5FU, adriamycin, and bleomycin during XRT. Similar to all of the other series, there was marked enhancement of glossitis and mucositis and XRT was temporarily discontinued after about 2000–2500 rad. It is noteworthy that the combined treatment resulted in 6/36 (17%) fatality.

The other studies using two-drug combinations[6,22,49] also demonstrated no enhancement or equivocal enhancement of tumour response but enhanced normal tissue reaction. In the series reported by Seagren et al.,[49] although 16/34 (66.7%) patients were free of disease after combined cyclophosphamide and bleomycin, and the XRT ± interstitial implant or surgery; the response was of short duration and 11/16 recurred locoregionally with a median time to recurrence of 5 months and 7/11 patients developed distant metastases.

Thus, multi-drug chemotherapy concurrent

with XRT appeared to be associated with increased morbidity and with increased mortality. Although most studies showed enhanced locoregional tumour response, there was with one exception,[38] no significant increase in survival, and there was no evidence suggesting decreased incidence of distant metastases with adjuvant multi-drug chemotherapy programmes.

DISCUSSION

The main objectives of combined chemotherapy and XRT are to improve local control and survival, and decrease distant metastases without excessively increasing the injury to normal tissues. From the preceding review it is apparent that improved locoregional control has been shown with bleomycin, 5FU, MTX, HU, and multi-drug chemotherapy used concurrently with XRT for advanced head and neck cancer. Improved survival in randomized studies has been demonstrated only with bleomycin and 5FU, and only for oral cavity carcinomas.[31,51] There is no evidence of decreased incidence of distant metastases. Furthermore, enhanced normal tissue reactions, primarily radiation mucositis, has been seen with most single agents used concurrently with XRT.

When multi-drug chemotherapy was used concurrently with XRT, although there was usually an increased tumour response, severe local normal tissue reactions often led to interruptions of treatment and required intensive supportive care.[12,15,38,56] Systemic toxicities and fatal complications have been reported.[12,39,56] At the present time there is little, if any, evidence to suggest any improved therapeutic ratio with concurrent multi-drug chemotherapy and XRT.

One of the obstacles to progress in this area of clinical research may be the lack of methods for selecting active drugs for the individual patients. Experimental combined modality studies suggest that no enhanced tumour response can be expected when drugs are combined with XRT unless the drugs are active against the tumour by themselves. Ideally, it would be more rational to first determine which drugs are most effective for the individual patient before combining them with XRT. Although stem cell assay for the selection of optimal chemotherapy has become available, its usefulness in the treatment of solid tumours is limited at the present time.[46] Future technical improvements in this area of research may potentially improve the results of combined chemotherapy and XRT.

Although a large number of chemotherapeutic drugs are currently used in the treatment of a variety of malignant neoplasms, only a limited number of drugs have been evaluated in combination with XRT for advanced head and neck cancer. Further exploration of currently available, but heretofore untested, drugs for combined use with XRT may be worthwhile. Drugs such as DDP and mitomycin C in combination with XRT for head and neck cancer are currently under clinical evaluation.[9,19,20]

One other aspect of combined modality treatment which has not been adequately evaluated clinically is the optimal timing of drug and radiation administration. In most studies reported, the time of drug administration in relation to XRT has not been specified. It is possible that certain schedules of drug and radiation administration, exploiting differences in proliferative kinetics between tumour and normal tissues, would yield the optimal therapeutic ratio. Further research into this aspect of combined modality studies in the laboratory, as well as in the clinic, might prove fruitful.

Most data available suggest that multi-drug chemotherapy concurrent with XRT is poorly tolerated. Enhanced normal tissue effects are most often seen with concurrent chemotherapy and XRT, and are less likely to occur when they are administered sequentially.[14] Unless true enhancement of tumour effects occurs only with concurrent use of XRT and chemotherapy, it would be more preferable to administer the two modalities in a sequential fashion to avoid excessive injury to the normal

tissues, especially when multiple drugs are used. Recent reports suggest induction chemotherapy given prior to XRT and/or surgery can be well tolerated with good tumour response, without increasing the morbidity of subsequent XRT and/or surgery.[1,16,34,64]

One of the reasons for the incidence of improved locoregional control without improved survival for combined therapy may be that most patients treated for advanced squamous cell carcinoma of the head and neck are chronic alcoholic and tobacco abusers and are in a poor nutritional state. They are further debilitated or compromised by their disease and/or the aggressive treatment. Thus, more intensive supportive care directed towards the improvement of the nutritional status of the patient may be necessary to achieve the ultimate goal of combined modality treatments which is improved survival.

In spite of the improved locoregional control, the problem of distant metastases remains unresolved. Combination chemotherapy using different regimens both before and after XRT may be necessary to eradicate microscopic distant metastases. Experience from recent clinical trials suggests poor patient compliance with maintenance chemotherapy. For practical purposes, any maintenance programme should not be too toxic and should preferably be administered on an outpatient basis. Here again, intensive supportive care may be necessary for the full implementation of long-term administration of chemotherapy after completion of the primary treatments.

Finally, other new treatment modalities such as hyperthermia, radiosensitizers, and radioprotectors may be combined with chemotherapy and XRT to further improve the therapeutic ratio. The potential efficacy of combining these new modalities will need further exploration.

REFERENCES

1. Al-Sarraf, M., Drelichman, A., Jacobs, J., Kinzie, J., Hoschner, J., Loh, J.J.-K., and

Weaver, A. (1981). Adjuvant chemotherapy with cis-platinum, oncovin, and bleomycin followed by surgery and/or radiotherapy in patients with advanced previously untreated head and neck cancer: Final report. In S.E. Salmon and S.E. Jones (Eds), *Adjuvant Therapy of Cancer*, vol. III, Grune and Stratton, New York, pp.145–152.

2. Bagshaw, M.A., and Doggett, R.L.S. (1969). A clinical study of chemical radiosensitization. *Front. Radiat. Ther. Oncol.*, **4**, 164–173.

3. Bakowski, M.T., Macdonald, E., Mould, R.F., Cawte, P., Sloggem, J., Barrett, A., Dalley, V., Newton, K.A., Westbury, G., James S.E., and Hellmann, K. (1978). Double blind controlled clinical trial of radiation plus razoxane (ICRF 159) versus radiation plus placebo in the treatment of head and neck cancer. *Int. J. Radiat. Oncol. Biol. Phys.*, **4**, 115–119.

4. Berdal, P. (1976). Head and neck carcinoma treatment with bleomycin and radiation. *Gann Monograph on Cancer Research*, **19**, 133–149.

5. Bezwoda, W.R., de Moor, N.G., and Derman, D.P. (1979). Treatment of advanced head and neck cancer by means of radiation therapy plus chemotherapy – a randomized trial. *Med. Pediatr. Oncol.*, **6**, 353–358.

6. Bitter, K. (1977). Bleomycin–methotrexate chemotherapy in combination with telecobalt radiation for patients suffering from advanced oral carcinoma. *J. Maxillofac. Surg.*, **5**, 75–81.

7. Cachin, Y., Jortay, A., Sancho, H., Eschwege, F., Madelain, M., Desaulty, A., and Gerard, P. (1977). Preliminary results of a randomized E.O.R.T.C. study comparing radiotherapy and concomitant bleomycin to radiotherapy alone in epidermoid carcinomas of the oropharynx. *Eur. J. Cancer*, **13**, 1389–1395.

8. Condit, P.T. (1968). Treatment of carcinoma with radiation therapy and methotrexate. *Mo. Med.*, **65**, 832–835.

9. Coughlin, C.T., Grace, M., LeMarbre, P., O'Donnell, J., Douple, E.B. (1982). Combined modality therapy for advanced head and neck cancer. *Proc. Am. Soc. Clin. Oncol.*, **1**, 200.

10. De-la-Garza, J.G., Garcia Olivares, F., Armendariz, C., and Flores-F, A.M. (1976). Simultaneous use of bleomycin and radiotherapy in malignant tumors of the head and neck. *J. Int. Med. Res.*, **4**, 158–164.

11. Douple, E.B., and Richmond, R.C. (1979). A review of platinum complex biochemistry suggests a rationale for combined platinum-radiotherapy. *Int. J. Radiat. Oncol. Biol. Phys.*, **5**, 1335–1339.

12. Fu, K.K., Silverberg, I.J., Phillips, T.L., and Friedman, M.A. (1979). Combined radiotherapy and multidrug chemotherapy for advanced head and neck cancer: Results of a radiation therapy oncology group pilot study. *Cancer Treat. Rep.*, **63**, 351–357.

13. Fu, K.K., Phillips, T.L., Silverberg, I.J., Friedman, M.A., Kohler, M., Carter, S.K. (1983). Combined bleomycin and radiotherapy in advanced inoperable head and neck cancer – an NCOG randomized study. *Proc. Am. Soc. Clin. Oncol.*, **2**, 159 (C-622).

14. Fu, K.K. (1979). Normal tissue effects of combined radiotherapy and chemotherapy for head and neck cancer. *Front. Radiat. Ther. Oncol.*, **13**, 113–132.

15. Glick, J.H., Fazekas, J.T., Davis, L.W., Rominger, J.C., Breen, F.A., and Brodovsky, H.S. (1979). Combination chemotherapy – radiotherapy for advanced inoperable head and neck cancer. A RTOG pilot study. *Cancer Clin. Trials.*, **2**, 129–136.

16. Glick, J.H., Marcial, V., Richter, M., and Velez-Garcia, E. (1980). The adjuvant treatment of inoperable stage III and IV epidermoid carcinoma of the head and neck with platinum and bleomycin infusions prior to definitive radiotherapy: an RTOG pilot study. *Cancer*, **46**, 1919–1924.

17. Goepfert, H., Jesse, R.H., and Lindberg, R.D. (1973). Arterial infusion and radiation therapy in the treatment of advanced cancer of the nasal cavity and paranasal sinuses. *Am. J. Surg.*, **126**, 464–468.

18. Goldsmith, M.A., and Carter, S.K. (1975). The integration of chemotherapy into a combined modality approach to cancer therapy. *Cancer Treatment Rev.*, **2**, 137–158.

19. Harwood, A.R., Princess Margaret Hospital, Toronto, Canada (personal communications).

20. Haselow, R.E., Adams, G.S., Oken, M.M., Goudsmit, A., Lerner, J.H., and Marsh, J.C. (1983). Cis-platinum (DDP) and radiation therapy (RT) for locally advanced unresectable head and neck cancer. *Proc. Am. Soc. Clin. Oncol.*, **2**, 160.

21. Heidelberger, C., Griesbach, L., Montag, B.J., *et al.* (1958). Studies on fluorinated pyrimidines II. Effects on transplanted tumors. *Cancer Res.*, **18**, 305–317.

22. Hollmann, K., Jesch, W., Kuehboeck, J., and Dimopoulos, J. (1979). Combined intra-arterial chemotherapy and radiation therapy of tumors in the maxillofacial region. *J. Maxillofac. Surg.*, **7**, 191–197.

23. Hussey, D.H., and Abrams, J.P. (1975). Combined therapy in advanced head and neck

cancer: Hydroxyurea and radiotherapy. *Prog. Clin. Cancer*, **6**, 79–86.

24. Jesse, R.H., Helmuth, G., Lindberg, R.D., *et al.* (1969). Combined intra-arterial infusion and radiotherapy for the treatment of advanced cancer of the head and neck. *Am. J. Roentgenol.*, **105**, 20–25.

25. Jörgensen, S.J. (1972). Time-dose relationships in combined bleomycin treatment and radiotherapy. *Eur. J. Cancer*, **8**, 531–534.

26. Kapstad, B. (1978). Treatment of squamous cell carcinomas of the head and neck region with cobalt and bleomycin. *Int. J. Radiat. Oncol. Biol. Phys.*, **4**, 91–94.

27. Kapstad, B., Bang, G., Rennaes, S., and Dahler, A. (1978). Combined preoperative treatment with cobalt and bleomycin in patients with head and neck carcinoma – a controlled clinical study. *Int. J. Radiat. Oncol. Biol. Phys.*, **4**, 85–89.

28. Komiyama, S., Hiroto, I., Ryu, S., Nakashima, T., Kuwano, M., and Endo, H. (1978). Synergistic combination therapy of 5-fluorouracil, vitamin A and cobalt-60 radiation therapy upon head and neck tumors. *Oncology*, **35**, 253–257.

29. Kramer, S. (1969). Use of methotrexate and radiation therapy for advanced cancer of the head and neck. *Front. Radiat. Ther. Oncol.*, **4**, 116–125.

30. Lerner, J.H. (1977). Concomitant hydroxyurea and irradiation. Clinical experience with 100 patients with advanced head and neck cancer at Pennsylvania Hospital. *Am. J. Surg.*, **134**, 505–509.

31. Lo, T.C., Wiley, A.L. Jr., Ansfield, F.J., Brandenburg, J.H., Davis, J.L., Jr., Gollin, F.F., Johnson, R.O., Ramirez, G., and Vermund, H. (1976). Combined radiation therapy and 5-fluorouracil for advanced squamous cell carcinoma of the oral cavity and oropharynx: a randomized study. *Am. J. Roentgenol.*, **126**, 229–235.

32. Lustig, R.A., DeMare, P.A., and Kramer, S. (1976). Adjuvant methotrexate in the radiotherapeutic management of advanced tumors of the head and neck. *Cancer*, **37**, 2703–2708.

33. Malaker, K., Robson, F., and Schipper, H. (1980). Combined modalities in the management of advanced head and neck cancers. *J. Otolaryngol.*, **9**, 24–30.

34. Marcial, V.A., Vélez-Garcia, E., Figueroa-Vallés, N.R., Cintrón, J., and Vallecillo, L.A. (1980). Multidrug chemotherapy (vincristine-bleomycin-methotrexate) followed by radiotherapy in inoperable carcinomas of the head and neck: Preliminary report of a pilot

study of the Radiation Therapy Oncology Group. *Int. J. Radiat. Oncol. Biol. Phys.*, **6**, 717–721.

35. Mason, J., and Ediger, A. (1970). Infusion chemotherapy. *Proc. Sixth Natl. Cancer Conf.*, **621**, 625.

36. Matsuzawa, T., Onozawa, M., Morita, K., and Kakehi, M. (1972). Radiosensitization of bleomycin on lethal effect of mouse cancer cells in vitro. *Strahlentherapie*, **144**, 614–616.

37. Morita, K. (1980). Clinical significance of radiation therapy combined with chemotherapy. *Strahlentherapie*, **156**, 228–233.

38. O'Connor, A.D., Clifford, P., Dalley, V.M., Durden-Smith, D.J., Edwards, W.G., and Hollis, B.A. (1979). Advanced head and neck cancer treated by combined radiotherapy and VBM cytotoxic regimen – four-year results. *Clin. Otolaryngol.*, **4**, 329–337.

39. O'Connor, D., Clifford, P., Edwards, W.G., Dalley, V.M., Durden-Smith, J., Hollis, B.A., and Calman, F.M. (1982). Long-term results of VBM and radiotherapy in advanced head and neck cancer. *Int. J. Radiat. Oncol. Biol. Phys.*, **8**, 1525–1531.

40. Phillips, R.A., and Tolmach, L.J. (1966). Repair of potentially lethal damage in x-irradiated HeLa cells. *Radiat. Res.*, **29**, 413–432.

41. Richards G.J., and Chambers, R.G. (1969). Hydroxyurea: a radiosensitizer in the treatment of neoplasms of the head and neck. *Am. J. Roentgenol. Radium Nucl. Med.*, **55**, 555–565.

42. Richards, G.J., and Chambers, R.G. (1973). Hydroxyurea in the treatment of neoplasms of the head and neck: a resurvey. *Am. J. Surg.*, **126**, 513–518.

43. Rominger, C.J. (1971). Hydroxyurea and radiation therapy in advanced neoplasms of the head and neck. *Am. J. Roentgenol.*, **111**, 103–108.

44. Rygard, J., and Hansen, H.S. (1979). Bleomycin as adjuvant in radiation therapy of advanced squamous cell carcinoma in head and neck. *Acta Otolaryngol.* (Suppl.) (Stockh.) **360**, 161–166.

45. Sakamoto, K., and Sakka, M. (1974). The effect of bleomycin and its combined effect with radiation on murine squamous carcinoma treated in vivo. *Br. J. Cancer*, **30**, 463–468.

46. Salmon, S.E., Alberts, D.S., Meyskens, F.L., Durie, B.G.M., Jones, S.E., and Moon, T.E. (1981). Tumor stem cells and adjuvant chemotherapy: perspectives in 1981. In S.E. Salmon and S.E. Jones (Eds), *Adjuvant Therapy of Cancer III*, Grune & Stratton, New York, pp.13–23.

47. Sato, Y., Morita, M., Takashi, H.O.,

Watenabe, N., and Kirkae, I. (1970). Combined surgery, radiotherapy and regional chemotherapy in carcinoma of the paranasal sinuses. *Cancer*, **25**, 571–579.

48. Seagren, S.L., Byfield, J.E., Nahum, A.M., and Bone, R.C. (1979). Treatment of locally advanced squamous cell carcinoma of the head and neck with concurrent bleomycin and external beam radiation therapy. *Int. J. Radiat. Oncol. Biol. Phys.*, **5**, 1531–1535.

49. Seagren, S.L., Byfield, J.E., Terence, M.D., and Thomas, R.S. (1982). Bleomycin, cyclophosphamide and radiotherapy in regionally advanced epidermoid carcinoma of the head and neck. *Int. J. Radiat. Oncol. Biol. Phys.*, **8**, 127–132.

50. Shah, P.M., Shukla, S.N., Patel, K.M., Patel, N.L., Baboo, H.A., and Patel, D.D. (1981). Effect of bleomycin-radiotherapy combination in management of head and neck squamous cell carcinoma. *Cancer*, **48**, 1106–1109.

51. Shanta, V., and Krishnamurthi, S. (1980). Combined bleomycin and radiotherapy in oral cancer. *Clin. Radiol.*, **31**, 617–620.

52. Shigematsu, Y., Sakai, S., and Fuchihata, H. (1971). Recent trials in the treatment of maxillary sinus carcinoma, with special reference to the chemical potentiation of radiation therapy. *Acta Otolaryngol.*, **71**, 63–70.

53. Silverberg, I.J., Phillips, T.L., Fu, K.K., and Chan, P.Y. (1981). Combined radiotherapy and bleomycin for advanced head and neck cancers: Results of a phase I pilot study. *Cancer Treat. Rep.*, **65**, 697–698.

54. Sinclair, W.K. (1968). The combined effect of hydroxyurea and x-rays on Chinese hamster cells in vitro. *Cancer Res.*, **28**, 190–206.

55. Sinclair, W.K. (1965). Hydroxyurea: differential lethal effects on cultured mammalian cells during the cell cycle. *Science*, **150**, 1729–1731.

56. Smith, B.L., Franz, J.L., Mira, J.G., Gates, G.A., Sapp, J., and Cruz, A.B. Jr. (1980). Simultaneous combination radiotherapy and multidrug chemotherapy for stage III and stage IV squamous cell carcinoma of the head and neck. *J. Surg. Oncol.*, **15**, 91–98.

57. Steel, G.G., and Peckham, J.M. (1979). Exploitable mechanism in combined radiotherapy-chemotherapy: The concept of additivity. *Int. J. Radiat. Oncol. Biol. Phys.*, **5**, 85–91.

58. Stefani, S., Eells, R.W., and Abbate, J. (1971). Hydroxyurea and radiotherapy in head and neck cancer. *Radiology*, **101**, 391–396.

59. Tanaka, Y., Wada, T., Fuchihata, H., Makino, T., and Inoue, T. (1976). Combined treatment with radiation and bleomycin for intra-oral carcinoma. A preliminary report. *Int. J. Radiat. Oncol. Biol. Phys.*, **1**, 1189–1193.

60. Terasima, T., Takabe, Y., and Yasukawa, M. (1975). Combined effect of x-ray and bleomycin on cultured mammalian cells. *Gann*, **66**, 701–703.

61. Vermund, H., Hodgett, J., and Ansfield, F.J. (1961). Effects of combined roentgen irradiation and chemotherapy on transplanted tumors in mice. *Am. J. Roentgenol.*, **85**, 559–567.

62. Vietti, T., Eggerding, F., and Valeriote, F. (1971). Combined effect of x radiation and 5-fluorouracil on survival of transplanted leukemic cells. *J. Natl. Cancer Inst.*, **47**, 865–870.

63. Weichselbaum, R.R., Posner, M.R., Ervin, T.J., Fabian, R.L., and Miller, D. (1981). Toxicity of aggressive multimodality therapy including cis-platinum, bleomycin and methotrexate with radiation and/or surgery for advanced head and neck cancer. *Int. J. Radiat. Oncol. Biol. Phys.*, **8**, 909–913.

64. Wittes, R., Heller, K., Randolph, V., Howard, J., Vallejo, A., Farr, H., Harrold, C., Gerold, F., Shah, J., Spiro, R., and Strong, E. (1979). Cis-dichlorodiammineplatinum(II) based chemotherapy as initial treatment of advanced head and neck cancer. *Cancer Treat. Rep.*, **63**, 1533–1538.

65. Young, C.N., and Hodas, S. (1964). Hydroxyurea: inhibitory effect on DNA metabolism. *Science*, **146**, 1172–1174.

Chapter 16

Immunology and Immunotherapy

Elias Y. Hilal* and Carl M. Pinsky†
* *Mercy Hospital, Pittsburgh, PA. USA*
† *Memorial Sloan – Kettering Cancer Center, New York, NY, USA*

INTRODUCTION

The relationship between the immune system and malignant disease, though extensively investigated in the last quarter-century, still has many unexplained aspects and poses many unanswered questions. Evidence has accumulated that the three main components of the immune response – namely the humoral or B-cell mediated, the T-cell mediated, and the macrophage systems – are involved in the normal reaction to malignant transformation.

The theory of immunological protection against cancerous transformation of normal tissues, termed immunological surveillance, derives support from several laboratory and clinical observations:

(1) neonatal thymectomy, administration of anti-lymphocyte serum or immunosuppressive drugs, or total body irradiation, predispose laboratory animals to increased susceptibility to induction of malignant tumours;

(2) similarly, some human immunodeficiency diseases are associated with increased incidence of malignancy;

(3) therapeutic immunosuppression, as in transplant recipients, increases the incidence of malignant tumours;

(4) the decline of immunocompetence with ageing is concomitant with the increased incidence of cancer in older people;

(5) occasional spontaneous tumour regressions have been documented in humans;

(6) the intense lymphocytic infiltration found in some tumours has been associated with improved prognosis;

(7) there are some reports of increased survival following infectious complications of surgical cancer treatment;

(8) many carcinogens are immunosuppressive.

The mechanisms of escape from, or failure of, immunological surveillance are thought to include:

(1) weak antigenicity of tumours;

(2) excess antigen in the tumour producing 'immune paralysis';

(3) immunosuppression of the host induced by tumour products or by endogenous suppressor cells;

(4) blocking antibodies.

Patients with squamous carcinoma of the head and neck have been found to have significant impairment of immunological reactivity. In the following discussion the general make-up of the immune system will be outlined, as well as the results of immunological investigations in head and neck cancer. The various factors involved in the impaired immune reactivity in patients with this cancer will be considered, and the results of recent immunotherapeutic trials in head and neck cancer will be summarized.

PHYSIOLOGY OF THE IMMUNE SYSTEM

The immune system can be subdivided into three main components: the T-cell system, the B-cell system, and the reticuloendothelial or macrophage system. B-lymphocytes are primarily involved with antibody production as they mature to form plasma cells. This function is regulated in at least two ways: first, excess formation of antibody activates a feedback mechanism; and second, suppressor T-cells inhibit antibody production.

The T-cells, or thymus-derived lymphocytes, make up about 70–90% of circulating lymphocytes and are also formed in the deep cortical regions of lymph nodes, the white pulp of the spleen, Peyer's patches, and bone marrow. Their function includes delayed hypersensitivity reactions to microbial and other antigens, allograft rejection, and formation of lymphokines including interferon, macrophage activating factors, transfer factor, LIF, etc. T-cells are also postulated to be effectors of immunological surveillance, i.e. the recognition, inhibition, and destruction of tumour cells. Subpopulations of T-cells play a regulatory function as they interact with B-cells. Some are helper T-cells, helping B-cells in antibody production; others, termed suppressor T-cells, suppress B-cell proliferation as mentioned earlier.

Macrophages and monocytes are involved with phagocytosis and destruction of microbes. *In vitro* evidence suggests a role for these cells in tumour cell destruction and in initiating and regulating T and B cell responses. These cells are also believed to be a source of interferon. In order to evaluate the function of these cells, a number of *in vivo* and *in vitro* tests can be used. Some of these tests are listed in Table 16.1.

TABLE 16.1 EVALUATION OF IMMUNOCOMPETENCE

I B-cells
  (a) *In vivo*:
    (1) Humoral immunity: primary and secondary antibody responses to antigenic stimulus.
  (b) *In vitro*:
    (1) Number (surface I_gG, EAC rosettes).
    (2) Immunoglobulin levels (immunoelectrophoresis, quantitative immunodiffusion).
    (3) Complement system (total complement and complement components C_{1q}, C_3).

II T-cells
  (a) *In vivo* tests – cutaneous delayed hypersensitivity reactions:
    (1) Primary: DNCB, KLH (Keyhole limpet haemocyanin).
    (2) Recall: microbial antigens, homograft rejection.
  (b) *In vitro* tests:
    (1) Total lymphocyte count (WBC and differential).
    (2) T-lymphocyte levels (SRBC rosettes, monoclonal antibodies).
    (3) Lymphocyte transformation: mitogens (PHA, ConA, PWM), specific microbial antigens, alloantigens (mixed lymphocyte culture).
    (4) Lymphokine production (soluble mediators, e.g. MIF).
    (5) Cytotoxicity assays: direct, antibody-dependent.

III Monocyte–macrophage system;
  (a) Chemotactic response.
  (b) Phagocytosis.
  (c) Cytotoxicity (direct, ADCC).
  (d) T-cell suppressor activity (MLC).

IV Granulocyte function:
  (a) Nitroblue tetrazolium test.
  (b) Phagocytosis.

IMMUNE COMPETENCE IN CANCER PATIENTS

Deficits of cell-mediated immunity have been demonstrated in many human cancers. Originally the attention of investigators was focused on lymphoid malignancies because of the direct involvement of the cells of immunity by the malignant process.[1,2] Interest in these investigations was further stimulated by the observation that lymphoid malignancies account for most of the cancers developing in patients with congenital immunodeficiency diseases or those under therapeutic immunosuppression.[3]

As patients with various other solid tumours were studied, it became apparent that immunological impairment is a common finding in cancer patients,[4,5] even in early stages of disease; as the cancer progresses, immune responses decline.[6] Further evaluations and follow-up showed that immune deficiency correlated with poor prognosis in cancer patients.[6-8]

IMMUNOLOGICAL ABNORMALITIES OF HEAD AND NECK CANCER PATIENTS

Comparison of immunological abnormalities in patients with various solid tumours highlighted the fact that patients with squamous carcinoma of the head and neck exhibited a higher incidence of immunosuppression than patients with tumours of other histological types.[6,8,9] This generated enormous enthusiasm for the investigation of the immunobiological aspects of head and neck cancer. This was done through the study of several parameters.

Delayed Hypersensitivity Reactions

The ability of the DNCB response to test both the afferent and efferent limbs of the immune system *in vivo* made it a particularly attractive investigative tool.[10] Several authors found that a significant proportion of patients with head and neck cancer had weak or absent reactions to DNCB when tested preoperatively[11] even at early stages[12,13] and many showed this immunosuppression to correlate with poor prognosis.[10,12] Impaired reactivity to DNCB has also been found in patients cured of squamous carcinoma.[14] This raised the question of a possible pre-existing immune defect in these patients predisposing them to the development of the malignancy.

Eilber *et al.*[11] observed a high incidence of recurrent disease in patients who converted from positive to negative reactivity during follow-up. Our own investigation of immunological reactivity in 183 patients with head and neck cancer showed that the negative

DNCB reaction could identify patients in early stages of disease who will do poorly despite adequate therapy. This prognostic value did not hold up with advanced stages of disease.[15] Other investigators did not find a useful prognostic value in DNCB reactivity, and hence caution was emphasized in interpreting and applying the results of these studies to individual clinical situations.[16,17]

One major limitation of DNCB testing is the 2-week interval required between sensitization and challenge. During this period any therapeutic intervention (surgery, radiation therapy, or chemotherapy) could affect the results of the test in a way not necessarily reflecting the interaction between the tumour and the immune system.

Enumeration of T-Lymphocytes

The absolute numbers and proportions of circulating T-lymphocytes were found to be significantly reduced with increasing size of the primary tumour.[18] The appearance of lymph node metastasis, however, was not associated with further decreases in the number of T-cells.[19] Olkowski and Wilkins observed a return of the number of circulating T-cells to normal about 2 weeks after surgical removal of the tumour.[20] Mason *et al.* found that enumeration of T-cells did not extend prognositc abilities beyond those based on clinical staging of disease.[21]

Lymphocyte Reactivity *in vitro*

Lymphocyte responses *in vitro* to mitogens (PHA, ConA, and PWM) and microbial antigens were studied. In general these showed progressive depression with advancing disease.[15,19] The prognostic significance of these decreased responses was not consistently observed.[15,22]

Macrophage Function

Berlinger *et al.*, using the mixed lymphocyte culture (MLC), found that macrophages inhibted lymphocyte responses to alloantigens *in vitro*. This suppression correlated with stage of disease and with short-term prognosis.[23]

Golub *et al.*[24] compared *in vivo* and *in vitro* tests of immune competence and found MLC responses to correlate best with DNCB reactivity.

Serum Factors

Several studies have attempted to elucidate the mechanism of immunosuppression in head and neck cancer. Sera from cancer patients inhibited responses of normal lymphocytes to PHA and to alloantigens in mixed lymphocyte culture; the degree of inhibition increased with progression of disease.[25] Hattler and Soehalen[26] described an inhibiting factor which could be eluted from leucocytes and suggested that it was an antigen-antibody complex. Maxim *et al.*[27] found evidence of soluble immune complexes in 80% of sera of head and neck cancer patients compared to 10% of control sera. These complexes persisted following treatment and were thought to act as blocking factors resulting in the anergy observed in these patients.

The immunoglobulin IgA has been implicated in the formation of these antigen–antibody complexes. Elevated levels of IgA have been found in sera of patients with head and neck cancer.[28] IgA has also been shown to have immunosuppressive properties *in vitro*.[29] Elevated levels of IgA antibody to the viral capsid antigen of Epstein–Barr virus were found to correlate with poor prognosis in patients with nasopharyngeal carcinoma.[30]

Wolf *et al.* demonstrated increased serum levels of specific acute phase proteins in head and neck cancer patients and these levels correlated better with tumour stage than cellular immune parameters. Levels of α_2-HS glycoprotein decreased with increased tumour stage. These glycoproteins have been found to suppress lymphocyte function *in vitro*, possibly by masking antigen receptor sites and by coating antigenic determinants on tumour cells.[31]

Lymph Node Morphology

Tsakraklides *et al.*[32,33] studied sections of lymph nodes draining malignant tumours of the breast and uterine cervix. They found improved survival in patients with lymph nodes exhibiting a lymphocytic predominance pattern, and poor prognosis in patients whose lymph nodes draining the area of malignancy had a lymphocyte depletion pattern. Berlinger *et al.*[34] applied this methodology to patients with head and neck squamous carcinoma and found significantly improved survival in patients whose regional lymph nodes had expanded inner cortices or increased numbers of germinal centres, denoting active immunological responses.

VIROLOGICAL ASPECTS OF HEAD AND NECK CANCER

The aetiological role of viruses in human cancers has long been suspected. Interest was directed to the Epstein–Barr virus following demonstration of this virus in cultured lymphoblasts from Burkitt's lymphomas.[35] Antibodies to EBV were then demonstrated in human sera to a variety of EBV-related antigens. IgA antibody titres to the viral capsid antigen of EBV were found to correlate with tumour burden and the clinical course of patients with nasopharyngeal carcinoma, but not with other squamous carcinomas of the head and neck.[30]

Positive IgA anti-herpes virus-induced antigens were found in the sera from 61% of patients with squamous carcinoma of the head and neck, and 57% of heavy smokers. Only a small percentage of patients with non-squamous malignant lesions and non-smokers had positive titres. No herpes virus antigens have been demonstrated in the nucleus, cytoplasm, or surface of epidermoid carcinoma cells.[36]

Another virus associated with head and neck neoplasia is the adenopapilloma virus demonstrated in conjunction with laryngeal papillomas, verruca vulgaris, and condylomata acuminata. The association here is believed to be one of coexistence, and evidence for causation of neoplasms in humans by viruses is still lacking.

TUMOUR-ASSOCIATED ANTIGENS

The concept of immunological reactivity against tumours rests on the assumption that tumours do exhibit certain specific antigens which can be recognized by the host lymphocytes and result in an immune reaction. Specific tumour antigens have been demonstrated in experimental animals; however detection of antigens in human malignant tumours has not been forthcoming.

Identification of antigens related to herpes virus in head and neck cancer patients and to EBV in nasopharyngeal carcinoma suggests a possible role of these viruses as aetiological agents.

Lymphocytes from patients with epidermoid carcinomas of various sites in the head and neck have been shown to react *in vitro* with tumour cells cultured from a laryngeal primary. This suggested the possible presence of a common antigen to all squamous carcinomas.[37]

Krause *et al.*[38] found that patients with epidermoid carcinoma developed a typical delayed hypersensitivity when injected intradermally with cell-free extracts of their own tumours, but not when injected with extracts of their normal tissues. This technique has potential applications in the diagnosis and prognosis of cancer; greater precision and sensitivity, however, would be expected from *in vitro* testing.

Demonstration of lymphocyte cytotoxicity against tumour cells *in vitro* depends on the successful establishment of cultured cell lines from epidermoid carcinomas. This type of tumour has unfortunately not been easily amenable to propagation in tissue culture. Recently, Aust and co-workers, using a collagenase or trypsin dispersion method, reported improved success in culturing head and neck tumours.[39] The tumour cells were then used to demonstrate specific lymphocyte cytotoxicity. This advance holds promise for the study of tumour antigenicity *in vitro*.

Another tumour antigen extensively investigated in gastrointestinal cancers, and particularly colon cancer – i.e. the carcinoembryonic antigen – was studied in 439 patients with squamous cancer of the head and neck by Silverman *et al.*[40] This tumour marker was not found to have useful applications in this disease.

FACTORS INFLUENCING GENERAL IMMUNOCOMPETENCE IN HEAD AND NECK CANCER

Several factors commonly considered to have significant aetiological associations with epidermoid carcinoma of the head and neck appear to have demonstrable effects on general immunocompetence.

Effect of Smoking

Studies on the effects of chronic inhalation of tobacco on immunocompetence in experimental animals and in man showed changes in both cellular and humoral systems. The early changes consist of increased T-cell levels and increased reactivity to PHA and tumour-specific cytotoxicity. Chronic changes with heavier tobacco consumption consist of progressive decline of reactivity to PHA.[41]

Investigations of the effect of chronic smoking on the humoral immune system show an elevation in serum IgA with specificity for herpes simplex virus-induced antigens. The frequency and magnitude of these increased IgA titres are similar to those seen in patients with squamous carcinoma of the head and neck. Antibodies in the IgA class have also been implicated in impairment of cell-mediated cytotoxicity by acting as blocking antibodies.[41]

Wolf *et al.* analysed glycoprotein levels in chronic smokers, non-smokers, and head and neck cancer patients. They found increased levels of antitrypsin and decreased levels of pre-albumin in smokers, both changes also seen in cancer patients.[31] The implication of these findings on the aetiology and pathogenesis of epidermoid carcinoma of the head and neck remains to be elucidated.

Alcohol Intake

The association between alcohol abuse and cancer of the head and neck has been observed in several epidemiological studies. Based on these observations, certain hypotheses have been suggested to explain this association. Alcohol may act as an immunosuppressant and thus enhance malignant transformation by failure of the immune surveillance mechanisms; or alcohol may act directly as a carcinogen or indirectly by enhancing the carcinogenic potential of other substances. The nutritional consequences of chronic alcoholism and cirrhosis could also be contributing factors.

The existence of impaired delayed hypersensitivity reactions in chronic alcoholics with cirrhosis parallels that found in patients with epidermoid carcinoma.[42]

Lundy *et al.* evaluated the acute and chronic effects of alcohol on the immune system.[43] They found no impairment of *in vivo* reactivity among alcoholic patients as measured by skin testing with DNCB and recall antigens. However, depression of T-cell counts in *in vitro* responses were observed in acute alcoholic states; the deficiency usually reversed with recovery from the alcoholic insult. Serum levels of immunoglobulins IgA, IgG, and IgM were significantly elevated among alcoholics.

Nutritional Status

Malnutrition and weight loss are known to be prevalent in patients with head and neck cancer due primarily to the local effects of the tumours. Poor nutritional status prior to any therapeutic intervention was highly correlated with immunosuppression, as evidenced by absence of delayed cutaneous reactivity to DNCB and low total lymphocyte counts. Furthermore, malnutrition was shown to have an adverse effect on prognosis, perhaps by causing a secondary immunodeficiency.[44] Serial studies of immune parameters in cancer patients undergoing hyperalimentation show improvement in lymphocyte functions. However, a beneficial effect of hyperalimentation on survival following cancer therapy still needs to be established.

Effect of Ageing

Malignant neoplasms in general, and head and neck carcinomas in particular, are far more common in older people than in the young. Paralleling this observation is the demonstration of gradual impairment of immune competence with ageing in humans. It has been shown that the incidence of negative tuberculin reactions increases markedly after the fifth decade. A significantly lower proportion of healthy persons over 70 develop delayed hypersensitivity reaction to DNCB (69%) compared to the group younger than 70 (94%).[45] Numbers and *in vitro* responses of lymphocytes also decrease with ageing. The relationship of this immunological 'senescence' to the development of cancers is still not clear.

IMMUNOLOGICAL EFFECTS OF CONVENTIONAL THERAPY

Effects of Anaesthesia and Operation

Suppression of immune function has been demonstrated following general anaesthesia and/or major surgical procedures. Several *in vivo* and *in vitro* tests of cell-mediated immunity have shown impairment starting immediately postoperatively and lasting up to 14 days.[46] Tarpley *et al.*[47] reported increased incidence of anergy to DNCB in cancer patients who have their 2-week period of sensitization interrupted by anaesthesia or surgery.[47] This observation emphasizes the need to have immunological evaluation completed prior to surgical intervention in cancer patients.

Effects of Radiation Therapy

Despite few reports that have shown no significant change or even an increase in lymphocyte responses *in vitro* following radiation therapy,[48] most investigators have shown suppression of immune parameters during and immediately after radiation therapy, primarily involving the T-cell system.[49,50] This suppression seems to be rather prolonged; up to several years in some reports.[51] The degree of suppression also appears to depend on the volume of tissue irradiated, and is particularly pronounced when the thymus or large portions of bone marrow are included in the field of radiation.[52]

Effects of Chemotherapy

Specific studies on the effect of chemotherapeutic agents on immune responses in patients with head and neck cancer have not been reported. However, inferences could be made from observations with other malignancies. In general, most chemotherapeutic agents are known to be immunosuppressive, mostly through bone marrow suppression and the observed absolute lymphopenia. These effects are both dose- and time-related and usually recover in a few days, hence the immunological advantage of intermittent chemotherapy.[53] Recovery of immune responses to a level higher than pretreatment values was found to be associated with prolonged survival.[54]

IMMUNOTHERAPY

The inability of conventional therapy to control disease in a significant proportion of patients with head and neck cancer has prompted the search for effective adjuvant therapy. With the observed impairment of immunocompetence in these patients even at an early stage of disease, several approaches to the correction of the immune defect have been considered.

Active Non-specific Immunotherapy

This method involves generalized non-specific stimulation of the immune system to improve non-specific anti-tumour host defence mechanisms. The most extensively investigated agents in this category are BCG, levamisole, and *Corynebacterium parvum*.

BCG (Bacillus Calmette–Guerin) has been the oldest and most widely used form of immunotherapy in humans. Studies in experimental animals have demonstrated significant immunological effects of BCG. These include increased reticuloendothelial system function,

namely increased clearance of bacteria and carbon particles from circulation; augmentation of the antibody response; increased delayed hypersensitivity responses to a variety of antigens; increased activity of peritoneal macrophages including cytotoxicity against tumour cells. It was postulated that these mechanisms could be operative in the anti-tumour activity of BCG.[55]

The initial clinical trials with BCG were conducted by Mathé in children with acute lymphocytic leukaemia. The results suggested an increase in disease-free survival.[56] Subsequent trials gave encouraging results in ovarian carcinoma, non-Hodgkin's lymphoma, and following resection of Stage I lung carcinoma.[57] Intra-lesional injection of BCG into cutaneous and subcutaneous melanoma nodules produced regressions that sometimes included non-injected nodules.[58]

In 1972 Donaldson reported his experience with the combination of methotrexate, isoniazid, and BCG in patients with advanced or recurrent squamous cell carcinoma of the head and neck. There was a 50% or greater decrease in the size of the lesions in 13 of 16 patients (81%) on this regimen. Isoniazid was used as an adjuvant chemotherapeutic agent (not as an anti-BCG agent) based on one observation of complete tumour regression in a tuberculous patient with recurrent squamous carcinoma of the floor of the mouth, who was receiving isoniazid concurrently with methotrexate and cyclophosphamide.[59]

Further follow-up yielded somewhat less impressive results but these still appeared to be better than with methotrexate alone.[60] This study provided the impetus for further controlled investigation of BCG as an adjuvant in head and neck cancer. Most of the subsequent results did not live up to the optimism generated by the study of Donaldson. Thus, Richman and associates found that the addition of weekly BCG by scarification to chemotherapy had no effect on the response rate or response duration, but significantly prolonged survival in patients with head and neck cancer having distant metastases.[61]

Subsequent randomized studies using methotrexate, BCG, and INH, or methotrexate and methanol-extraction residue (MER) of BCG in patients with advanced head and neck cancer showed no beneficial effect of BCG in the palliation of these patients.[62] Similarly, Suen *et al.*[63] compared various treatment regimens using combination chemotherapy and BCG in patients with advanced disease, and found that response rates, median duration of response, and median survival times were not significantly different from those reported with chemotherapy alone. In 1978 Papac *et al.*[64] reported the results of a prospective randomized study comparing methotrexate alone with methotrexate and BCG in patients with advanced inoperable squamous carcinoma of the head and neck. No benefit from BCG was observed in this trial.

The use of BCG following curative therapy was evaluated in a controlled randomized study by Taylor *et al.*[65] Patients with Stage III or IV head and neck cancer, rendered free of disease by surgery and/or radiation therapy, were randomized to receive either methotrexate alone or methotrexate and BCG. Some patients in this latter group received neuraminidase-treated autologous tumour cell vaccine whenever available. The results showed reduced recurrence rate in the chemo-immunotherapy group, but the difference was not statistically significant.

Results of serial immunological testing in the patients undergoing BCG immunotherapy in this trial failed to show any significant change. One possible explanation is that most of these patients had advanced disease, and in this situation many factors contribute to a profound depression of the immune system rendering it non-responsive to stimulation.

Levamisole is a phenylimidothiazole and had been widely used as an antihelminthic agent. Interest was raised in its immunotherapeutic potential by the discovery in 1971 that it augments the response to *Brucella* vaccination in mice.[66] Subsequent investigation showed that levamisole increased both antibody production and delayed

hypersensitivity reactions. The main activity of levamisole in experimental animals is its ability to restore impaired immune reactivity to normal.[67] This provided the rationale for a number of immunotherapeutic trials using levamisole in cancer patients.

Encouraging results were obtained in lung[68] and breast cancer.[69] Our own prospective randomized trial with levamisole following conventional therapy for head and neck cancer patients initially showed no overall advantage, but did suggest improved disease-free survival in the subgroup of patients with Stage II oral cavity epidermoid carcinoma.[70] Further follow-up is necessary to substantiate these results. A similar study by Olivari and co-workers[71] showed no difference in overall recurrence and survival rates at 36-month follow-up; Stage I and II patients treated with levamisole, however, had a significantly higher incidence of recurrence than the placebo-treated patients. In neither of these studies was evidence of immunological enhancement or reconstitution observed.

Corynebacterium parvum was also extensively investigated as a non-specific immunostimulant in cancer patients. *C. parvum* is administered as phenol-killed bacteria and exerts its major immunopotentiating effect by activating macrophages and stimulating the reticuloendothelial system.[67] Only a few studies using *C. parvum* in head and neck patients have been published. Cheng and co-workers injected *C. parvum* intralesionally and into cervical lymph nodes and intravenously in 21 patients with oral cavity cancers, prior to conventional therapy. No differences were observed in the survival of these patients compared to historical controls.[72]

In another trial, patients with oral cavity cancers were randomized to receive either *C. parvum* alone, combination chemotherapy, or observation following definitive surgery or radiotherapy. The results did not show differences in recurrence or survival rates between the different treatment arms when all the patients were considered. However, there was a significantly increased survival in surgically treated patients with Stage I or II tumours who received either *C. parvum* or chemotherapy compared with controls.[73]

Recently encouraging observations have been made with other synthetic immunomodulators both in laboratory studies and in limited clinical trials. Indomethacin and cimetidine have shown some promise in this regard[74,75] and their wider application awaits further evidence.

Active Specific Immunotherapy

This approach involves challenging the host with tumour cells or tumour cell components to produce an immune response to tumour-specific antigens. The problem with this method in head and neck cancers has been the difficulty in establishing tissue culture lines of these tumours, and in identifying or isolating specific tumour antigens. One attempt along this line has been the trial by Cunningham *et al.* in which neuraminidase-treated autogenous tumour cells, plus BCG and methotrexate, were administered to a small group of patients with advanced head and neck tumours following conventional therapy. Recurrences occurred in five of 11 patients on methotrexate alone, and in two of 11 patients on chemoimmunotherapy. No improvement in immune parameters was noted following this therapy, though no cytotoxicity studies were done.[76]

Immunotherapy with cytokines

This method of therapy is based on the administration of immunologically active materials to immunodeficient patients in order to reconstitute their immune responses. Examples are thymosin, interferon, and transfer factor.

Thymosin

The thymus gland is known for its role in the development of T-cells, the effectors of cell-mediated immunity. Experimental evidence has accumulated that this function is due in part to a hormonal mechanism. Thymectomized animals receiving transplanted thymus or thymic epithelium, in a cell-impermeable chamber, undergo reconstitution of their T-lymphocyte number and function. Children with certain immunodeficiency diseases involving thymus dysfunction, such as ataxia – telangiectasia and the Nezelof syndrome, had improved cellular immune responses with administration of thymosin, a fetal calf thymus extract.[77]

The rationale for treating cancer patients with thymosin rests on the observation that immune deficiency associated with malignant disease is primarily a T-cell deficiency. Following treatment with thymosin, patients had increased number of T-cells in circulation and increased delayed cutaneous hypersensitivity responses to recall antigens.[78] Kenady *et al.*[79] found that incubation with thymosin *in vitro* increased T-cell levels in patients undergoing radiation therapy for mediastinal malignancies, but not for head and neck or pelvic malignancies. Wara and co-workers demonstrated recovery of radiation-induced immunosuppression as evidenced by increased PHA stimulation and MLC responses following thymosin administration to head and neck cancer patients. In a randomized study these authors found that 64% of the thymosin-treated patients remained free of disease compared to 45% of the controls after a median follow-up period of 2 years ($P = 0.08$).[80] Further studies on the biological and therapeutic effects of thymosin in cancer patients are needed.

Interferon

Interferon refers to a family of glycoproteins produced by lymphocytes and other cells in response to viruses and other inducers, and acts intracellularly to inhibit viral replication. Three main types of interferon have been described:

(1) fibroblast interferon, released by fibroblasts in response to viral stimulation *in vitro*;

(2) leucocyte interferon, produced *in vitro* by cultures of buffy coat cells in response to viruses;

(3) immune interferon, released by T-cells following stimulation by specific antigens or mitogens.

The antiviral activity of interferon is species-specific. This has presented a major limitation on the supply of interferon for clinical investigation. Immunological effects of interferon include enhancement of T-cell and macrophage function.

Interferon has been shown to have anti-tumour activity in experimental animals against virus-induced tumours, as well as those with no known viral aetiology. The mechanism of anti-tumour action of interferon appears to be through inhibition of tumour cell division, and by alteration of the surface properties of tumour cell membranes.

Beneficial effects of interferon in human malignancies have been reported initially with osteogenic sarcoma, then with multiple myeloma. These reports sparked considerable interest in interferon as an immunotherapeutic agent. Treuner et al.[81] recently reported regression of nasopharyngeal carcinoma in an adolescent male. These authors also demonstrated a direct cytotoxic effect of interferon on tumour cells of the same patient grown in tissue culture. Interferon-induced regression of juvenile laryngeal papillomas have also been reported.[82,83] Currently several trials are being conducted to evaluate the effect of interferon on human cancer, including head and neck carcinoma.

Transfer factor

The successful transfer of tuberculin skin test reactivity with 'disrupted leucocytes' by Lawrence[84] started the interest in what became known as transfer factor. This consists of a dialysate of lysed leucocytes and contains molecular components of less than 10 000 molecular weight. Using its demonstrated ability to transfer delayed hypersensitivity reactions, several investigators used transfer factor to treat various chronic infectious diseases as well as congenital and acquired immunodeficiency states with significant improvements reported.

Trials of transfer factor immunotherapy in malignant diseases produced only sporadic successes or regressions. Vetto et al.[85] treated 35 patients with various advanced malignancies with transfer factor and observed a 'clinical effect' in 13 patients, mostly as short-lasting arrest of metastatic disease or pain relief. Immunological effects in another group of head and neck cancer patients consisted of increased T-cell levels in eight of 38 patients and decreased lymphocyte responses to PHA in 12 of 38.[86]

The major problem in treating malignant disease with transfer factor has been the selection of appropriate donors. Individuals with demonstrable high levels of immunity to tumour-specific antigens would theoretically be ideal donors of transfer factor to treat patients with the same kind of tumour. Using this approach, Goldenberg and Brandes[87] reported tumour regression in one of two patients with nasopharyngeal carcinoma who were treated with transfer factor from donors with previous infectious mononucleosis.

THE FUTURE OF IMMUNOTHERAPY OF CANCER

Results of conventional therapy of head and neck cancer are still primarily determined by stage of disease and remarkably unaffected by recent 'advances' in surgical or radiotherapeutic modalities. Several studies have now shown no significant difference in survival between preoperative and postoperative radiation therapy. The enthusiasm for preoperative chemotherapy with active agents, though promising a few years ago, has now yielded to more scepticism and the need for further investigation as the results of larger series and longer follow-ups begin to accumulate.

The theoretical considerations of immune modulation as adjuvant therapy in head and neck cancer remain attractive. The failure of immunotherapy trials in this disease could be ascribed to several factors:

(1) first and foremost, the nature and aetiology of immunosuppression associated with head and neck cancer is still not completely understood;

(2) the mechanism of action of many of the immunotherapeutic agents is not well elucidated;

(3) the earlier trials were conducted in patients with advanced disease and therefore a large tumour load, whereas one of the basic postulates of immunotherapy is its effectiveness in situations with minimal residual disease;

(4) only few prospective randomized trials have been carried out.

Recently the development of monoclonal antibodies appears to be promising. These antibodies showing very high specificity to certain tumour determinants could conceivably be used as therapeutic tools in their own right or as carriers of toxic components such as chemotherapeutic agents or radioisotopes to be delivered specifically to the tumour cells.

REFERENCES

1. Aisenberg, A.C. (1962). *J. Clin. Invest.*, **41**, 1964–1970.
2. Brown, R.S., Haynes, H.A., Foley, H.T., Godwin, H.A., Barnard, C.W., and Carbone, P.B. (1967). *Ann. Intern. Med.*, **67**, 291–302.
3. Penn, I., and Starzl, T.E. (1972). *Transplantation*, **14**, 407.
4. Catalona, W.J., and Chretien, P.B. (1973). *Cancer*, **31**, 353.
5. Catalona, W.J., Sample, W.F., and Chretien, P.B. (1973). *Cancer*, **31**, 65.
6. Pinsky, C.M., El-Domeiri, A., Caron, A.S., Knapper, W.H., and Oettgen, H.F. (1974). *Recent Results Cancer Res.*, **47**, 37.
7. Eilber, F.R., and Morton, D.L. (1970). *Cancer*, **25**, 362.
8. Pinsky, C.M., Wanebo, H.J., Mike, V., and Oettgen, H.F. (1976). *Ann. N.Y. Acad. Sci.*, **276**, 407.
9. Lichtenstein, A., Zighelboim, J., Dorey, F., Brossman, S., and Fahey, J.L. (1980). *Cancer*, **45**, 2090.
10. Pinsky, C.M. (1976). *Clinical Immunobiology*, **3**, 97.
11. Eilber, F.R., Morton, D.L., and Ketcham, A.S. (1974). *Am. J. Surg.*, **128**, 534.
12. Lundy, J., Wanebo, H., Pinsky, C., Strong, E., and Oettgen, H. (1974). *Am. J. Surg.*, **128**, 530.
13. Olivari, A., Pradier, R., Feierstein, J., Guardo, A., Glait, H., and Rojas, A. (1976). *J. Surg. Oncol.*, **8**, 287.
14. Twomey, P.L., Catalona, W.J., and Chretien, P.B. (1974). *Cancer*, **33**, 435.
15. Hilal, E.Y., Wanebo, H.J., Pinsky, C.M., Middleman, P., Strong, E.W., and Oettgen, H.F. (1977). *Am. J. Surg.*, **134**, 469.
16. Mandel, M.A. (1976). *Plastic Reconstr. Surg.*, **57**, 621.
17. Gilbert, H.A. *et al.* (1978). *J. Surg. Oncol.*, **10**, 73.
18. Deegan, M.J., and Coulthard, S.W. (1977). *Cancer*, **39**, 2137.
19. Wanebo, H.J., Jun, M.Y., Strong, E.W., and Oettgen, H.F. (1975). *Am. J. Surg.*, **130**, 445.
20. Olkowski, Z.L., and Wilkins, S.A. (1975). *Am. J. Surg.*, **130**, 440.
21. Mason, J.M. *et al.* (1977). *Arch. Otol.*, **103**, 223.
22. Maisel, R.H., Ogura, J.H. (1976). *Ann. Otol.*, **85**, 517.
23. Berlinger, N.T., Hilal, E.Y., Oettgen, H.F., and Good, R.A. (1978). *Laryngoscope*, **88**, 470.
24. Golub, S.H., O'Connell, T.X., and Morton, D.L. (1974). *Cancer Res.*, **34**, 1833.
25. Suciu-Foca, N., Buda, J., McManus, J., Thiem, T., and Reemtsma, K. (1973). *Cancer Res.*, **33**, 2373.
26. Hattler, B.G., and Soehalen, B. (1974). *Science*, **184**, 1374.
27. Maxim, P.E. *et al.* (1978). *Otolaryngology*, **86**, ORL 428.
28. Katz, A.E. (1980). *Otol. Clin. N.A.*, **13**, 431.
29. Hughes, N.R. (1971). *J. Natl. Cancer Inst.*, **46**, 1015.
30. Neel, H.B. *et al.* (1980). *Laryngoscope*, **90**, 1981.
31. Wolf, G.T. *et al.* (1979). *Am. J. Surg.*, **138**, 489.
32. Tsakraklides, V. *et al.* (1973). *Cancer*, **31**, 860.
33. Tsakraklides, V. *et al.* (1974). *Cancer*, **34**, 1259.
34. Berlinger, N.T. *et al.* (1976). *Cancer*, **37**, 697.
35. Old, L.J. *et al.* (1966). *Proc. Natl. Acad. Sci.*, **56**, 1699.
36. Smith, H.G., Chretien, P.B. *et al.* (1976). *Am. J. Surg.*, **132**, 541.
37. Kennedy, J.T. (1975). *Laryngoscope*, **85**, 806.
38. Krause, C.J., Nysather, J., and McCabe, B.F. (1975). *Ann. Otol.*, **84**, 787.
39. Aust, J.C. (1977). *Trans. Am. Acad. Ophthalmol. Otol.*, **84**, ORL 602.
40. Silverman, N.A., Alexander, J.C., and Chretien, P.B. (1976). *Cancer*, **37**, 2204.

41. Chretien, P.B. (1978). *Laryngoscope*, **88**, Suppl. 8, 11–13.
42. Palmer, D.L. (1978). *Laryngoscope*, **88**, Suppl. 8, 13–17.
43. Lundy, J. *et al.* (1975). *Surg. Gynecol. Obstet.*, **141**, 212.
44. Brookes, G.B., and Clifford, P. (1981). *J. Roy. Soc. Med.*, **74**, 132.
45. Gross, L. (1965). *Cancer*, **18**, 202.
46. Roth, J.A. *et al.* (1976). *Surgery*, **79**, 46.
47. Tarpley, J.L. *et al.* (1977). *J. Surg. Res.*, **22**, 195.
48. McCredie, J.A., Inch, R., and Sutherland, R.M. (1972). *Cancer*, **29**, 349.
49. Jenkins, V.K. *et al.* (1980). *Arch. Otol.*, **106**, 414.
50. Stefani, S.S., Kerman, R., and Abbate, J. (1976). *Am. J. Roentgenol.*, **126**, 880.
51. Tarpley, J.L., Potvin, C., and Chretien, P.B. (1975). *Cancer*, **35**, 638.
52. Nordman, E., and Toivanen, A. (1978). *Acta Radiol. Oncol.*, **17**, 3.
53. Cheema, A.R., and Hersh, E.M. (1971). *Cancer*, **28**, 851.
54. Hersh, E.M. *et al.* (1971). *N. Engl. J. Med.*, **285**, 1211.
55. Hersh, E.M., Gutterman, J.U., and Mavligit, G.M. (1977). *Ann. Rev. Med.*, **28**, 489.
56. Mathe, G. (1969). *Br. Med. J.*, **4**, 7.
57. McKneally, M.F. *et al.* (1976). **Lancet**, **1**, 377.
58. Pinsky, C.M., Hirshaut, Y., and Oettgen, H.F. (1973). *Natl. Cancer Inst. Monograph*, **39**, 225.
59. Donaldson, R.C. (1972). *Am. J. Surg.*, **124**, 427.
60. Donaldson, R.C. (1973). *Am. J. Surg.*, **126**, 507.
61. Richman, S.P. *et al.* (1976). *Cancer Treat. Rep.*, **60**, 535.
62. Donaldson, R.C., Banda, F., and Keehr, R. (1977). In R.G. Crispen (Ed.), *Neoplasm Immunity: Solid Tumor Therapy*, Franklin Institute Press, Chicago, p.243.
63. Suen, J.Y. *et al.* (1977). *Am. J. Surg.*, **134**, 474.
64. Papac, R. *et al.* (1978). *Cancer Res.*, **38**, 3150.
65. Taylor, S.G., Sisson, G.A., and Bytell, D.E. (1978). *Recent Results Cancer Res.*, **68**, 297.
66. Renoux, G., Renoux, M., and Hebdomadaires, C.R. (1971). *Séances Acad. Sci. Paris*, **272**, 349.
67. Oettgen, H.F., Pinsky, C.M., and Delmonte, L. (1976). *Med. Clin. N.A.*, **60**, 511.
68. Amery, W.K. (1975). *Br. Med. J.*, **3**, 461.
69. Rojas, A.F. *et al.* (1976). *Lancet*, **1**, 211.
70. Wanebo, H. *et al.* (1978). *Cancer Treat. Rep.*, **62**, 1663.
71. Olivari, A.J. *et al.* (1979). *Cancer Treat. Rep.*, **63**, 983.
72. Cheng, V.S.T. *et al.* (1978). *Cancer*, **42**, 1912.
73. Szpirglas, H., Chastang, C., and Bertrand, J.C. (1979). *Recent Results Cancer Res.*, **68**, 309.
74. Maca, R.D., and Panje, W.R. (1982). *Cancer*, **50**, 483.
75. Talapaz, M. *et al.* (1982). *Clin. Immunol. Immunopathol.*, **24**, 155.
76. Cunningham, T.J. *et al.* (1976). *Ann. N.Y. Acad. Sci.*, **277**, 339.
77. Goldstein, A.L. *et al.* (1976). *Med. Clin. N.A.*, **60**, 591.
78. Berlinger, N.T. (1980). In M. Paparello, and M. Schumrick (Eds), *Otolaryngology*, W.B. Saunders Co., Philadelphia, p.731.
79. Kenady, D.E. *et al.* (1977). *Cancer*, **39**, 642.
80. Wara, W.M. *et al.* (1981). In S. Salmon and S. Jones (Eds), *International Conference on the Adjuvant Therapy of Cancer*, III. Grune & Stratton, New York, p.169.
81. Treuner, J. *et al.* (1980). *Lancet*, **1**, 817.
82. Haglund, S. *et al.* (1981). *Arch. Otol.*, **107**, 327.
83. Schouten, T.J. *et al.* (1982). *Laryngoscope*, **92**, 686.
84. Lawrence, H.S. (1955). *J. Clin. Invest.*, **34**, 219.
85. Vetto, R.M. *et al.* (1976). *Cancer*, **37**, 90.
86. Vetto, R.M., and Burger, D.R. (1978). *Laryngoscope*, **88**, Suppl. 8. 79.
87. Goldenberg, B.J., and Brandes, L.J. (1972). *Clin. Res.*, **20**, 947.

Chapter 17

Nutrition

Barbara E. Hearne* and
John M. Daly†
* Co-Ordinating Clinical Research
Dietitian, Nutrition and Metabolism
Research Unit
† Associate Attending Surgeon, Memorial
Sloan–Kettering Cancer Center and
Associate Professor of Surgery, Cornell
University Medical College, New York
Department of Surgery, Memorial
Sloan–Kettering Cancer Center, New
York, NY, USA.

Patients with head and neck malignancies often present with significant nutritional deficits prior to treatment. This may be due to dietary indiscretions associated with a history of alcohol and tobacco abuse which is common to this population.[1] In addition, the presence of a tumour in the oropharynx or upper alimentary tract with concomitant dysphagia or odynophagia, oedema, ulceration, and bleeding may interfere with the patient's ability to chew and swallow a balanced diet, making adequate nutritional intake impossible. Finally, communication of the diagnosis of head and neck cancer to the patient, with the prospective treatments and prognosis, may contribute to anxiety and loss of appetite with further compromise of the patient's nutritional status.

NUTRITIONAL COMPLICATIONS OF CANCER TREATMENT

Radiation Therapy

Multimodality treatment of head and neck tumours using radiation, chemotherapy, and surgery, either singly or in combination, produces toxicities and/or complications which interfere with the patient's ability to ingest and absorb adequate nutrients. Radiation therapy to the head and neck produces toxicities to normal tissues which greatly interfere with oral alimentation. After radiotherapy of 1000–2000 rads, salivary glands produce thickened secretions and usually cease to function after 3000–4000 rads.[2] The resulting xerostomia limits food palatability and necessitates selection of moist foods and abundant use of liquids. Patchy mucositis which appears at 2000–3000 rads becomes confluent, erythematous, inflamed mucositis after 4000–5000 rads.[2] With severe mucositis the patient may be unable to swallow solids or ingest liquids by mouth. Taste alterations may appear at 2000–3000 rads, which may progress to complete absence of taste sensation at higher dosages. Taste recovery may not occur until several months following radiation treatment and may compromise nutrient intake during this time. Nausea, gastric bloating, and severe constipation have been documented in patients with advanced, inoperable head and neck cancer during radiation therapy[3] and may be related, in part, to reduced fibre intake due to dysphagia, pain on mastication, and xerostomia. Post-irradiation caries, osteoradionecrosis, buccal oedema, and trismus, as well as slow recovery of taste and salivary function, may preclude adequate nutient intake for several months after radiotherapy has been completed.[4]

Chemotherapy

Chemotherapeutic agents used in the treatment of head and neck cancer patients may produce severe toxicities which interfere with adequate oral intake. Stomatitis and mucositis produced by chemotherapy may cause pain on food ingestion. Other toxicities such as anorexia, nausea, vomiting, diarrhoea, constipation, and paralytic ileus may result in diminished oral intake.[5,6] Alterations in taste sensations such as aversion to meat or intolerance to sweets may cause the elimination of flesh foods or simple carbohydrates from the diet, which may contribute to protein–calorie undernutrition. These toxicities may appear from immediately post-therapy to 7–14 days after therapy; other toxicities may appear with cumulative drug dosages.

Surgery

Surgery remains the primary mode of therapy for the majority of head and neck tumours. Interruption of oral intake and increased metabolic requirements caused by operative therapy compromises the nutritional status of the patient. In addition, radical ablative therapy such as partial or total glossectomy or mandibulectomy severely interferes with the patient's mastication and deglutition. Even patients with less ablative surgery have been shown to have major swallowing disorders postoperatively.[7]

Each of these antineoplastic therapies used singly or in combination (radiation, chemotherapy, and surgery) interferes with the patient's ability to maintain adequate oral intake. With increased use of combined sequential treatment, each phase further compromises the patient's nutritional status. Because many patients with head and neck malignancies present with malnutrition, these patients should be nutritionally assessed and aggressively nourished prior to and following therapy to promote wound healing, minimize the incidence and severity of complications, and maximize the opportunity to complete planned treatment to improve tumour response.[8]

ASSESSMENT OF NUTRITIONAL STATUS

Subjective Assessment

At the time of tumour diagnosis and treatment planning, the patient with head and neck cancer should undergo a complete nutritional assessment by a registered dietitian. A nutrition history reveals the economic, cultural, and social influences on patient's eating habits and aids in the development of a care plan. Included in the nutrition history is a food-frequency questionnaire which may provide information on nutrient deficits by noting omissions of foods or food groups in the patient's usual diet. A carefully taken 24-hour dietary recall or 3-day diet diary may yield important information about the patient's recent dietary habits. The patient should also be interviewed about taste alterations and chewing or swallowing problems which may affect food selections and nutrient intake.

The patient's weight history (weight 1 year,

6 months, and 2 months prior to diagnosis obtained from the medical record, patient or primary-care physician) provides important information about the patient's nutritional status. Recent weight loss, even in the obese or normal weight-for-height patient, may be accompanied by nutrient deficits.

Objective Assessment

Following assessment of dietary habits and weight history, the patient should undergo anthropometric and biochemical assessment of nutritional status. Anthropometric measurements (height, weight, mid-arm circumference, triceps skinfold thickness) may be compared to normal values by age and sex to document deficits in body fat or lean body mass. These measurements may also be compared serially throughout the treatment course to indicate nutritional improvement or debilitation. Arm muscle strength, an indicator of nutritional status, can be measured using hand-grip dynamometry and compared with normal values for age and sex. This simple measurement has been described as a useful modality in assessing nutritional status which may be repeated serially throughout the patient's clinical course.[9,10]

Laboratory indices such as serum albumin, transferrin, and pre-albumin concentration provide information on the patient's visceral protein status. In addition, the creatinine height index obtained from a 24-hour urine collection for creatinine can be compared with normal values to indicate the status of lean body mass. Delayed cutaneous hypersensitivity to recall antigens such as mumps and candida may indicate T-cell immune deficits either to protein–calorie malnutrition or the presence of tumour.

Finally, a thorough clinical examination of the skin, oral cavity, and musculature by the physician completes the nutrition assessment. At this time the patient's ability to masticate and swallow is evaluated, as well as the ability to take nutrients by mouth, nasointestinal tube, or vein. Knowledge of the stage of disease, the present nutritional status, and the expected oncological treatment, along with the estimated time the patient will be unable to achieve adequate oral intake, are mandatory in planning optimal nutritional therapy to assure maximal therapeutic results with minimal morbidity.[11]

NUTRITIONAL THERAPY

Oral Nutritional Support

In the mildly depleted patient who is able to ingest liquids and solid foods, and who is undergoing mild to moderate stress, the first step to nutritional therapy is aggressive dietary counselling by a registered dietitian. Patients with head and neck cancer frequently require modification in the texture and consistency of foods due to decreased ability to chew and swallow. Pre-surgery chemotherapy or radiation therapy and their side-effects may make adequate intake of solid foods impossible, necessitating the use of liquid supplements. A wide variety of nutritionally complete liquid formulas are commercially available either unflavoured or in a variety of flavours. Many patients experiencing taste alterations during radiation therapy prefer the unflavoured forms. If adequate oral nutritional intake cannot be achieved due to dysphagia, anorexia, or increased requirements, supplemental feedings by nasointestinal tube should be considered next (Table 17.1).

Nutritional Support by Tube

In the moderately to severely malnourished patient undergoing moderate to high-magnitude therapy who cannot eat enough by mouth, feeding by tube should be initiated unless contraindicated. Contraindications to tube feeding include intestinal obstruction or abnormal gastrointestinal function.

Formula selection should be based on the patient's nutritional needs and gastrointestinal function, as well as ease of preparation and cost considerations. Ready-to-use commercially prepared liquid formulas are sterile,

TABLE 17.1   SELECTION OF NUTRITIONAL THERAPY IN HEAD AND NECK CANCER

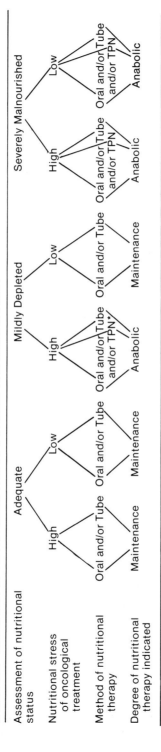

Assessment of nutritional status	Adequate		Mildly Depleted		Severely Malnourished	
Nutritional stress of oncological treatment	High	Low	High	Low	High	Low
Method of nutritional therapy	Oral and/or Tube	Oral and/or Tube	Oral and/or Tube and/or TPN*	Oral and/or Tube	Oral and/or Tube and/or TPN	Oral and/or Tube and/or TPN
Degree of nutritional therapy indicated	Maintenance	Maintenance	Anabolic	Maintenance	Anabolic	Anabolic

* TPN = Total Parenteral Nutrition

nutritionally complete, and convenient to use. They are, however, more expensive than blenderized formulas prepared at home. A blenderized formula, on the other hand, requires preparation time and proper kitchen facilities for preparation and storage. In addition, blenderized diets are more viscous and require larger-bore catheters for administration.

Enteral formula compositions have been widely described.[11-14] When a commercially prepared liquid formula is selected an isotonic formula with an intact protein source is well tolerated in most patients.[3] When symptoms or gastric bloating limit the volume of formula tolerated, additional calories may be provided either through the addition of glucose polymers (Polycose, Ross Laboratories; Moducal, Mead Johnson) or through a high caloric density formula which provides two kilocalories per millilitre. These increase the osmotic load of the feeding and may require adjustments in rate or volume of formula delivery.

A wide variety of soft, small-bore (8–10 French) catheters are available in inert (silicone rubber or polyurethane) materials which are comfortable and well-accepted by patients (Keofeed, Hedeco; Entriflex, Biosearch; Health Care Group, American Pharmaseal; Duo-Tube, Argyle) for long-term use. These are preferred over the red rubber catheters which become stiff and uncomfortable with prolonged use. Stylets are available to aid tube passage in patients with mild swallowing problems. Lubrication of the stylet prior to insertion allows its easy withdrawal. With proper care these tubes remain patent for extended periods and are not affected by radiation. In addition, patients can comfortably feed by mouth with the tube in place. Larger-bore catheters (No. 12, 14 and 16 French) are also available in these materials which can be used in patients with more severe swallowing problems in whom passage of a smaller catheter cannot be achieved. They may also be used for those who wish to use a thicker, blenderized formula at home.

Prior to tube insertion, the patient is placed in a Fowler's position and the patient's gag reflex tested with a tongue blade. The patency of each nostril is tested and any nasal septal deviation evaluated. Lubrication of the tip and first several centimetres of the tube with water-soluble lubricant allows easier passage. The tube is passed gently into the nostril and along the floor of the nasal passageway aiming downward and backward. This is facilitated by having the patient rest his/her chin on the chest. Unless contraindicated the swallowing of the tube is facilitated by allowing the patient to sip small amounts of water through a straw. When using a stylet it should be withdrawn *slowly* when the 50 centimetre marking is at the nares to prevent gagging. Tube placement is confirmed by aspirating stomach contents and injecting 10 millilitres of air and listening over the stomach with a stethoscope. If placement cannot be confirmed by this method, the most accurate method is a chest–upper abdominal roentgenogram if the tube is mercury-tipped or radio-opaque.

Gastrostomy and jejunostomy feeding may be used in patients with complete oral or upper gastrointestinal obstruction or fistula, or in patients who require chronic nutrition support. Oesophagostomy is a seldom-used technique in patients who have had a subtotal gastrectomy or oesophagogastrectomy with the stomach in the chest.[15] These methods require surgical placement using local, regional or general anaesthesia with minimal operative risk.

Tube feeding may be administered by intermittent bolus feedings; intermittent or continuous gravity drip; and intermittent or continuous pump infusion. Bolus is the simplest, but is accompanied by increased incidence of cramping, bloating, and diarrhoea. Intermittent or continuous gravity drip through a bottle or bag attached to a drip regulator allows greater control over flow rate. Patient tolerance is greater with this method. Pump infusion, though more costly, is the best-tolerated method and is useful in patients who have gastrointestinal complications which are not managed by alterations in feeding volumes, intervals, or rates.

For outpatients receiving tube feeding, formula delivery schedules and methods of formula delivery should be designed within the patient's living and treatment schedules and tolerance of the formula. Highly motivated patients with good swallowing function may be taught to pass the tube themselves. In a prospective randomized trial at Memorial Sloan – Kettering Cancer Center of the tube versus oral feeding in patients with advanced, inoperable head and neck cancer who were receiving radiation therapy,[3] 14 of 17 patients randomized to the tube were tube-fed exclusively as outpatients. Patients were fed an isotonic, commercially prepared formula with 1 kilocalorie per millilitre. Patients were begun on half-strength formula administered via intermittent gravity drip with 500 millilitres administered per feeding with a minimum of 4 hours between feedings. Three patients were hospitalized because of their treatment and not solely for the tube feeding. The method of tube passage and formula administration is summarized in Table 17.2. Four patients passed their own tubes either via nares or oral cavity using 90 centi-

metre No. 8 or 10 French silicone or polyurethane tubes. Two patients used orogastric because of tumour burden in the nasal cavity; the remaining two patients used nasogastric passage but left the tube in place near the completion of therapy because of dysphagia and throat soreness. Two patients opted for continuous nocturnal feeding to prevent interference with their daily activities. Of 14 patients managed primarily on intermittent feedings and formula gravity drip, five required change to intermittent pump infusion near the end of therapy, which resolved symptoms of gastric bloating, nausea, and diarrhoea. On initiation of tube feeding at the beginning of radiation therapy, tube feeding was used in combination with oral feeding to achieve desired calorie and protein goals. As toxicities to radiation limited oral intake, protein and calorie intake from tube feeding increased. Table 17.3 summarizes the transition from oral to tube feeding as radiation therapy progressed. Patients began tube feeding with an isotonic 1 kilocalorie per millilitre formula with intact protein source. Six patients who were unable to achieve their caloric requirements with the tolerated maximum volume of this formula achieved their

TABLE 17.2   PRIMARY METHOD OF TUBE PLACEMENT AND FORMULA DELIVERY DURING RADICAL RADIATION THERAPY

Mode of administration	Total	Daily self-passage by patient	Tube placement for duration of therapy
Intermittent gravity drip	14	3	11
Intermittent pump infusion	1	—	1
Continuous nocturnal pump infusion	2	1	1
	—	—	—
Total	17	4	13

TABLE 17.3   METHOD OF NUTRITION THERAPY DURING RADICAL RADIATION THERAPY (XRT)

Method of enteral support	Week 1–2 XRT	Week 3–4 XRT	Week 5–end XRT
PO + tube (PO > 50% total calories)	9	3	3
PO + tube (PO < 50% total calories)	5	5	2
Tube only (100% total calories)	2	8	11

needs when changed to a high caloric density commercially prepared formula with 2 kilocalories per millilitre administered via pump or gravity drip. The more concentrated and viscous formula required a larger nasointestinal catheter (No. 10 or 12 French) to achieve the desired flow rates and prevent clogging of the tube lumen. These experiences have shown tube feeding to be a flexible, easily managed mode of nutritional support during radiation therapy which can be used in combination with oral feeding to achieve adequate nutritional intake when toxicities to therapy limit oral intake.

Parenteral Nutritional Support

The most commonly used parenteral solution for total parenteral nutrition consists of a hypertonic mixture of the following: 20–25% dextrose; 4–5% crystalline amino acids or protein hydrolysate; minerals; vitamins (Table 17.4).[16] Each unit of solution in 1000–1100 millilitres of water provides approximately 900–1000 kilocalories with 5.25–6.0 grams of nitrogen. The specific fluid and electrolyte requirements, as well as caloric and nitrogen needs, of each patient must be individualized to prevent metabolic imbalances during therapy. Electrolytes and vitamins are added to the base solution for maintenance require-

ments as well as to correct any existing deficits. The preparation of these solutions for patients with head and neck cancer has been widely described.[11,16,17]

Hypophosphataemia, which occurs in patients receiving parenteral nutrition, probably occurs secondary to phosphorus uptake in newly synthesized protein rather than through urinary losses. Thus, patients with severe protein–calorie malnutrition as may be found in head and neck cancer, are at high risk for developing hypophosphataemia. Trace elements such as copper, cobalt, iodine, magnesium and zinc are not routinely added to the nutritional solution of patients with head and neck cancer unless nutritional needs require total parenteral nutrition for more than 3 weeks. Water-soluble vitamins should be added to each litre of solution and administered daily with a fat emulsion. Folic acid and vitamins B_{12} and K should be given in appropriate dosages as they are not included in the commercially prepared vitamin preparations.

Due to hyperosmolarity of the nutrient solution (1800–2000 milliosmoles per litre) they should be administered into a high-flow blood vessel, preferably the superior vena cava. Polyvinyl, silastic, or Teflon catheters may be directed into the superior vena cava following percutaneous cut-down insertion into the subclavian vein, or cephalic or basal veins. Cancer of the head and neck usually precludes use of the internal or external jugular veins. Silastic catheters inserted percutaneously through a peripheral vein have a lower incidence of thrombophlebitis and pyophlebitis than earlier polyvinyl catheters. Infraclavicular, percutaneous, subclavian venous catheterization is the safest and most effective method for long-term infusion of parenteral nutrition solutions in adults.

Unless contraindicated by the presence of a radiation portal, either subclavian vein may be safely used. Following catheter placement, a broad-spectrum antimicrobial ointment or povidine–iodine antiseptic ointment is applied to the puncture site. An occlusive, sterile dressing is fixed to the skin with tincture of benzoin

TABLE 17.4   COMPOSITION OF AMINO ACID
SOLUTION FOR TOTAL
PARENTERAL FEEDING

500 ml 50% dextrose

plus

500 ml 8.5% Crystalline amino acids

plus

30–50 mEq	Sodium chloride
20–30 mEq	Potassium acetate
15–20 mEq	Potassium acid phosphate
15 mEq	Magnesium sulphate
5 ml	Multivitamins* (MVI)†
1 g	Calcium gluconate*
5 mg	Zinc
0.5 mg	Copper

* Added to only one unit of solution daily.
† MVA – USV Pharmaceutical Corp. Tuckahoe, New York.

and adhesive tape. Patients with pharyngo-cutaneous and/or tracheostomy stomas may require an adherent plastic sheet over the dressing site to prevent contamination from stomal secretions. For patients receiving radiation therapy the catheter entry site is placed outside of the radiation field, tunnelling subcutaneously if necessary to exit outside the radiation site. Tape should not be applied to skin in the radiation field, to prevent the development of skin bullae. Following catheter insertion, prior to infusion, a chest roentgenogram is obtained to verify the placement of the catheter tip in the mid-portion of the superior vena cava.

Aseptic management of the subclavian vein catheter is paramount in patients treated for head and neck cancer because secretions from pharyngocutaneous and tracheostomy stomas often contaminate catheter dressings. As a result, dressings are changed as frequently as required, often twice daily. The skin catheter site is meticulously cleansed with acetone or ether and the skin prepared with povidone–iodine. Antimicrobial ointment is applied around the catheters and occlusive sterile dressings replaced. The parenteral nutrition catheter and surrounding site should be used exclusively to infuse nutrient solution to prevent catheter-related infection. Any febrile episodes are assumed to be catheter-related. If no other aetiology is identified the catheter should be removed. Clinical management of parenteral feeding has been widely described.[11,16,17]

Parenteral nutrition solutions are usually initiated at 1000 millilitres over 24 hours administered at a constant rate via infusion pump; or with micro-drip administration coupled with careful monitoring of rate by nursing staff. Once the patient is stable the rate may be increased by 1000 millilitres every 12 hours. The average adult will tolerate 3000 millilitres of parenteral solution over 24 hours by the third to fifth day. Extremely malnourished patients, however, may not tolerate large fluid volumes initially and should be advanced conservatively.

Osmotic diuresis is prevented by maintaining a rate which does not allow quantitative urinary glucose to exceed 2 grams per 100 millilitres (greater than 3 + nitroprusside reaction) or blood glucose greater than 200 milligrams per decilitre. Crystalline insulin may be added to intravenous dosage of patients with diabetes mellitus or persistent glycosuria. Dosages of 5–60 units per 1000 kilocalories are required to control blood sugar. Frequent monitoring of blood and urinary glucose is necessary as insulin requirements may change abruptly with the patient's condition. Abrupt discontinuance of parenteral feeding may result in 'rebound hyoglycaemia'.[16] Tapering off over a 24-hour period, or rapid tapering followed by a 10% glucose infusion, may prevent this complication. Total parenteral feeding is discontinued prior to surgery or general anaesthesia to prevent any unrecognized complications. Conscientious adherence to technique in catheter placement, aseptic catheter care, and clinical management should ensure successful central venous catheterization and feeding.

RESULTS OF NUTRITIONAL ASSESSMENT AND SUPPORT

Pre-treatment Assessment

Numerous studies of general surgical patients have demonstrated a significant correlation between objective measures of nutritional status and increased operative morbidity and mortality.[18–21] The relationship of protein–calorie under-nutrition to the development of postoperative complications has increased awareness and aggressiveness of nutritional intervention in the clinical setting. The variety of techniques for nutritional assessment allow objective definition of nutritional parameters which predict postoperative morbidity and thus indicate the need for preoperative nutritional therapy.

A prognostic nutritional index was recently developed and validated[20] in a group of heterogeneous surgical patients. Patients were evaluated preoperatively utilizing the following parameters: triceps skinfold thickness, serum albumin and transferrin concentrations, and delayed cutaneous hypersensitivity. Post-operative evaluation of patient complications was done by an observer with no patient-care responsibilities or knowledge of preoperative nutritional status. All complications were defined by rigid, objective criteria. The results were used to develop a linear, predictive model to predict the occurrence of postoperative complications based on preoperative nutritional parameters.

This prognostic nutritional index was pro-spectively tested for validity at the Cleveland Clinic in 29 head and neck cancer patients undergoing surgery following preoperative radiotherapy of 5000–5500 rads.[22] Preliminary results in this trial indicated the prognostic nutritional index to be an important predictor of major postoperative complications. It did not, however, predict for minor complications in this population of patients. Further exami-nation of this index, or development of models using additional assessment techniques, may provide guidelines for decisions as to when to initiate preoperative nutritional support.

Weight loss has been well documented as a complication of radiation treatment for head and neck cancer.[23] A recent prospective trial in Toronto examined the pathogenesis of weight loss in 31 patients receiving radiation therapy for head and neck cancer.[24] Patients received nutritional assessments before and after radio-therapy. Toxicities to therapy were evaluated and body weight changes recorded from pre-treatment to 6 months post-therapy. Pre-treatment nutritional status as indicated by serum albumin concentrations, absolute lymphocyte count, serum creatinine level, creatinine height index, or anthropometric measurements did not predict for weight loss. Patients receiving radiotherapy to the oral cavity or oropharynx experienced the greatest weight loss. Patients receiving radiotherapy to the larynx with the oropharynx/oral cavity blocked lost significantly more weight with field sizes greater than 8 by 8 (64 square centi-metres) compared with smaller field sizes. Continued weight loss post-therapy was related to the presence of treatment-related morbidity rather than the persistence of tumour. This study suggests that planning of nutritional therapy during radiation be related to know-ledge of field site, size, and toxicities to therapy.

These studies indicate a rational basis for planning nutritional therapy either pre-surgery or pre-radiotherapy based on nutritional status and planned treatment modality and site. Further studies are needed to refine parameters for other disease sites, stages, and treatment modalities to assure optimal results of therapy.

NUTRITIONAL THERAPIES

Enteral Nutrition

Nasointestinal tube feeding has been shown to reverse negative nitrogen balance and promote body weight gain in hospitalized patients with a variety of diseases.[25–28] Haffejee and Angorn[29] fed 20 unresectable oesophageal carcinoma patients who had documented protein–calorie malnutrition with negative nitrogen balance. Nitrogen balance and immune response were evaluated pre- and post-nutritional repletion by tube. Positive nitrogen balance was attained in all patients. In addition, pre-therapy immune response parameters such as depressed T-lymphocyte counts and *in vitro* mitogenic response to phytohaemagglutinin improved significantly as negative nitrogen balance was reversed. The DNCB skin test, however, remained unreactive both pre- and post-repletion. Achievement of nitrogen balance using tube feeding improved some aspects of cell-mediated immunity in these patients with oesophageal carcinoma without reduction in tumour burden.

In a prospective trial of tube versus oral feeding at Memorial Hospital,[3] patients with unresectable Stage III and IV head and neck carcinoma were randomized to either treat-ment group for 11 weeks during and after radiotherapy. Patients were stratified by site, first treatment (radiation alone versus chemo-therapy alone or combined with radiation) and previous head and neck surgery (yes versus no). Prior to and during therapy, anthropometric measurements (height, weight, mid-arm circumference, and triceps skinfold thickness), serum albumin and performance status were evaluated. Pre-treatment taste changes, dysphagia, xerostomia, nausea, vomiting, constipation, and diarrhoea were graded on a four-point scale. Toxicities were documented biweekly throughout therapy. A nutritional care plan was devised for each patient using 40 kilocalories per kilogram and 1.0 gram protein per kilogram body weight. Patients randomized to oral nutrition received extensive counselling and oral supplements throughout radiation. Patients randomized to tube feeding received tube and oral feedings to achieve caloric goals. Additional caloric intake was prescribed to maintain weight or to achieve weight gain. Oral patients characteristically were unable to maintain their caloric and protein intakes when toxicities to therapy were fully manifest at week 4 to end of radiotherapy (4000–7000 rads dosage).

Table 17.5 summarizes presenting body weight changes for Group A with the oral cavity or oropharynx partially or fully irradiated and Group B with the oral cavity/oropharynx blocked during radiotherapy. Group A presented with significantly greater loss of pre-illness weight than Group B ($P = 0.001$). This is probably due to lack of tumour burden in the oral cavity or oropharynx in Group B, whose primary disease was nasopharyngeal or laryngeal carcinoma. Group B showed no difference in body weight change at the end of radiotherapy in the tube and oral groups. Group A, however, whose primary tumours included oral cavity, oropharynx, hypopharynx, and recurrent nasopharyngeal carcinoma had significantly less weight loss if fed by tube ($P = 0.02$) compared with oral feeding. There was no significant difference between mean field size or radiation dosage for either nutrition therapy. Toxicities to therapy show no difference between either group. Preliminary results show no difference in tumour response or patient survival for either the tube or oral group. These results confirm Johnston's results[24] that patients receiving radiation to the oral cavity/oropharynx are at greater nutritional risk. In addition, based on improved

TABLE 17.5   (a) MEAN INITIAL BODY WEIGHT CHANGE

Site irradiated	n	Percentage of usual weight Mean	SD	
Group A (oral cavity irradiated)	15	− 10.5	±7.6	p = 0.001
Group B (oral cavity blocked)	9	− 1.3	±2.1	

TABLE 17.5   (b) MEAN BODY WEIGHT CHANGE AT END OF RADIATION THERAPY

Site irradiated	n	Percentage of Initial weight Tube mean	SD	n	Oral mean	SD	
Group A (oral cavity irradiated)	10	− 0.7	±6.3	5	− 7.8	±4.2	p = 0.02
Group B (oral cavity blocked)	4	− 2.5	±1.9	5	− 3.4	±2.5	

body weight during tube feeding, these results indicate the need for tube feeding in patients receiving radiation therapy when the oral cavity/oropharynx is not blocked.

Parenteral Nutrition

Several studies have demonstrated the beneficial effects of total parenteral nutrition in head and neck cancer patients prior to, during, and following therapy.[8,11] Use of parenteral nutrition therapy in 70 patients with head and neck cancer patients were recently described.[11] These patients received total parenteral nutrition perioperatively, during chemotherapy, radiation, during convalescence, or for enterocutaneous fistulas (Table 17.6). Of the 29 patients (mean age, 61.1 years) receiving perioperative support, 19 underwent laryngopharyngectomy (16 with a radical neck dissection) and 10 had a thoracoacromial flap repair (Table 17.7). These patients received parenteral nutrition therapy for a mean period of 36.6 days. Fifteen received therapy both pre- and postoperatively with a mean weight gain of 5.1 kilograms. This group showed an

increase in mean serum albumin from 3.2 to 3.5 grams per decilitre. Preoperative parenteral feeding was used for an average of 16.1 days to achieve adequate nutritional rehabilitation prior to a high-stress, extensive surgical procedure. No patients exhibited tumour growth during this preoperative support. Postoperative parenteral nutrition therapy was required for an average of 20.3 days until adequate enteral intake could be achieved.

Postoperative parenteral nutrition therapy only was used in 14 patients for a mean period of 36.8 days. The mean serum albumin levels in these patients rose from 2.8 to 3.1 grams per decilitre with a mean body weight gain of 3.6 kilograms. Total parenteral nutrition was initiated in these patients because of nutritionally related complications such as poor wound healing, pneumonia, and malabsorption of enterally administered feedings. These resolved during parenteral nutrition. In addition, healthy granulation tissue appeared and skin grafts were used to close fistula openings and cover denuded wounds. Weight gains, increased muscle strength, and increased serum albumin concentrations were achieved more rapidly in patients receiving nutritional therapy preoperatively rather than postoperatively. Thus, pre-surgical repletion is indicated in malnourished patients undergoing ablative surgery.

Nine patients received parenteral nutrition therapy for an average of 34.8 days while receiving radiation therapy for head and neck cancer.[30] These patients (mean age 51.2 years; mean cumulative dosage 4900 rads) gained an average of 3.4 kilograms body weight. All patients experienced improvement in mucositis and pharyngitis during nutritional therapy; five patients experienced a greater than 50% reduction in tumour size.

Ten patients receiving total parenteral nutrition therapy during convalescence from surgery or radiation gained an average of 4.0 kilograms. Four patients underwent transition to nasoenteric tube feedings by discharge, two patients went to gastrostomy feedings for chronic ambulatory therapy and three patients

TABLE 17.6   TOTAL PARENTERAL NUTRITION IN PATIENTS WITH HEAD AND NECK CANCER

Indications for TPN	Number of patients
Perioperative support	29
Chemotherapy	16
Convalescent support	10
Radiation therapy	9
Enterocutaneous fistulas	6
	70

TABLE 17.7   PERIOPERATIVE TOTAL PARENTERAL NUTRITION THERAPY

Operative procedure	Number of patients
Laryngopharyngectomy	19
Radical neck dissection	16
Thoracoacromial flap	10
	(1 bilateral)
Mandibulectomy	3
Glossectomy	3
Forehead flap	2

were able to make the transition to oral feedings following head and neck musculature rehabilitation. Improved muscle strength was noted following intravenous therapy.

Sixteen patients receiving chemotherapy underwent parenteral therapy for an average period of 27 days with a mean body weight gain of 4.5 kilograms. All patients tolerated chemotherapy well with minimal nausea, vomiting, diarrhoea, and stomatitis. Thirty per cent of the patients experienced a greater than 50% reduction in tumour mass. These clinical experiences in parenteral nutrition therapy demonstrate its effectiveness in improving tolerance and recovery from oncological therapy.

Sako *et al.* compared parenteral feeding with tube feeding in a randomized trial at Roswell Park.[31] Sixty-nine patients were entered and randomized to postoperative parenteral nutrition (n = 35) or enteral alimentation by tube (n = 33). Patients were stratified by percentage of pre-illness body weight loss and prognosis. Hyperalimentation was given for a minimum of 14 days. Patients were assessed by complete blood counts, blood chemistries, anthropometric measurements, and delayed cutaneous hypersensitivity tests. Measurement of nitrogen balance revealed more patients in positive nitrogen balance with a higher mean nitrogen balance in the parenteral compared with the tube group ($P < 0.02$). There were no significant differences in serum protein levels, lymphocyte determinations, skin tests, postoperative complications, and patient survival between the two groups.

The results of this study indicate enteral nutrition to be as effective as parenteral nutrition based on these parameters. The ease of enteral feeding on an outpatient basis,[3] as well as cost savings, favours the use of enteral nutrition support when the gastrointestinal tract is functional.

RESEARCH QUESTIONS

Many questions need to be addressed in the nutritional management of head and neck cancer patients. The first is the proper means for assessing patients at nutritional risk. Parameters for identifying patients at risk by disease site, stage, and planned treatment modality are needed. The second is identifying the most effective method of nutritional therapy to coincide with the disease and treatment modality (oral, tube, or parenteral). This issue requires prospective randomized trials of various nutritional therapies. Third, the specific nutrient requirements of patients with head and neck cancer need to be identified. Increased caloric needs caused by the tumour or treatment with radiation, chemotherapy, or surgery have not been established despite improved technology in indirect calorimetry. In addition, protein requirements as well as vitamin, mineral, and micronutrient requirements during therapy and convalesence, have not been examined.

Finally, the measure of effectiveness of nutritional therapy must include objective measures of quality of life. Present studies indicate improved body weight and muscle strength but show no difference in tumour response or patient survival.

In summary, patients with head and neck cancer are often malnourished when they present for diagnosis of their disease. Oncological therapy using radiation, chemotherapy, and/or surgery often leads to progressive weight loss and protein–calorie malnutrition. Careful definition of populations treated with optimal therapy may yield improved response, duration, and quality of life in patients with head and neck malignancies.

REFERENCES

1. Feldman, J.G., Hazan, M., Nagorajan, M., and Kisin, B. (1975). *Prev. Med.*, **4**, 444–463.
2. Mossman, A. and Scheer, A. (1977). *Ear, Nose, Throat J.*, **56**, 90–95.
3. Daly, J.M., Hearne, B.E., Dunaj, J.M., Strong, E., Vikram, B., and DeCosse, J.J. (1982). Unpublished data.
4. Lederman, M. (1981). In J.J. Conley (Ed.), *Complications of Head and Neck Surgery*, W.B. Saunders, Philadelphia, pp. 329–352.
5. Ohnuma, T. and Holland, J.F. (1977). *Cancer Res.*, **37**, 2395.

6. Capizzi, R. (1981). In J.J. Conley (Ed.), *Complications of Head and Neck Surgery*, W.B. Saunders, Philadelphia, pp. 317 – 328.

7. Logemann, J., and Bytell, D. (1979). *Cancer*, **44**, 1095 – 1105.

8. Copeland, E.M., MacFayden, B.V. Jr., and MacComb, W.S. (1975). *Cancer*, **35**, 606 – 611.

9. Archer, T., Klidjian, A.M., and Karran, S.J. (1981). *J. Parent. Ent. Nutr.*, **5**, 570.

10. Fleeman, C., Rodgers, L., Miller, B., and Wright, R.A. (1981). *J. Parent. Ent. Nutr.*, **5**, 581.

11. Daly, J.M., Dudrick, S.J., and Copeland, E.M. (1981). In J.Y. Suen and E.N. Myers (Eds), *Cancer of the Head and Neck*, Livingstone, New York, p. 63 – 89.

12. Shils, M.E., Bloch, A.S. and Chernoff, R. (1979). In *Liquid Formulas for Oral and Tube Feeding*, Memorial Sloan – Kettering Cancer Center, New York, p. 1 – 9.

13. Shils, M.E. (1977). *Cancer Res.*, **37**, 2432 – 2439.

14. Chernoff, R. (1981). *J. Am. Dietet. Assoc.*, **79**, 426 – 430.

15. Graham, W.P. III, and Royster, H.P. (1967). *Surg. Gynecol. Obstet.*, **125**, 127 – 128.

16. Daly, J.M., Dudrick, S.J., and Copeland, E.M. (1979). *Cancer*, **43**, 925.

17. Copeland, E.M., Guillamondequi, O.M., and Dudrick, S.J. (1981). In J.J. Conley (Ed.), *Complications of Head and Neck Surgery*, W.B. Saunders, Philadelphia, pp. 308 – 316.

18. Kaminski, M., Fitzgerald, M., and Murphy, R. (1977). *J. Parent. Ent. Nutr.*, **1**, 27.

19. Meakins, J., Pietsch, J., and Bubenik, O. *et al.* (1977). *Ann. Surg.*, **186**, 241 – 250.

20. Mullen, J., Buzby, G., and Waldman, T. (1979). *Surg. Forum*, **30**, 80 – 82.

21. Mullen, J., Buzby, G., Matthews, D., Smale, B., and Rosato, E. (1980). *Ann. Surg.*, **192**, 604 – 613.

22. Flores, T.C., Levine, H., Hooley, R., Wheeler, T., and Steiger, E. (1982). In Program, *Meeting of American Society of Head and Neck Surgery*.

23. Donaldson, S. (1979). *Cancer Res.*, **37**, 2407.

24. Johnston, C.A., Keane, T.J., and Prudo, S.M. (1982). *J. Parent. Ent. Nutr.*, **6**, 399 – 402.

25. Page, C.P., Ryan, J.A., and Haff, R.C. (1976). *Surg. Gynecol. Obstet.*, **142**, 184 – 188.

26. Heymesfield, S.B., Bethel, R.A., Ansley, J.D., Nixon, D.W., and Rudman, D. (1979). *Ann. Intern. Med.*, **90**, 62.

27. Hill, G.L., Pickfod, I., Young, G.A., Schorak, C.J., Blackett, R.L., Burkenshaw, L., and Warren, J.V. (1977). *Lancet*, **1**, 689.

28. Yeng, C., Smith, R.C., and Hill, G.L. (1979). *Gastroenterology*, **77**, 652 – 657.

29. Haffejee, A.A., and Angorn, I.B. (1979). *Ann. Surg.*, **189**, 475 – 479.

30. Copeland, E.M., Daly, J.M., and Dudrick, S.J. (1979). *Head Neck Surg.*, **1**, 350 – 363.

31. Sako, K., Lore, J.M., Kaufman, S., Razack, M.S., Bakamjian, V., and Reese, P. (1981). *J. Surg. Oncol.*, **16**, 391 – 402.

Chapter 18

Chemoprevention

Frank L. Meyskens,
Department of Internal Medicine, and Cancer Center, University of Arizona, Tucson, Arizona, USA

Epidemiological studies strongly implicate exogenous factors in the development of head and neck cancers (Table 18.1). The evidence supporting the participation of these items as complete or co-carcinogens has been recently summarized by several investigators and will not be reviewed here.[1-4] The epidemiological data are compelling, showing that elimination of exposure to these agents would dramatically lower the incidence of lip, oropharynx, tongue, nasopharynx, and laryngeal cancers.[1,2,5-7] However, social modification of smoking and alcohol habits seems unlikely, and other agents contribute only a minor role. Alternative approaches are needed as the morbidity and mortality of head and neck cancers

is very high. An increased understanding of the mechanisms underlying the development of tumours in the last two decades, and the identification of a number of different types of compounds which can modify this process, allow rational formulation of an approach to prevention of cancer.

PROCESS OF CARCINOGENESIS

Extensive investigations in animal models has identified two major steps in the development of cancers[8] (Figure 18.1). These include initiation and promotion phases, each of which has several discrete characteristics. The initiation phase is generally regarded as irreversible as this step involves a genotypic alteration. However, recent experiments indicate that in some cases the presence of co-carcinogens is needed to 'fix' this damage.[9] Additionally, recent advances in our understanding of DNA and carcinogenesis may allow manipulation of genetic material, at least in the early stages of transformation.[10] Although mechanisms underlying the process of initiation have been only recently defined, a number of compounds have been found to modify or alter this step of carcinogenesis (Table 18.2).

The phenomenon of promotion has been

TABLE 18.1 ENVIRONMENTAL FACTORS IMPLICATED IN THE DEVELOPMENT OF HEAD AND NECK CANCERS

Tobacco and alcohol
Tobacco
Ultraviolet light radiation
Heavy metals — nickel, chromium, arsenic, asbestos, radium
Dust (aflatoxin)
Nitrosamines/polycyclic aromatic hydrocarbons (in air)
Vitamin deficiencies
Viruses

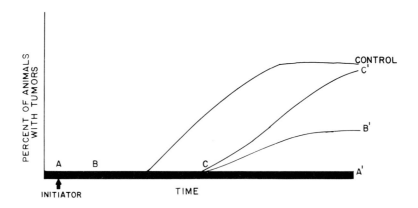

Figure 18.1   Idealized presentation of carcinogenesis and chemoprevention. A complete carcinogen is given at time A. If a strong antipromotor (arrow) is given before or simultaneously with the initiator, the formation of tumours is completely blocked (A′). If the antipromotor is started later (B), but before the development of tumours, the appearance of tumours will be delayed and the number of tumours decreased (B′). The antipromotor must be given continuously. If the antipromotor is removed at any time (C), tumours rapidly appear, and the incidence of tumours reaches that of the control (C′).

TABLE 18.2   INHIBITORS OF
CARCINOGENESIS

Antioxidants (BHTA, BHT, selenium, ascorbate, vitamin E)
Protease inhibitors
Retinoids (and vitamin A)
Protease inhibitors
Anti-inflammatory steroids

easier to approach experimentally, and therefore more is known about this stage of carcinogenesis. The key feature of the promotion phase is that it is reversible. A number of phenotypic alterations routinely accompany promotion, including cellular hyperplasia, enhancement of proliferation, and progressive loss of differentiation. These biological changes are accompanied by profound biochemical alterations;[11] the most important may be transient induction of the key regulatory enzyme ornithine decarboxylase.[12] The promotion phase has been further dissected into several discrete steps and inhibitors for each substage identified.[13] An

extremely important conclusion from these studies is that the role of weak co-promotors becomes more important as the dose or concentration of a strong promotor is decreased. One can easily envision that either a combination of several weak promotors or a weak promotor and a suboptimal dose of a strong promotor may lead to phenotypic transformation. This may be particularly germane to head and neck cancer in which the facilitating role of alcohol in enhancing smoking-induced cancers has been appreciated for some time.

TYPES OF PREVENTION

A number of different types of prevention can be defined based on our knowledge of the carcinogenesis process (Table 18.3). Clearly the most important approach is primary prevention. Although epidemiological observations suggest that head and neck cancer would nearly disappear in a decade if smoking were to stop, social and political considerations make dim the prospects for primary prevention. Secon-

TABLE 18.3   TYPES OF PREVENTION IN HUMANS

Type	Description	Example
Primary	Remove source of carcinogen	Stop smoking
	Block exposure to carcinogen	Apply sunscreen
Secondary	Modify interaction of carcinogen with host	Normalize vitamin A and selenium levels, include ascorbate in diet
Tertiary	Suppress or reverse established preneoplasia	Effect of retinoids on leukoplakia (or other antipromotors)

dary prevention is largely related to efforts to modulate the initiation or early promotion phase of carcinogenesis by dietary modification and ingestion of natural inhibitors or supplementation with pharmacological inhibitors of initiation or promotion. The epidemiological evidence is strong that individuals with low serum levels of vitamin A or β-carotene, or histories of low ingestion of vegetables, are at increased risk for epithelial malignancies.[14] The poor nutritional status and the heavy smoking and alcohol history of many patients who develop head and neck cancer undoubtedly provide an optimal milieu for a malignant event to develop.

Two stages of tertiary prevention should be considered in patients at risk for head and neck cancer. These include an early stage when no preneoplasia can be clinically identified and a later stage when preneoplastic events (such as leukoplakia) have already occurred. Most investigators postulate that the earlier the stage of phenotypic alteration the less potent the antipromotor required to effect a positive permanent change.[15,16] On the other hand, the later the stage of preneoplasia, the more potent the antipromotor required, and the change produced will only be partial and temporary.

ANTI-INITIATORS AND ANTI PROMOTORS

As the process of initiation and promotion and the mechanisms of action of compounds which block these processes have been more extensively studied, the distinction between anti-initiators and antipromotors has become blurred and investigators now frequently refer to these compounds as 'inhibitors of carcinogenesis'.[13] Nevertheless, there is heuristic value in considering these two classes of compounds separately.

Examples of classical inhibitors of initiation include antioxidants and protease inhibitors while anti-inflammatory steroids and retinoids are generally thought to function as antipromotors. Antioxidants maintain a reducing atmosphere and thereby inhibit the conversion of many carcinogens to their active moiety.[17] A large number of compounds are considered to function as antioxidants but BHA (butylated hydroxyanisole), BHT (butylated hydroxytoluene), sodium selenide, and vitamin E may be the most important. BHA and BHT are both widely used as additives in food and they clearly alter carcinogen metabolism in a favourable way.[18] Selenium is a key regulator of the proliferation of normal and tumour cells[19,20] and an increasing number of studies indicate that both salts of selenium and vitamin E can function as antipromotors.[21,22] However, all these compounds are toxic at high doses and combinations of these agents at low doses may be a preferred approach to the prevention of cancer because of their different biochemical points of action.

Intracellular proteases are proteins that catalyse the hydrolysis of peptide bonds at specific sites.[23] These enzymes may function to derepress specific genes and accelerate the process of promotion. Proteases have been shown to inhibit the promotional step of carcinogenesis as well as inflammation and metastases in a number of systems. The mechanism of action of proteases is clearly complex, and the use of inhibitors of these enzymes remains in the future.

Anti-inflammatory steroids have been shown to be very active inhibitors of tumour-promoting phorbol esters,[24] but investigations in other promotion models remain to be performed. Nevertheless, the results indicate that a combination of anti-inflammatory steroids and vitamin A derivatives (see below) may provide potent antipromotion.

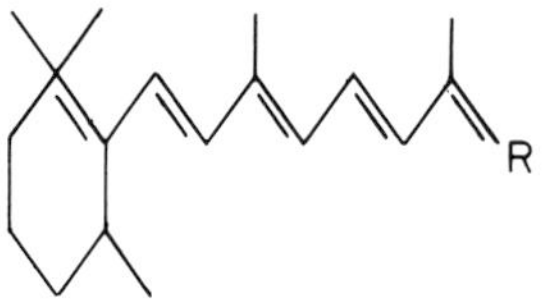

R = COH   retinol
    CO   retinal
    COOH trans retinoic acid

Figure 18.2   Structure of retinoids.

RETINOIDS AS CHEMOPREVENTIVE AGENTS

Biochemical Features

Knowledge about vitamin A and its natural and synthetic derivatives (retinoids) as potential chemopreventive agents far surpasses our knowledge about all other compounds combined. The basic structure of vitamin A is shown in Figure 18.2. Several hundred modifications of the basic structure of vitamin A have been performed in an attempt to improve the therapeutic ratio.[25,26] Several of these derivatives are in a variety of clinical trials in Europe and the United States including retinyl palmitate, 13 *cis*-retinoic acid, and an aromatic retinoic acid ethyl ester analogue (RO-10-9359). The mechanisms of retinoid action have been intensively studied over recent years. The identification of highly specific intracellular retinol and retinoic acid binding proteins has suggested that the process for the mediation of retinoid action may be similar to that of steroids.[27,28] However, several important differences from steroid receptors have

been discovered.[29] Additionally, retinoids have been found to have other biochemical sites of action,[30] including alteration of membranes via incorporation into glycoproteins[31] and direct inhibition of induced ornithine decarboxylase activity.[32] Nevertheless, the detection of intracellular retinoic acid binding proteins in a number of human cancers,[33] including head and neck cancers[34] suggest that these malignant cells can be modulated by retinoic acid, inasmuch as cultured cells which contain intracellular retinoic binding protein are favourably modulated by retinoic acid derivatives in most cases.[29,35]

Biological Features

A large number of biological actions for retinoids have been proposed,[30] but only two major areas have been well characterized: (a) alteration of various immunological parameters, and (b) interactions with epithelial cells.

Investigations of the effects of retinoids on immunological function are relatively recent and therefore limited in scope. Nevertheless, in various systems retinoids have stimulated both humoral and cell-mediated immunity.[36,37] The basis of these responses is not known but Sidell has postulated that retinoids alter early lymphoid maturation.[38] Further studies in this area will be of considerable interest since many malignancies, including head and neck cancers, are accompanied by deficiences or alterations in immune function.

Two major aspects of the interaction of retinoids and epithelial cells have been well characterized. These include (a) suppression of phenotypic transformation initiated by chemical, physical, and viral carcinogens,[15] and (b) inhibition of proliferation of malignant cells; this action of retinoids is frequently accompanied by induction of differentiation, particularly in epithelial tissues.[35,39] A large number of investigators have reported on the interaction of carcinogens and normal tissues *in vitro* and *in vivo* in animal models. The results of these studies can be summarized as follows:

(1) Retinoids can function as antipromotors and inhibit the phenotypic development of cancer whether initiated by chemical, physical, or viral carcinogens.[15]

(2) The maximal antipromotion effect is obtained if the retinoid is given at the time of initiation (or before) or soon thereafter. In most cases little effect by antipromotors is seen after tumours begin to develop.[8,40]

(3) The effectiveness of retinoids is determined by the nature of the carcinogen and the type of cancer, even in the same animal species.[41]

(4) Different retinoids may have widely diverse effects in the same system, ranging from ineffectiveness to complete suppression of the malignant phenotype.[41]

These results have important implications for studies in humans since it is likely that the general principles of carcinogenesis and anticarcinogenesis can be applied to humans. These findings imply that the particular retinoid (or other antipromotor) which will be effective in humans is unlikely to be predicted by animal studies, since the carcinogen(s) responsible for specific human cancers is infrequently known and the histology of the tumours in animals and humans is frequently different. The effect of retinoids on transformed cells has also been studied.[36,37,42-45] The results of these studies can be summarized as follows:

(1) The growth of a large number of different animal and human cells can be inhibited *in vitro* by retinoids. This is frequently accompanied by evidence for differentiation, a feature best studied in malignant melanoma,[39] neuroblastoma,[42] and leukaemia[43,45] cells.

(2) The effect of retinoids on growth is non-cytotoxic and totally reversible.

(3) A large subpopulation of tumour cells is resistant to the effect of retinoids except in unusual cases.

(4) Differential responses of tumour cells to different retinoids are evident.

These results also have important implications

for human studies of retinoids as they indicate that these compounds may inhibit the growth of frankly transformed cells also.

Clinical Potential

A number of investigations support the use of retinoids as anti-cancer agents in humans. These include evidence from epidemiological, dermatological, and oncological studies and can be summarized as follows:

(1) A number of large epidemiological investigations suggest that low serum vitamin A or β-carotene levels or a history of low vegetable intake correlates inversely with the development of a number of epithelial cancers.[14]

(2) Retinoids can inhibit the growth of a number of dysplastic skin lesions and tumours,[46] including actinic keratoses,[47] and basal[48] and squamous[49] cell carcinomas.

(3) We have conducted a large phase II trial of 13 *cis*-retinoic acid in 105 patients with advanced cancer. Objective responses were seen in patients with carcinomas of head and neck and lung, as well as in patients with melanoma. In all cases the responses were confined to skin and subcutaneous sites and were of short duration.[50]

(4) We have initiated a carefully stratified, randomized adjuvant trial of BCG ± vitamin A (100 000 units/day) in Stage I and II malignant melanoma.[51] Therapy was administered for 18 months. One hundred patients have been accrued to date and after a median follow-up of 56 weeks a slight trend ($P = 0.20$) for the combined arm was evident. Toxicity of the vitamin A was mild and no evidence of liver damage was evident.

(5) We have also conducted a phase I–II trial of locally applied β-*trans*-retinoic acid against cervical intraepithelial neoplasia I (mild) and II (moderate).[52] This trial has afforded us with the opportunity to deal with problems related to local delivery

systems and the local side-effects of retinoic acid on vaginal mucosa. Our results indicate that the limiting side-effects were vaginal toxicity (no cervical toxicity was seen) and that even with short (4 days) applications of retinoid reversal of dysplasia was seen in some cases.

HEAD AND NECK CANCER AS A UNIQUE OPPORTUNITY FOR CHEMOPREVENTION INTERVENTION

The number of cancers in which chemoprevention in humans in conceptually possible is large, but the practical limitations are considerable (Table 18.4). Head and neck cancers present a singular opportunity to investigate the role of chemoprevention in

TABLE 18.4   MALIGNANCIES IN HUMANS WHICH MAY BE CANDIDATES FOR LOCAL CHEMOPREVENTION

Head and neck cancer
Bladder cancer
Cervical cancer
Lung cancer

humans. In most cases the initiator (carcinogens in smoke) and promotor (carcinogens in smoke or alcohol) are known. Identification and serial examination of the suspected disease sites can be done easily and without invasive techniques. Additionally, for sites where local drug delivery is possible, systemic delivery (and consequent toxicity) of the chemopreventive agent should not be necessary. There are a number of different unrandomized and randomized chemoprevention trials which can be considered for head and neck cancers.

Dietary Supplementation of Individuals at High Risk

The practical problems notwithstanding, identification of individuals who both smoke and drink heavily would be the first part of this study. Measurement of serum or tissue levels of substances such as vitamin A, β-carotene,

and selenium in these patients would then be determined. Patients would be stratified for amount of smoking, alcohol ingestion, and baseline serum levels of natural chemopreventive inhibitors and randomized in a double-blind control fashion into a placebo and treatment (natural inhibitor, ?retinoid, ?other) groups. Such a trial presents several formidable problems including patient compliance, occult ingestion of chemoprevention agents (particularly of non-prescription items), monitoring for incidence of cancer events, and long-term follow-up. Such a study will have to be multi-institutional and involve multidisciplinary teams with epidemiologists, otolaryngologists, oncologists, and pharmacologists.

Treatment of Oral Leukoplakia

Leukoplakia represents a situation in which initiation and at least early promotion has occurred and therefore presents a unique opportunity in which to test retinoids, as these compounds have been postulated to work at the late stages of promotion.[13] Additionally, a controlled trial may not be necessary as spontaneous reversal of leukoplakia is rare and the lesion easily measured. A number of studies from Europe indicate that leukoplakia can be reversed by systemic administration of retinoids.[53,54] However, as the cutaneous and mucosal side-effects of retinoic acid derivatives may be unacceptable for patients undergoing preventive treatment, local delivery would be desirable. Several methods should be considered including retinoic acid impregnated in gum or lozenge or delivered via a spray, or perhaps even simultaneously with cigarette smoke. One major theoretical disadvantage of this approach is that retinoids have been found to function as promotors in some cases when delivered at high doses in a local environment. The pros and cons of this issue have recently been cogently discussed.[55]

Treatment of Viral-associated Conditions

Evidence has been presented that retinoids can

inhibit the growth of rabbit papilloma virus *in vitro* and *in vivo*,[56] and we have seen complete regression of laryngeal papillomatosis (a disease clearly associated with human papilloma virus) in one patient and partial regression in an additional patient (S. Coulthard, D. Alberts, and F. Meyskens, unpublished observation). Limited data also indicate that the proliferation of other DNA viruses can also be blocked by retinoids (W. Meinke, personal communication). Although further laboratory work in this area is needed, a large-scale trial of retinoids in individuals at high risk for nasopharyngeal cancers may be a reasonable goal in the future as the population at risk has been clearly defined and the association of DNA viruses strongly suspected.[57,58]

CONCLUSIONS

Our knowledge about carcinogens related to the development of head and neck cancers has become well defined in the past several decades. Laboratory advances have provided a clearer understanding of the process of carcinogenesis leading to established malignancies, and retinoids have been identified as powerful antipromotors of this process. The local nature of most head and neck cancers suggests that this malignancy offers a unqiue opportunity in which to explore the interaction of chemopreventive agents and carcinogenesis in humans and the results of clinical and epidemiology trials will be eagerly anticipated.

ACKNOWLEDGEMENTS

We thank R. Markmann for excellent secretarial assistance and J. Mertz for graphics preparation. Supported in part by grant CA-27502 from the National Institute of Health.

REFERENCES

1. Williams, R.R. and Horm, J.W. (1977). Association of cancer sites with tobacco and alcohol consumption and socioeconomic status of patients: interview study from the third national cancer survey. *J. Natl. Cancer Inst.*, **58**, 525–547.

2. Wynder, E.L., Bross, I.J., and Feldman, R.M. (1957). A study of the etiological factors in cancer of the mouth. *Cancer (Phila.)*, **10**, 1300–1323.

3. Keane, W.M., Atkins, J.P., Wetmore, R., and Vidas, M. (1981). Epidemiology of head and neck cancer. *Laryngoscope*, **91**, 2037–2044.

4. Decker, J., and Goldstein, J.C. (1982). Risk factors in head and neck cancer. *N. Engl. J. Med.*, **306**, 1151–1155.

5. McCoy, G.D., and Wynder, E.L. (1979). Etiological and preventive implications in alcohol carcinogenesis. *Cancer Res.*, **39**, 2844–2850.

6. Bross, I.J., and Coombs, J. (1976). Early onset of oral cancer among women who drink and smoke. *Oncology (Basel)*, **23**, 136–139.

7. Vincent, R.G., and Marchetta, F. (1963). The relationship of the use of tobacco and alcohol to cancer of the oral cacity, pharynx or larynx. *Am. J. Surg.*, **106**, 501–505.

8. Farber, E. (1981). Chemical carcinogenesis. *N. Engl. J. Med.*, **305**, 1379–1389.

9. Becker, F.F., and Stout, D.L. (1980). Progressive DNA damage in hepatic nodules during 2-acetylaminofluorene carcinogenesis. *Cancer Res.*, **40**, 1269–1273.

10. Klein, G. (1981). The role of gene dosage and genetic transpositions in carcinogenesis. *Nature*, **294**, 313–318.

11. Miller, E.C. (1978). Some current perspectives on chemical carcinogenesis in humans and experimental animals: Presidential address. *Cancer Res.*, **38**, 1479–1496.

12. Boutwell, R.K. (19). The role of the induction of ornithine decarboxylase in tumor promotion. In H. Hiatt *et al.* (Eds), *Origins of Human Cancer*, Book B., Cold Spring Harbor Laboratory, New York, pp.49–58.

13. Slaga, T.J., Fischer, S.M., Nelson, K., and Gleason, G.L. (1980). Studies on the mechanisms of skin tumor promotion: evidence for several stages of promotion. *Proc. Natl. Acad. Sci.*, **77**, 3659–3663.

14. Peto, R., Doll, R., Buckley, J.D., and Sporn, M.B. (1981). Can dietary beta-carotene materially reduce human cancer rates? *Nature*, **290**, 201–208.

15. Sporn, M.B. (1977). Retinoids and carcinogenesis. *Nutr. Rev.*, **35**, 65–69.

16. Meyskens, F.L. Jr. (1981). Modulation of abnormal growth by retinoids: a clinical perspective of the biological phenomenon. *Life Sci.*, **28**, 2323–2327.

17. Chow, C.K. (1979). Nutritional influence on cellular antioxidant defense systems. *Am. J. Clin. Nutr.*, **32**, 1066–1081.

18. Wattenberg, L.W. (1978). Inhibitors of chemical carcinogenesis. *Adv. Cancer Res.*, **26**, 197–223.

19. Coombs, G.F., Noguchi, T., and Scott, M.L. (19   ). Mechanisms of action of selenium and vitamin E in protection of biological membranes. *Fed. Proc.*, **34**, 2090–2095.

20. Griffin, A.C. (1979). Role of selenium in cancer chemoprevention. *Adv. Cancer Res.*, **29**, 419–443.

21. Ip, C., (1981). Prophylaxis of mammary neoplasia by selenium supplementation in the initiation and promotion phases of chemical carcinogenesis. *Cancer Res.*, **41**, 4386–4390.

22. Bright-See, E., and Newmark, H.L. (1982). Potential and probable role of vitamin C and E in the prevention of carcinogenesis, In Frank L. Meyskens, Jr. and Kedar N. Prasad (Eds), *Proceedings of the First International Symposium on the Modulation and Mediation of Cancer by Vitamins*, Karger, New York, pp.000–000.

23. Rossman, T.G., and Troll, W. (1980). Prolease inhibitors in carcinogenesis: possible sites of action, in T. Slaga (Ed.), *Carcinogenesis*, vol. 5: *Modifiers of Chemical Carcinogenesis*, Raven Press, New York, p.127.

24. Slaga, T.J., and Scribner, J.D. (1973). Inhibition of tumor initiation and promotion by antiinflammatory agents. *J. Natl. Cancer Inst.*, **51**, 1723–1725.

25. Sporn, M.B., Dunlop, N.M., Newton, D.L., and Henderson, W.R. (1976). Relationship between structure and activity of retinoids. *Nature*, **263**, 110–113.

26. Mayer, H., Bollag, W., Hanni, R., and Ruegg, R. (1978). Retinoids, a new class of compounds with prophylactic and therapeutic activities in oncology and dermatology. *Experientia*, **34**, 1105–1119.

27. Ong, D.E., and Chytil, F. (1975). Specificity of cellular retinol-binding protein for compounds with vitamin A activity. *Nature*, **255**, 74–75.

28. Ong, D.E., Page, D.L., and Chytil, F. (1975). Retinoic acid binding protein: occurrence in human tumors. *Science*, **90**, 60–61.

29. Trown, P.W., Palleroni, A.V., Bohoslawec, O., Richelo, B.N., Halpern, J.M., Gizzi, N., Geiger, R., Lewenski, C., Machlin, L.J., Jetten, A., and Jetten, M.E.R. (1980). Relationship between binding affinities to cellular retinoic acid-binding protein and *in vivo* and *in vitro* properties for 18 retinoids. *Cancer Res.*, **40**, 212–220.

30. DeLuca, L.M., and Shapiro, S.S. (Eds), (1981). Modulation of cellular interactions by vitamin A and its derivatives (retinoids). *Ann NY Acad. Sci.*, **359**, 000.

31. Lotan, R., Kramer, R.H., Neumann, G., Lotan, D., and Nicolson, G.L. (1980). Retinoic acid-induced modifications in the growth and cell surface components of a human carcinoma (HeLa) cell lines. *Exp. Cell Res.*, **130**, 401–414.

32. Verma, A.K., and Boutwell, R.K. (1977). Vitamin A acid (retioic acid), a potent inhibitor of 12-0-tetradecanoyl-phorbol-13-acetate-induced ornithine decarboxylase activity in mouse epidermis. *Cancer Res.*, **37**, 2196–2201.

33. Ong, D.E., page, D.L., and Chytil, R. (1975). Retinoic acid binding protein: occurrence in human tumors. *Science*, **190**, 60–61.

34. Ong, D.E., Goodwin, J., Jesse, R.H., and Griffin, A.C. (1982). Presence of cellular retinol and retinoic-acid binding proteins in epidermal carcinoma of the oral cavity and oropharynx. *Cancer*, **49**, 1409–1412.

35. Lotan, R. (1980). Effects of vitamin A and its analogs (retinoids) on normal and neoplastic cells. *Biochem. Biophys. Acta*, **605**, 33–91.

36. Lotan, R., and Dennert, G. (1979). Stimulatory effects of vitamin A analogs on induction of cell-mediated cytotoxicity *in vivo*. *Cancer Res.*, **39**, 55–58.

37. Abb, J., Deinbardt, F. (1980). Effects of retinoic acid on the human lymphocyte response to mitogens. *Exp. Cell Biol.*, **48**, 169–179.

38. Sidell, N., Famatiga, E., and Golub, S.H. (1981). Augmentation of human thymocyte proliferative responses by vitamin A (retinoic) acid. *Exp. Cell Biol.*, **49**, 239–245.

39. Meyskens, F.L. Jr., and Fuller, B.B. (1980). Characterization of the effects of different retinoids on the growth and differentiation of a human melanoma cell line and selected subclones. *Cancer Res.*, **40**, 2194–2196.

40. Stinson, S.F., Reznik, G., and Donahoe, R. (1981). Effect of three retinoids on tracheal carcinogenesis with N-methyl-N-nitrourea in hamsters. *J. Natl. Cancer Inst.*, **66**, 947–951.

41. Lowe, G.M. Jr., and Kamarek, M.S. (1981). Retinoids, urinary bladder carcinogenesis, and chemoprevention: a review and synthesis. *Nutr. Cancer*, **3**, 109–114.

42. Sidell, N. (1982). Retinoic acid-induced growth inhibition and morphologic differentiation of human neuroblastoma cell in vitro. *J. Natl. Cancer Inst.*, **68**, 589.

43. Breitman, T.R., Selonick, S.E., and Collins, S.J. (1980). Induction of differentiation of the

human promyelocytic leukemia cell lines (HL-60) by retinoic acid. *Proc. Natl. Acad. Sci., USA*, **77**, 2936–2940.

44. Meyskens, F.L. Jr., and Salmon, S.E. (1979). Inhibition of human melanoma colony formation by retinoids. *Cancer Res.*, **39**, 4055–4057.

45. Douer, D., and Koeffler, H.P. (1982). Retinoic acid: inhibition of the clonal growth of human myeloid leukemic cells. *J. Clin. Invest.*, **69**, 277–283.

46. Clamon, G.H. (19). Retinoids for the prevention of epithelial cancers: current status and future potential. *Med. Ped. Oncol.*, **8**, 177–185.

47. Moriarty, M., Dunn, J., Dawagh, A., Lambe, R., and Brick, I. (1982). Etretinate in treatment of actinic keratosis. *Lancet*, **1**, 364–365.

48. Peck, G.L. (1981). Chemoprevention of cancer with retinoids. *Gynecol. Oncol.*, **12**, 5331–5340.

49. Bollag, W. (1976). Vitamin A and vitamin A acid in the prophylaxis and therapy of epithelial tumors. *Int. J. Vit. Res.*, **40**, 299–314.

50. Meyskens, F.L., Gilmartin, E., Alberts, D.S., Levine, N.S., Brooks, Salmon, S.E., and Surwit, E.A. (1982). Activity of isotretinoin against squamous cell cancers and preneoplastic lesions. *Cancer Treat. Rep.*, **66**, 1315–1319.

51. Meyskens, F.L., Aapro, M., Voakes, J.B., Moon, T.E., and Gilmartin, E. (1981). A stratified randomized adjuvant study of BCG ± high dose vitamin A in stage I and II malignant melanoma, In S.E. Salmon and S.E. Jones (Eds), *Adjuvant Therapy of Cancer*, vol. III, Grune & Stratton, New York, pp.217–224.

52. Surwit, E.A., Graham, V., Droegemueller, W., Alberts, D., Chvapil, M., Dorr, R.T., Davis, J.R., and Meyskens, F.L. Jr. (1982). Evaluation of topically applied trans-retinoic acid in the treatment of cervical intraepithelial lesions. *Am. J. Obstet. Gynecol.*, **143**, 821.

53. Koch, H.F. (1978). Biochemical treatment of precancerous oral lesions: the effectiveness of various analogues of retinoic acid. *J. Max. Fac. Surg.*, **6**, 59–63.

54. Ryssel, M.J., Brunner, K.W., and Bollag, W. (1971). Die perorale Anwendung von Vitamin A-saure bei leukoplakien, hyperkeratosen, und plastenepithelkarzinomen; Ergebnisse und Wertraglichkeit. *Schweiz Med. Wochenschr.*, **101**, 1027–1030.

55. Schroder, F.W., and Black, E.W. (1980). Retinoids: tumor preventers or tumor enhancers. *J. Natl. Cancer Inst.*, **65**, 671–674.

56. Ito, Y. (1980). Effect of an aromatic retinoic acid analog (RO-10-9359) on growth of virus-induced papilloma (Shope) and related neoplasia of rabbits. *Europ. J. Cancer*, **17**, 35–42.

57. de-The, G., and Ito, Y. (Eds), (1978). *Nasopharyngeal Carcinoma: Etiology and Control*. International Agency for Research on Cancer, Lyon.

58. Hirayama, T., and Ito, Y. (1981). A new view of the etiology of nasopharyngeal carcinoma. *Prev. Med.*, **10**, 614–622.

D
CELLS IN CULTURE

Chapter **19**

Establishment of Epidermoid Carcinoma Cell Lines

Thomas E. Carey
Departments of Otorhinolaryngology and Microbiology/Immunology, The University of Michigan School of Medicine, Ann Arbor, MI, USA

INTRODUCTION

Epidermoid carcinoma or squamous cell carcinoma (SCC) is a prominent form of cancer at many sites in the body and is the most common human malignancy capable of metastasis.[1] Squamous carcinomas account for over 90% of cancers arising in the larynx and oral cavity.[2] Of the epidemic of malignant cancers arising from the lung and bronchial tree, nearly one-half are squamous cell carcinomas.[3] In addition, squamous cell cancers make up about one-fifth to one-third of all skin cancers[1] and account for 90% of cancers arising from the uterine cervix.[4] Presumably, epidermoid cancer is so prevalent because squamous epithelial cells line the surfaces most frequently exposed to environmental carcinogenic agents. Factors implicated in the origins or causes of SCC are numerous and include viruses, chemical carcinogens, and electromagnetic radiation.[1,5,6] In addition, there is an increased risk of squamous cell cancer in immunosuppressed individuals.[7] Aetiological factors are discussed

in more detail in other chapters of this book.

In spite of the prevalence of this human cancer type, relatively little is known of the cell biology and growth regulatory factors affecting squamous cell carcinoma. This chapter will discuss examples of successful culture of squamous cell carcinomas, the difficulties that have arisen from cross-contamination of cell lines, the current methods for culture of squamous carcinoma, and the identification of features which distinguish SCC cells *in vitro*.

EPIDERMOID CARCINOMA IN CULTURE: HISTORICAL REVIEW

There has been a widespread belief that epidermoid or squamous cell cancers are particularly difficult to establish in culture, and although epidermoid carcinomas are among the most common of human cancers, relatively few representative lines were in existence until recently. In fact squamous cell carcinomas have been successfully grown in culture since the early 1950s, but no large series were established until recently.

Successful culture of human tumours began with the pioneering studies in the early 1900s by Alexis Carrel,[8] who used clots of plasma as the growth medium to cultivate a human fibro-sarcoma line. By the mid-1950s the development of well-defined liquid media and refinements in tissue culture methodology by the Geys, Parker *et al.*, Weymouth, Earle, Eagle, and others, resulted in an improved success rate for the development of permanent human tumour cell lines.[9-14]

HeLa: Epidermoid Carcinoma or Adenocarcinoma

One of the earliest and perhaps one of the most famous and widely used cultured human tissue culture lines is the HeLa cell line, established in 1952 by George Gey and his co-workers.[15] HeLa was established from a biopsy of a tumour of the uterine cervix which was initially reported to be an epidermoid carcinoma[15] and was referred to as such in many publications.[16-20] In one later publication Gey described the tumour as a transitional cell carcinoma.[21] However, 20 years after establishment of the HeLa line in culture, the patient's history was reviewed and the histology of the original specimen was reassessed. The patient was a 31-year-old black woman who began to experi-ence intramenstrual spotting several months after giving birth to her fifth child. She was found to have a friable lesion of the uterine cervix which was biopsied and placed in culture. On the basis of a retrospective review of the original histology slides of this lesion, Jones *et al.* concluded that the original cancer was an adenocarcinoma.[22] Recent serological studies in my laboratory tend to support this conclu-sion, since HeLa cells fail to express the squamous cell antigens found on all of the SCC cell lines (30/30) we have tested to date.[23,24] The HeLa line we tested was obtained from the human tumour bank of J. Fogh at the Sloan–Kettering Institute. Our vial was labelled HeLa P-3 and had been in frozen

storage from March 1972 until 1982 when it was tested. Since the HeLa line was already 20 years old in 1972, the P-3 most likely refers only to the number of passage transfers performed in the Sloan–Kettering laboratory before it was frozen. The HeLa cells we tested express human HLA polymorphic determinants and the β_2 microglobulin antigen, but do not react with antibodies to pemphigus, pemphigoid, and blood group antigens (Carey *et al.*, unpublished data).

The HEp and KB Lines

The remarkable usefulness of the HeLa line for many kinds of *in vitro* studies[19-21,25,26] stimu-lated other investigators to attempt to develop additional human cancer cell lines. In 1953 Helene Toolan and her co-workers[27] success-fully established transplantable xenografts of human epidermoid cancers by implanting fresh, finely minced tumour tissue in rats that had been immunosuppressed with cortisone and radiation. Several human tumours culti-vated in this way could be transplanted to other immunosuppressed animals and were established as the continuous transplantable carcinoma lines HEp 1, HEp 2, and HEp 3.[28]

HEp 1 was derived from a 52-year-old female patient with recurrent epidermoid carcinoma of the cervix. Tumour tissue was obtained from an inguinal lymph node containing metastatic cancer cells. This tumour line, subsequently transplanted through 40 generations within 1½ years, demonstrates the remarkable ability of a human tumour to grow in immunosuppressed animals.

HEp 2 was derived from a recurrent epider-moid carcinoma of the larynx in a 57-year-old white male. After two generations in suppressed rats HEp 2 was transferred to culture.[28] After 17 months of passage, cells from the *in vitro* culture were used to re-establish HEp 2 as a transplantable xenograft line. Histological features characteristic of epidermoid carcinoma were noted in photomicrographs of fixed sections of the xenografted HEp 2 tumour. These features were similar to those exhibited by the original tumour.

HEp 3 was established as a xenograft line from a cervical lymph node metastasis of a buccal epidermoid carcinoma in a 62-year-old black male. This was an aggressive tumour both in the patient, who died of his cancer within 3 months after this surgery, and in the animal hosts in which HEp 3 was capable of invasive growth and metastases. The remarkably aggressive growth of this human xenograft caused some suspicion that the transplantable tumours might not be of human origin. However, when extracts of the tumour transplants were tested by immunodiffusion against an antiserum to human tissues, lines of precipitation demonstrated that human antigens were present.[28] The authors also showed that even after several generations the tumours produced in the rats were histologically similar to the original patients' tumours.[28] Eventually all three of the HEp cell lines were established in *in vitro* culture as permanent cell lines, HEp 2 by Fjelde,[28,29] HEp 1 and HEp 3 by Alice Moore *et al.*[30]

At the same time that these studies were going on, Eagle developed a liquid culture medium that optimally supported the growth of HeLa.[31,32] He used this medium to establish a new epidermoid carcinoma line from a 54-year-old white male with buccal cancer. The new cell line, called KB, grew slowly at first but when trypsinized after 2 weeks in culture it suddenly began to grow rapidly with a doubling time of 30 hours.[33] It seemed from these studies that use of the appropriate growth medium would simplify the establishment of human epidermoid carcinoma cells in culture. In spite of these initial successes, very few additional epidermoid carcinoma lines were reported in the literature during the next 12 years, although numerous epithelial cell lines derived from other tissue types were reported.[34–37] However, a discovery of widespread cross-contamination called into question the identity of many epithelial cell lines, including the existing epidermoid carcinoma lines.

Cross-contamination of Cultured Lines

In 1967 Gartler used isozyme analysis to characterize and identify individual human cell lines. He made the surprising discovery that 18 different human cell lines all expressed the same relatively rare glucose-6-phosphate dehydrogenase (G6PD) phenotype.[38] Among the lines he tested were HeLa and the epidermoid carcinoma cell lines KB and HEp 2, as well as a presumed normal oesophageal epithelial cell line, Minnesota-EE.[36] In each case the G6PD activity in the cell extracts was associated with the more rapidly migrating type A electrophoretic band rather than the common but more slowly migrating type B band. According to Gartler, type A G6PD is not known to occur in Caucasians and is expressed in only 30% of the Negro population. Furthermore, all 18 lines also expressed the same isozyme of phosphoglucomutase (PGM type 1) which has a frequency of 65% in both Caucasion and Negro populations. On the basis of these observations Gartler concluded that the human epithelial cell lines he tested were all contaminated by a cell type that expressed the G6PD type A phenotype. He presumed that HeLa was the contaminating line because HeLa was so widely used and because, since the donor of HeLa was a black woman, there was a reasonable probability that she carried the gene for type A G6PD expression. Gartler's findings were extended and confirmed by Peterson *et al.*[39] who went on to show that genetic conversion (from type B to type A) *in vitro* was apparently not a plausible explanation for the high frequency of type A isozyme among cultured cell lines. To demonstrate this, Peterson *et al.*[40] established a new epithelial line, Detroit 562, from the cells of a pleural effusion from a Caucasian female with adenocarcinoma of the oesophagus. This cell line was shown to continue to express the type B isozyme over 2 years and 114 passages. Thus, the expression of the type A isozyme by all 18 of the previously tested cell lines most probably occurred by cross-contamination. This was certainly possible, since HeLa and the other human cancer lines were often present in the same laboratory simultaneously.

Gartler's findings cast doubt on the identity

of all the purported epithelial cancer cell lines then available. This controversy over cross-contamination was continued as Nelson-Rees and his co-workers[41] compared the chromosomal markers of HeLa and other established cell lines and revealed that HeLa characteristics were indeed present in many human lines, including KB, HEp 2, HEK (embryonic kidney), HBT-3, HBT-39B (breast carcinomas), and MA-160 (prostate adenoma). However, a different aspect of the cell line identity controversy was illustrated by a dialogue which developed as a result of this report. Nelson-Rees had reported, in a note added in proof, that the RT4 bladder carcinoma cell line they tested contained marker chromosomes associated with HeLa cells. Rigby and Franks,[42] the developers of the RT4 line, responded in a subsequent issue of the same journal that the cells of this line maintained in their own laboratory were, in fact, distinct from HeLa by multiple isozymes.[43] Thus, any cross-contamination must have occurred in other laboratories and it was these cells that eventually were tested by Nelson-Rees.

Further studies on the problem of cross-contamination have been detailed.[44] These reports include additional evidence on isozyme signatures,[45] as well as evidence for the expression of prostate-specific markers in prostate-derived cell lines reported to be HeLa contaminants.[46] The latter raises the possibility that cell–cell hybridization may have occurred in some contaminated cultures.

In any case, the evidence for widespread cross-contamination of human cell lines was so strong that in 1975 Rafferty[47] stated in his review on epidermal cell culture that: 'It is widely accepted that few examples of human carcinoma cell lines are in existence, despite numerous attempts to establish them. Among widely disseminated lines there may in fact be only one, the HeLa cell.' Rafferty's comment is now known to be an overstatement, but it serves as a caveat to cell culturists to characterize each new human cell line carefully and to maintain each as a pristine and unique biological reagent.

Epidermoid Carcinoma Lines of the Post-HeLa Era

Regardless of the cross-contamination problem, investigators continued through the 1960s and 1970s to develop new cell lines from epidermoid cancers at the rate of about one or two reports each year. In 1962 Norrby et al.[48] established paired normal and cancer lines from two patients, one with papillary carcinoma of the bladder and another with medullary epidermoid cancer of the cervix. The cervical tumour line was called C-3 II. However, a photomicrograph of the culture showed spindle-shaped cells and the absence of intercellular connections. These morphological features are not what is typically observed in squamous cell cultures, which tend to be epitheloid and cohesive to adjacent cells. The cultures were originally derived in chicken plasma and chicken embryo extract, and the authors noted the possibility that viral contamination from this source might have influenced the cells which became established in culture.

Auersperg and Hawryluk[49] also reported the establishment of two new permanent squamous carcinoma lines in 1962. In 20 other attempted cultures in their series the epithelial cells ceased to divide or were overgrown by fibroblasts. The C-4 I culture grew well, however, and was characterized by a hypodiploid karyotype with a stable modal chromosome number of 44-45.[50] In 1969 Auersperg[51] reported detailed morphological studies of the two clones (C-4 I and C-4 II) that had been derived 7 years before from a biopsy of an invasive cervical squamous cell carcinoma in a 41-year-old Caucasian woman.[49] The clones were characterized for features of epithelial cells. In spite of being in culture for several years the cultures continued to express clear evidence of their squamous derivation, including stratification into layers of cells and the formation of intercellular tight junctions (desmosomes). Hemicyst or pseudocyst formation in ageing *in vitro* cultures and abundant intercellular microvilli also indicative of squamous cell carcinomas were demonstrated. Considerable additional studies were made on C-4 I,[52,53] but no specific comparison to HeLa cells was presented at this time, presumably because the controversy over cell line identity was not yet widely known. However, in 1977 Herz, working with Auersperg and others,[54] reviewed the features of the C-4 I cell line, such as its expression of type B G6PD,[58] its ability to form desmosomes, and its content of chromosome markers, which distinguish C-4 I from HeLa.

In 1970 Friedl *et al.*[55] noted that, in spite of the usefulness of HeLa, very few other reports of new uterine cervix carcinomas had appeared. They tested 10 biopsies of uterine cancers from Japanese patients for *in vitro* growth: seven were diagnosed as squamous cell carcinomas and three as adenocarcinomas. A permanent cell line called SiHa was derived from one of these. The tumour was a squamous cell carcinoma grade II of the cervix that arose in a 55-year-old Mongoloid female. The cell line had epithelioid morphology and contained desmosomes and tonofilaments, ultrastructural features usually found in cells of squamous derivation.

In 1970 Sykes and co-workers reported the establishment of another cervical squamous cell carcinoma.[56] This cell line, ME-180, was derived from a 66-year-old Caucasian female and was also shown to have tonofilaments and desmosomes. Unfortunately, HeLa was in use in this laboratory at the time ME-180 was derived and a potential for contamination existed. Nevertheless, ME-180 has antigenic features such as the expression of blood group A[57] and pemphigus antigen (see Ref. 24 and Table 19.4 of this chapter) which distinguish it from HeLa and show that such an event did not occur. Furthermore, Fogh *et al.*[58] reported that ME-180 was among a group of 127 human cell lines which express the G6PD isozyme with type B electrophoretic mobility.

In 1973 Giard *et al.*, as a result of a multicentre study to assess the ability of a variety of solid human cancers to grow *in vitro*,[59] reported that of 200 culture attempts, 13 new human cancer cell lines were developed for an overall success rate of 6%. Of the 13 new lines, three were established from a total of five biopsies of epidermoid carcinomas. These cell lines, A-253, A-388 and A-431, were established from a 54-year-old male, an 86-year-old male, and an 85-year-old female, respectively. By the time this study was begun there was widespread awareness of the cross-contamination problem and the authors specifically pointed out that there was no possibility of contamination by HeLa since the latter was not present in their laboratory.

Similarly, when George Moore *et al.*[60] reported the development of the COLO 16 line in 1975, the authors were careful to point out that the new line was definitely not a HeLa contaminant. COLO 16 was established from a squamous cell carcinoma and arose from a burn scar in the skin of a 59-year-old black female. In culture COLO 16 was shown to grow in tight clusters and to have intercellular bridges, desmosomes, and tonofilaments, all squamous cell characteristics. Initially, COLO 16 was reported to lack G6PD. However, the line was later found to have the rare G6PD isozyme with type A electrophoretic mobility like that expressed by HeLa.[61] Nevertheless, Moore's contention that COLO 16 was distinct from HeLa was upheld since karyotype analyses showed that this cell line did express different marker chromosomes from those known to characterize HeLa substrains.[62]

In 1976 O'Toole *et al.*[63] derived the SCaBER cell line from a male patient with squamous cell carcinoma of the urinary bladder. Cells of this line contain the Y chromosome, express the HLA antigens 2, 5, and W17 (also expressed by the patient's lymphocytes) and contain a hypodiploid contingent of chromosomes including markers different from those of HeLa. At last a cell line from a squamous cell carcinoma had been shown from the outset to be unequivocally distinct from HeLa by multiple criteria.

In 1977 Morgan *et al.*[64] working in Moore's lab, reported the establishment of COLO 227 and COLO 219, a squamous cell carcinoma line and a lymphoid line respectively, both established from a 59-year-old Caucasian male. The squamous carcinoma cell line was derived from a tumour that arose in an old burn scar. The burn scar was being treated with a pedicle graft at the time of diagnosis and when the pedicle was replaced back in the donor site the tumour was inadvertently transplanted to the patient's opposite leg. The transplanted tumour was widely excised but nevertheless recurred at the implantation site. A specimen from this recurrent tumour was placed in culture. Peripheral blood monocytes were also placed in culture, from which a continuously dividing lymphoid line became established. Both the tumour line and the lymphoid line expressed the Y chromosome, as would be expected. The squamous carcinoma line contained a modal distribution clustered around 106 chromosomes, as well as a number of marker chromosomes, including some which had been noted to be present in other cancers of the same type. This suggested that some markers might be a common consequence of neoplastic transformation rather than a distinguishing feature of an individual cell line. The authors also reported that COLO 227 secreted measurable quantities of parathyroid hormone as detected by a radioimmune assay, a feature these investigators had noted before with COLO 16.[60] They suggested that the ability of squamous cancer cells to produce this hormone might be an explanation for the clinical symptoms of hypercalcemia sometimes noted in squamous cell carcinoma patients. In fact, the donor of COLO 16 died with severe hypercalcaemia. The donor of COLO 227, however, had not had detectable elevation of serum calcium levels. This finding of ectopic hormone production is an important observation, since the production of ectopic hormones and other factors may prove to be valuable both as a means of identifying individual cell lines and also as tools to study mechanisms of metabolic derangement related to tumour growth *in vivo* and *in vitro*.

During 1978 Porter *et al.*[65] reported the development of two new squamous cell carcinoma lines. The first, EC–82, was established from a vaginal carcinoma and the second,

EC–50, from a carcinoma of the uterine cervix. Both cell lines produced tumours in immunosuppressed animals that re-created the histology originally found in the patient. In addition, EC–82, the carcinoma of the cervix, was found to produce human chorionic gonadotropin, a feature not found in the EC–50 line.

Okabe *et al.*[66] also contributed a new squamous cell carcinoma cell line to the existing repertoire. While significant for other reasons, this cell line was also the first of many that were to be established from patients with head and neck cancer in the next several years. The line, T3M–1, was derived from a 33-year-old Japanese male patient with squamous cell carcinoma of the oral cavity. The patient was noted to have neutropenia and it thus was of great interest that the cell line produced large amounts of colony-stimulating factor (CSF) *in vitro* and induced neutropenia *in vivo* when it was implanted in nude mice. The significance of this observation with respect to the effect of the tumour on the host has not been elucidated. However, the ability of the cell line to produce the factor was a very stable property retained over many *in vitro* passages through more than $1\frac{1}{2}$ years of culture.

One year later, in 1979, Nishihira and co-workers[67] established the TE–1 and TE–2 cell lines from two patients with squamous cell cancer of the oesophagus. TE–1 was derived from tumour tissue of a 58-year-old Japanese male patient with a well-differentiated SCC, while TE–2 was established from tumour tissue of a 57-year-old Japanese male patient with poorly differentiated SCC of the oesophagus. The lines both expressed a male karyotype and produced measurable CEA levels.

Panels of Squamous Cell Carcinoma Lines from Head and Neck Cancer Patients

In the studies described above, the authors often mentioned the difficulty of establishing epidermoid carcinoma lines *in vitro*, but for the most part were unable to pinpoint the reasons for successful culture when it occurred. That the reports of new SCC lines up to this time were restricted to the establishment of only one or two lines attests to certain inherent difficulties in establishing squamous cell carcinoma lines. One problem frequently cited through the years has been loss of promising cultures due to overgrowth by fibroblasts. Edwards *et al.*[68] reported in 1980 an innovative approach to resolving this problem. They treated primary squamous carcinoma cultures that contained both fibroblasts and epithelial cells with a monoclonal antibody to a fibroblast surface antigen. The addition of rabbit complement selectively lysed the fibroblasts, leaving behind viable epithelial cell colonies. This method was used by Easty and her co-workers[69] to successfully establish 10 new squamous cell carcinomas, HN – 1 to HN – 10, from 36 patients with cancer of the tongue or larynx. In this 1981 report they credited their success to a relatively simple, straightforward approach of placing tumour explants in culture and assiduously removing fibroblasts either by use of the anti-fibroblast monoclonal antibody,[68] by mechanical detachment with a rubber policeman, or by selective removal with trypsin – versene. An additional clue to this group's high culture success rate was their persistence in maintaining cultures for prolonged periods of up to 27 weeks before subculture. We have noted similar long quiescent periods of certain cultures in our own laboratory before continuous doubling begins. This point will be discussed further below. Easty *et al.* also assessed individual lines for tumour production in nude mice, for growth in agar, and for the production of the beta subunit of human chorionic gonadotropin (β-HCG), carcinoembryonic antigen (CEA), and plasminogen activator (PA). Of the six tumour lines tested, HN – 2, HN – 5, and HN – 6 produced tumours in nude mice and HN – 1, HN – 4, and HN – 5 did not. Only HN – 1 and HN – 2 formed colonies in soft agars; thus the ability of these tumour cell lines to grow in soft agar did not correspond to

growth in immunosuppressed mice. All but one cell line, HN – 4, produced immunoreactive β-HCG while five of nine lines produced CEA in the range of from 40 to 900 ng/ml in 24 hours. Plasminogen activator release was variable, ranging from 0 to 100 plough units/ml of medium for individual lines.

In 1981 Rheinwald and Beckett[70] reported an alternative approach to the culture of head and neck squamous cell carcinomas. They developed a method for the cultivation of normal keratinocytes[71] which relied on the use of a mitomycin-C treated mouse 3T3 cell feeder layer and the use of Dulbecco's MEM with 20% fetal calf serum and 0.4 μg/ml of hydrocortisone added to the medium. Using this method, six squamous cancer lines were established from 22 biopsies of tongue, epidermis, and pharynx cancers. Like normal keratinocyte cultures, one of the tumour cell lines, SCC – 13, remained dependent on the 3T3 feeder layer cells for growth and survival. Nevertheless, all of the lines, including SCC – 13, formed tumours with squamous cell features in nude mice. The ability of the SCC lines to form colonies in methylcellulose varied from an efficiency rate of 2% for SCC – 25 to 0.02% for SCC – 12 and 13.

Krause *et al.*[23] reported the initial culture results from our laboratory in 1981. Three new squamous cell carcinoma lines were established from tumours in patients with head and neck cancer. At the time we were unaware of the studies of Nishihira *et al.*[67] and Easty *et al.*[69] but we also found that explants were a very satisfactory method of establishing new squamous cancer cell lines. UM-SCC-1, our first cell line, was derived from a recurrent squamous cancer of the floor of the mouth in a 73-year-old male patient. The cell line grew from a piece of tissue that apparently consisted entirely of tumour cells, since only tightly clustered, cohesive cells of epithelioid shape composed the expanding monolayer that appeared as a halo around the tissue fragment (Figure 19.1). The cells composing the island were difficult to trypsinize and, once detached, were found to have a low plating efficiency.

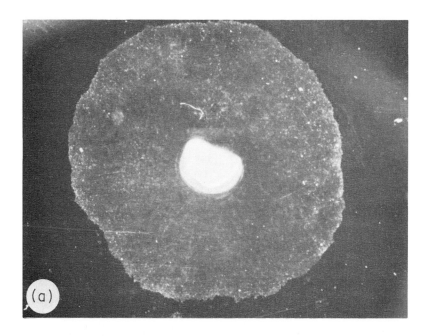

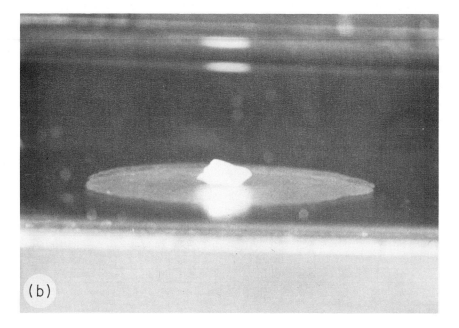

Figure 19.1   Photographs of the primary culture of UM-SCC-1. (**a**) Photograph of the flask from above. Shown are the tissue fragment and the expanding halo of tumour cells. No fibroblasts were found in this culture at any time. (**b**) Photograph of the UM-SCC-1 primary culture from an oblique angle showing the tissue fragment and rim of epithelial cells.

These are features, we soon learned, that were characteristic of many squamous cell cultures. The tissue fragment, which became detached during trypsinization, was transferred to a fresh flask where it gave rise to an additional monolayer. Eventually this fragment was used to establish monolayer cultures in five separate flasks from which, by using a high plating density, cells capable of reattaching to the substrate were isolated and grown as the UM-SCC-1 cell line. UM-SCC-1 has a morphology very typical of a large subset of squamous cancer cell lines. As shown in Figure 19.2 the cells are epithelioid or polygonal and tightly approximated to the adjacent cells of the culture. The nuclei are large, contain prominent nucleoli, and are well delineated from the granular cytoplasm. After the cells have been trypsinized they readily form into islands from which finger-like projections, formed by dividing cells, emerge (Figure 19.3a). Eventually the islands coalesce (Figure 19.3b) to form nearly confluent monolayers. In promising cultures, dividing cells are common

(Figures 19.2 and 19.3). In addition, multinucleated giant cells and cells undergoing dyskeratosis, as well as bizarre mitotic figures, are also frequently found in squamous cell carcinomas (Figure 19.3a, b). UM-SCC-1 has been carried continuously in culture since 1979 and has reached more than 50 passages several times over. The UM-SCC-1 cell line may be an *in vitro* representative of a moderately well-differentiated squamous carcinoma since it exhibited a low plating efficiency in early culture and since it will not produce tumours in nude mice.

UM-SCC-2 was established from a 63-year-old female patient with a recurrent metastatic squamous cell carcinoma of the alveolar ridge. The cell line was derived from tissue biopsied from an exophytic mass in the oral cavity. *In vitro* primary cultures of epithelial tumour cells were lost when fibroblasts overgrew the tumour cells. However, tissue from this biopsy was placed in a nude mouse where it gave rise to a progressively growing tumour with histological and ultrastructural features typical

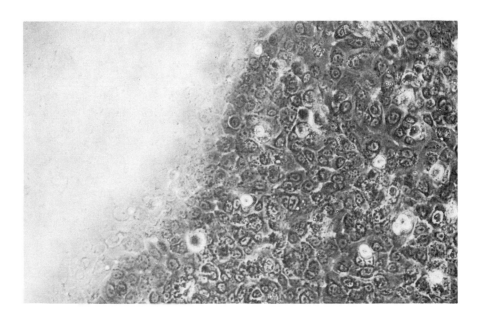

Figure 19.2   Phase contrast photomicrograph of the UM-SCC-1 culture. Shadows in the upper left portion of the photo are caused by the edge of the tissue fragment. Note that there are many mitotic cells in this field which appear as white or refractile circles above the plane of the cell monolayer ($\times$ 110).

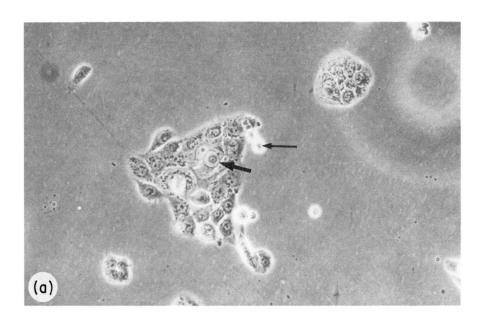

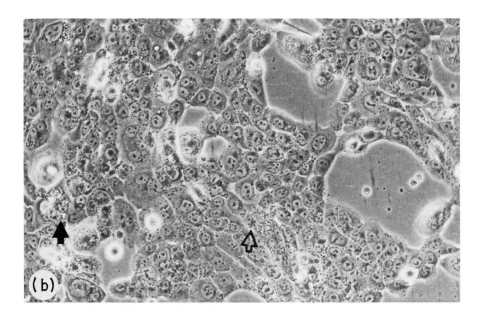

Figure 19.3   Phase contrast photomicrographs of early passages of UM-SCC-1. (a)
Three days after trypsinization cells have formed into islands and have begun dividing.
Note the mitotic cells at the edge of the centre island (small arrow). Individual cell
keratinization is shown by the large arrow (× 110). (b) Seven days after trypsinization
and transfer to a new flask, the islands of UM-SCC-1 cells are coalescing into a
monolayer. Giant cells, multinucleated cells (closed arrow) and bizarre mitoses are all
apparent in this field (open arrow) (× 110).

of squamous cell carcinoma (Figure 19.4a, b). Eventually this tumour was established *in vitro* where its morphological appearance was found to be very similar to UM-SCC-1 (Figure 19.4c). Cultured UM-SCC-2 cells will readily produce tumours in nude mice within 2–4 weeks after the inoculation of 10–20 million viable cultured cells. Electron micrographs of UM-SCC-2 cultured in the nude mouse clearly demonstrate the squamous cell ultrastructural features of interdigitating cell surface microvilli and intercellular desmosomes (Figure 19.5).

UM-SCC-3 taught us the value of patience and illustrated an inverse relation between the growth of fibroblasts and squamous carcinoma cells in primary culture. The tissue specimen used for culture was a cervical lymph node containing squamous cell carcinoma metastatic from a primary lesion that arose several years earlier in the nasal columella of a 73-year-old female patient. Initially, epithelial tumour cells grew out from the tissue fragments; however, fibroblasts began to grow rapidly and to surround all of the tumour cell islands. The fibroblasts were repeatedly removed by trypsinization and transferred to other flasks. The tumour islands grew very slowly for several months, while each week the fibroblasts rapidly proliferated, necessitating repeated trypsinizations. After nearly 6 months in culture the fibroblasts began to grow much more slowly, apparently as a result of *in vitro* senescence. During this time the islands of tumour cells in the primary flask began to show increased numbers of mitotic cells, and small two- and four-cell epithelial islands began to grow in the fibroblast-containing flasks (Figure 19.6). Individual islands began to enlarge and crowd the non-dividing fibroblasts until the primary flasks and the flasks containing trypsinized cells both reached confluence. At this point it was possible to transfer the epithelial cells to new flasks where they continued to grow. Cells of this line exhibit a morphological appearance which is representative of a different squamous cell carcinoma subset in which the cells are pleomorphic and will stratify if left as confluent cultures, as shown in Figure 19.7. In the nude mouse UM-SCC-3 produces tumours with features of well-differentiated squamous cell carcinomas, including extensive keratin pearl formation and individual cell keratinization

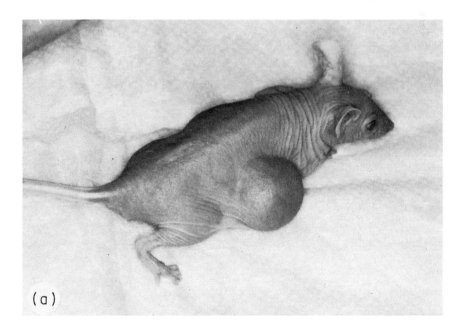

(a)

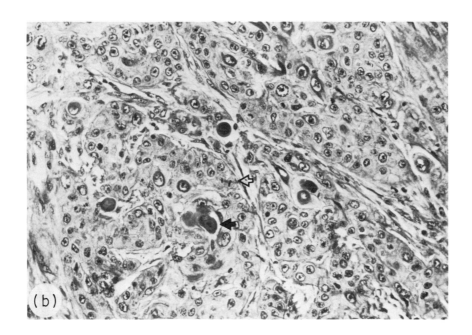

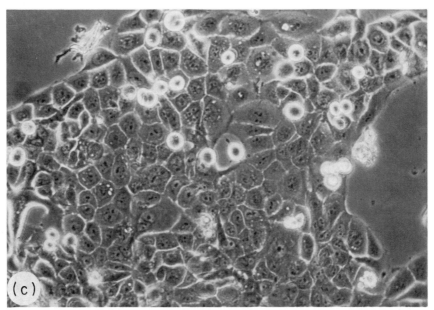

Figure 19.4   Establishment of the UM-SCC-2 squamous carcinoma cell line. (**a**) Fresh tumour fragments were implanted under the subcutaneous tissue of a nude mouse. The photograph shows the size of the tumour after 2 months *in vivo*. (**b**) Histological section of UM-SCC-2 tumour tissue from a nude mouse. Examples of individual cell keratinization are present (closed arrow) as are a number of mitotic cells (open arrow). Stained with haematoxylin and eosin (× 80). (Figure 19.4b is reprinted from Krause *et al.* (1981), *Arch. Otolaryngol.*, **107**., 703–710. Copyright 1981, American Medical Association. (**c**) Cells from passage 6 of UM-SCC-2 in nude mice were used to establish the UM-SCC-2 cell line. Many mitotic cells are present in this photomicrograph of the primary *in vitro* culture (× 210).

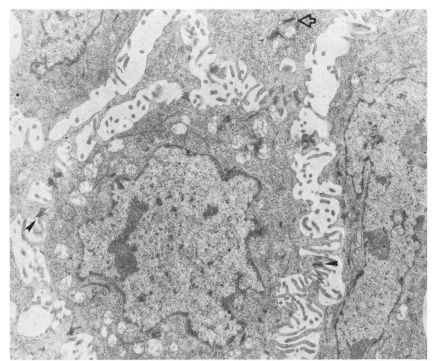

Figure 19.5   Electron micrograph of a section of UM-SCC-2 grown in the nude mouse. Abundant microvilli interconnecting adjacent cells and multiple desmosomes (closed arrowheads) are epithelial cell features. Occasional tonofilament bundles are present but difficult to discern in this photograph (open arrow). (Uranylacetate and lead citrate, × 8,800).

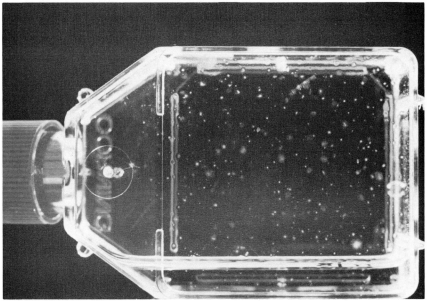

Figure 19.6   View of a tissue culture flask containing UM-SCC-3 cells and senescing fibroblasts. Opaque colonies of squamous carcinoma cells are visible. This photo was taken after the cells had been in this culture flask for nearly 6 months.

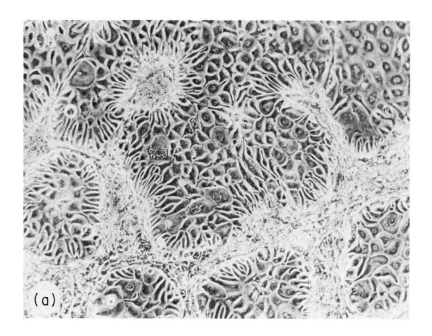

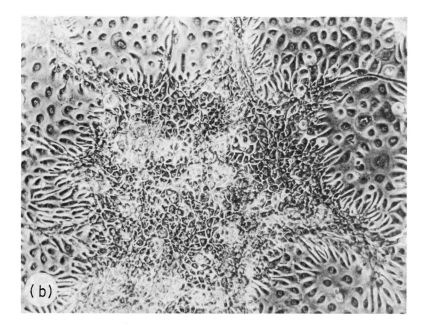

Figure 19.7   UM-SCC-3 cells after 12 passages in culture. The cells of this cell line are pleomorphic and range from large epithelioid cells in mono-layer to spindle-shaped cells surrounding areas of stratified cells. (a) and (b) are different fields in the same culture. In (a) the plane of the photograph is on the monolayer of cells on the flask surface. In (b) the cells in the stratified areas are shown in focus (× 210).

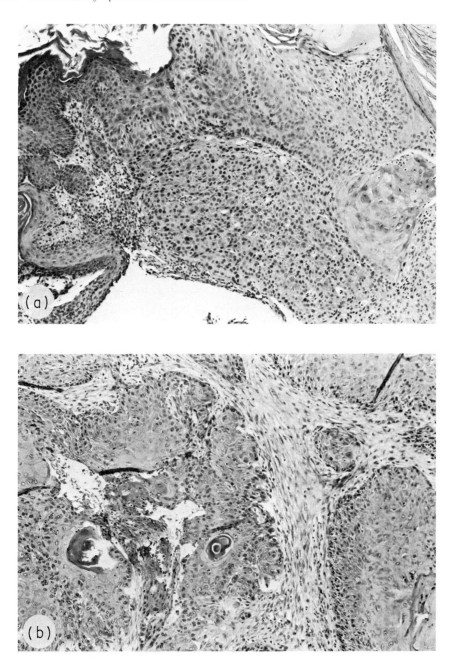

Figure 19.8   Photomicrographs of histology sections of UM-SCC-3 grown in the nude mouse (passage 31) (**a,c,e**) and the histology section of the tumour tissue from the patient from which the UM-SCC-3 cell line was derived (**b,d,f**). Low-power enlargements illustrate the striking similarity of the tumours from the cell line (**a**) and in the patient (**b**) (haematoxylin and eosin × 80). In both sections areas of keratinization and keratin pearl formation are present in sheets of proliferating cells. Under higher magnification nests of tumour cells in the patient (**d**) and nude mouse tumours (**c**) are indistinguishable (haematoxylin and eosin × 210). In some areas keratinization was extensive, resulting in keratin pearl formation in both the nude mouse tumour (**e**) (haematoxylin and eosin × 130) and the patient's tumour (**f**) haematoxylin and eosin × 210).

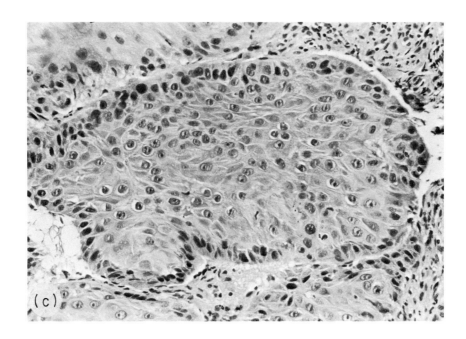

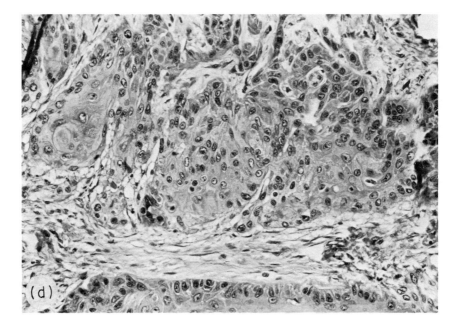

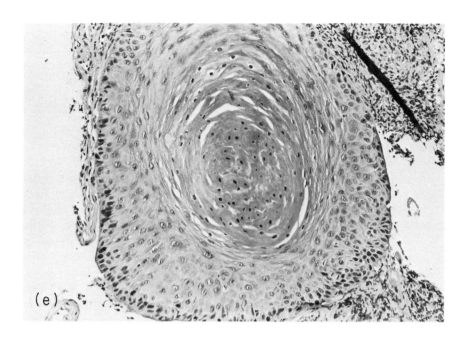

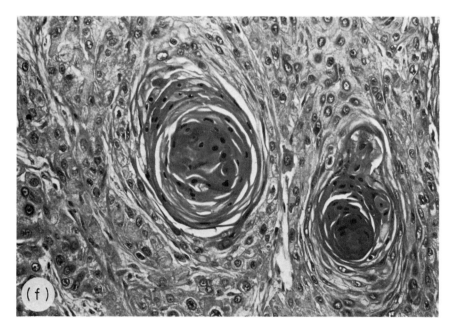

(Figure 19.8a, c, e) which are indistinguishable from those of the patient's original tumour (Figure 19.8b, d, f).

In 1982 Boukamp *et al.*[72] reported the establishment of SCL-1, a squamous carcinoma line derived from the skin of a 74-year-old woman with a poorly differentiated squamous cell carcinoma on her face. The tumour was minced and the fragments placed in plastic dishes and covered with a plasma clot. Later the dishes were covered with modified Eagle's MEM containing four times the usual concentration of ingredients and supplemented with 17% fetal calf serum. The SCL-1 cell line had typical squamous cell epithelioid morphology, with tightly clustered cohesive cells that would stratify. Keratin production was assessed by immunofluorescence and polyacrylamide gel electrophoresis. By electron microscopy the cells contained desmosomes, tonofilaments, and multiple interdigitating microvilli. The karyotype was initially hypodiploid but after 10 passages it became hypotetraploid. The authors noted two stable markers in all metaphases which led them to conclude that the tumour had a monoclonal origin. This relatively well-differentiated cell line had a long latency in nude mice and was unable to form colonies in soft agar.

Characterization of Squamous Cell Carcinoma Cell Lines

The cell lines described in this chapter are listed in Table 19.1. The donor's age and sex, the location of the primary tumour, and the type of tissue sample used to establish the culture are summarized together with the year reported, the author, and the reference number. Of the 40 lines listed the most common primary cancer site was the oral cavity, from which 15 cell lines were established. The second most common site was the uterine cervix with nine lines, followed by larynx and skin with five cell lines each. Two cell lines were established from epidermoid cancers of the oesophagus. One cell line each was derived from tumours of the vagina, urinary bladder,

salivary gland, and nose. Fifteen lines were derived from primary tumours, while the remainder were from recurrent or metastatic tumour deposits. Although there is some question about the identify of the cell lines established before 1962, the other lines listed here have been rather well characterized.

In addition to epidermoid carcinoma cell lines which may have been overlooked in this review, a substantial number of SCC lines have also been established in this laboratory. We have now developed 32 cell lines from 26 patients with squamous cell carcinoma of the head and neck. In five cases cell lines were established from separate tumour deposits in the same individual, i.e. from primary and metastatic lesions or from separate recurrences in the same individual. In one case three cell lines were developed from three separate recurrences in the same patient. Each of these cell lines has been carefully characterized for unique qualities and for qualities that identify each as a squamous cell cancer. Including the lines already published and our own panel, well over 50 examples of well-characterized squamous cell carcinoma cell lines are available for study. Thus, it is now clear that squamous cell cancers can be grown with a reasonable frequency.

The features typically used to describe squamous cell carcinomas are summarized in Table 19.2, and listed for individual lines in Table 19.3. In general, these traits can be grouped into five categories. The first category of cell line traits are those which are species-specific: karyotype, enzyme phenotype, and cell surface antigen expression can all be used to differentiate human cells from other species. The second category includes those features which identify a cell line according to properties representative of a broad tissue type. For example, epithelial cells typically have a polygonal or epithelioid shape and form tight junctions between adjacent cells. Such features do not, however, discriminate between different types of epithelial cells. A third category includes those features which are characteristic of a more narrow differentiation pathway.

TABLE 19.1 HUMAN CELL LINES REPORTED TO BE DERIVED FROM EPIDERMOID CARCINOMAS

Designation	Donor Sex	Age	Primary site	Tissue sample[a]		Originator and Reference
HeLa[b]	F	31	Uterine cervix	P	1953	Gey et al.[15]
ElCu[c]	F	?	Uterine cervix	?	1954	Gey et al.[17]
HEp 1[c]	F	52	Uterine cervix	P	1953–54	Toolan et al.[27–30]
HEp 2[d]	M	57	Larynx	M		
HEp 3[c]	M	62	Oral cavity	M–LN		
KB[d]	M	54	Floor of mouth	P	1955	Eagle[33]
C-3 11	F	36	Uterine cervix	P	1962	Norrby et al.[48]
C-4 1	F	41	Uterine cervix	P	1962	Auersperg and Hawryluk[49]
C-4 11						
SiHa	F	55	Uterine cervix	P	1970	Fried et al.[55]
ME–180	F	66	Uterine cervix	M	1970	Sykes et al.[56]
A–253	M	54	Submaxillary gland	?	1973	Giard et al.[59]
A–388[c]	M	86	?	?		
A–431[c]	F	85	?	?		
HT–3	F	58	Uterine cervix	M–LN	1975	Fogh[72]
COLO–16	F	59	Skin (burn scar)	M	1975	Moore et al.[60]
SCaBER	M	58	Urinary bladder	P	1976	O'Toole et al.[63]
COLO–227	M	59	Skin (burn scar)	R	1977	Moore et al.[64]
EC–50	F	57	Uterine cervix	M(AF)	1978	Porter et al.[65]
EC–82	F	42	Vagina	P		
T3M–1	M	33	Oral cavity	M(Pleura)	1978	Okabe et al.[66]
TE–1	M	58	Esophagus	P	1979	Nishihira et al.[67]
TE–2	M	57	Esophagus	P		
HN–1	M	51	Tongue	R	1981	Easty et al.[68]
HN–2	M	49	Larynx	R		
HN–3	M	63	Tongue	R		
HN–4	M	57	Larynx	R		
HN–5	M	73	Tongue	R		
HN–6	M	54	Tongue	R	1981	Easty et al.[68]
HN–7	M	57	Tongue	R		
HN–8	M	56	Larynx	R		
HN–9	F	67	Tongue	R		
HN–10	M	57	Larynx	R		
SCC–4	M	55	Tongue	R	1981	Rheinwald and Beckett[70]
SCC–9	M	25	Tongue	P		
SCC–12	M	60	Skin (face)	P		
SCC–13	F	56	Skin (face)	R		
SCC–15	M	55	Tongue	P		
SCC–25	M	70	Tongue	P		
UM–SCC–1	M	73	Floor of mouth	R	1981	Krause et al.[23]
UM–SCC–2	F	63	Alveolar ridge	M		
UM–SCC–3	F	73	Nasal columella	M–LN		
SCL–1	F	74	Facial skin	P	1982	Boukamp et al.[72]

[a] Tissue sample used for culture; P – primary lesion; M – metastasis; LN – lymph node; R – recurrent disease at the primary site or adjacent site after radiation, surgery, or chemotherapy; AF – ascites fluid.
[b] HeLa was later noted to be an adenocarcinoma as determined by a retrospective tissue review in 1971.[22]
[c] The author is uncertain whether these cell lines are still available. They are not listed in the American Type Culture Collection but may be available from individual laboratory repositories.
[d] The HEp 2 and KB cell lines have been identified as having HeLa characteristics. It is not known whether examples of these lines exist which are not contaminated by HeLa cells.

Thus, squamous cell carcinomas may be expected to express features that are unique to squamous epithelial cells. Features that seem to conform to this category are the ones marked by footnote a in Table 19.2. For example, keratinization is a feature of squamous cell differentiation; thus, individual cell dyskeratosis, keratin pearl formation, and the production of keratins by cell lines are all strongly indicative

of a squamous cell origin. In our laboratory we have used another feature that appears to be restricted to cells of squamous epithelial origin, namely the expression of squamous cell-specific antigens detected by antibodies from patients with the autoimmune skin diseases pemphigus vulgaris and bullous pemphigoid.[75-77]

The fourth category of distinguishing features are those which differentiate cell lines on the basis of the donor's genotype. Examples which can be used include isozyme markers, histocompatibility antigen expression, and blood group antigen expression.

The final category includes those features which are truly unique to an individual cell line and may even allow clear-cut discrimination between different tumour cell lines established from the same donor. For example, we have noted changes in the expression of membrane antigens detected by monoclonal antibodies that will distinguish between separate tumour cell lines established at different times from the same individual (Kimmel *et al.*, unpublished).

With these concepts in mind, the characteristics listed in Table 19.2 have different levels of importance depending on what point is being made. Thus, although microscopic features are both the first observable features and the ones most readily assessed in the tissue culture laboratory, only one – individual cell dyskeratosis – is considered to be squamous cell-specific. Ultrastructural features such as tonofilaments, desmosomes, and microvilli are usually expressed by squamous carcinomas. However, not all squamous carcinomas have abundant tonofilament formation and other epithelial cells such as well-differentiated adenocarcinomas may have microvilli and tight junctions. Keratinization is a feature that is used clinically to differentiate squamous carcinomas and it is also a feature that is useful for characterizing cultured lines. Thus, when a tumour cell line produces keratin pearls in the nude mouse or other immunosuppressed animal, it is very convincing evidence that the cell line is a

TABLE 19.2 CHARACTERISTICS OF SQUAMOUS CELL CARCINOMA CELL LINES

Microscopic features
  Tendency to form islands
  Intercellular bridges
  Polygonal to near spindle shape
  Prominent nucleoli
  Large nuclear to cytoplasmic ratio
  Cell size ranges from small, tightly packed to large cells with the appearance of cuboidal squamous cells.
  Individual cell dyskeratosis[a]
  Intracellular granules, granular cytoplasm

Karyotype
  Usually aneuploid
  Ranging from near diploid to tetraploid
  Fragments and markers common

In vivo *Xenografts*
  Keratin pearl formation[a]

Virus production
  Has not been reported

Ultrastructure
  Tonofilaments
  Desmosomes
  Microvilli

Membrane antigen expression
  Appropriate blood group[b]
  HLA, β_2 microglobulin
  Pemphigus vulgaris[a]
  Bullous pemphigoid[a]

Cell products
  Keratins[a]
  Ectopic hormones (PTH, β-HCG)
  CEA
  Plasminogen activator

---

[a] Denotes traits indicative of squamous cell differentiation.
[b] Blood group antigen expression is a common feature of squamous cell carcinoma lines but expression of blood group is not restricted to squamous cell tumours, since certain adenocarcinomas also express blood group antigens.

squamous cell carcinoma. However, keratin pearl formation is a feature that is associated both clinically and in tissue culture studies with well-differentiated tumours. Less well-differentiated tumours usually do not produce pearls, and may show only individual cell keratinization or even undetectable levels of keratinization. For this reason, and because not all tumour lines will produce tumours in *in vivo* models, it may prove useful to measure keratin production biochemically as reported by Boukamp *et al.*[72]

In my laboratory the method used to identify cell lines as squamous carcinomas has been to test for the expression of the pemphigus antigen.[75,76] As shown in Table 19.4, plasma from a pemphigus vulgaris patient reacts with squamous carcinoma cell lines in a highly specific manner. In this experiment only UM-SCC-1, UM-SCC-2, and ME-180 gave positive reactions with pemphigus sera. Normal fibroblast, breast carcinoma, ovarian carcinoma, colon carcinoma, bladder carcinoma, and melanoma cultures are all negative.[77] While the degree of pemphigus antigen expression varies greatly among different squamous carcinoma cell lines, all of the SCC lines we have tested are positive both by direct test and by absorption analysis (Carey, Diaz, Schwartz *et al.*, unpublished data). In contrast, none of a very large panel of cell lines derived from other tumour types express this antigen. In fact, only SCC lines and normal squamous cells in culture are positive. Our analysis of pemphigoid antigen expression is incomplete. However, initial results suggest that the pemphigoid antigen is present on only a subset of squamous carcinoma lines. As a result of these findings we consider the expression of the pemphigus antigen to be a cornerstone of cell line identification. In addition, as shown in Table 19.3, each cell line derived in our laboratory is tested for expression of blood group antigen, polymorphic HLA determinants, β_2 microglobulin (HLA light chain), and HLA-DR antigen. To date, all of our SCC lines express the blood group expressed by the donor, all have HLA and β_2

microglobulin, but they do not express HLA-DR antigens. To pursue further the precise identification of individual cell lines, and to examine the structures present on the squamous cell surface, we have developed a panel of monoclonal antibodies to squamous carcinoma cell surface antigens. However, the analysis of those antibodies is not yet complete.

METHODS FOR ESTABLISHING SQUAMOUS CELL CARCINOMAS *IN VITRO*

The methodolgy for developing new cell lines from epidermoid cancers has been alluded to in the foregoing historical review, and in this section the methods will be described in detail.

Microbial Contamination

Nearly all authors agree, and it is our experience, that a major problem in the *in vitro* cultivation of squamous carcinomas is the loss of promising cultures to microbial contamination. Most specimens from the skin or mucosal surface are likely to contain micro-organisms. If such tissue is placed in culture medium without first removing the organisms, abundant proliferation occurs and the cell culture is lost. The approach used in this laboratory is essentially the same as that described by other authors[69,70] and entails the following simple procedures. Specimens are collected immediately after removal in the operating room and placed in cold balanced salt solution containing penicillin and streptomycin to kill bacteria, and an antimycotic such as amphotericin B to suppress moulds and yeast, which are frequent contaminants of oral and skin lesions. Some authors have stressed the need to process the tissue immediately, but both our group and Easty *et al.*[69] have had good success even with specimens that are kept at 4 °C overnight, provided they are stored properly. In our experience the most important considerations are:

(1) to ensure that the specimens do not linger in the operating room at ambient temperature where tissue desiccation may occur;

TABLE 19.3   CHARACTERISTICS EXPRESSED BY INDIVIDUAL CELL LINES FROM EPIDERMOID CARCINOMAS

Cell line	Morphology[a]	Ultrastructure[b]	Karyotype[c]	*In Vivo* tumour production[d]	G6PD mobility
HeLa	E,D	D,TF(73)	XX; 71−90 markers		A(38)
EICu	E,D				
HEρ 1	E,C				
HEp 2	E,C		HeLa markers	+	A(38)
HEp 3	E,C		(44)	+	
KB	E,D	TF,D,HD(73)	HeLa marker (44)		A(38)
C−3 11	D,F		78		
C−4 1	E,C	D,TF,MV	45	+	B(58)
SiHa	E,C	D,TF		+ (58)	B(58)
ME−180	E,C	D,TF,MV	XX, markers aneuploid 48−130	+ (58)	B(58)
A−253	E,C,S			+ (58)	B(58)
A−388					
A−451					
HT−3			Near triploid with market ch.	+ (50)	B
COLO−16	E,C	TF	45−90		A
SCaBER	E,C	TF,D,MV	XY (55−80) Mode 50		
COLO−227	F,D,ICC	TF,D,MV	XY mode 105 with markers		B
EC−50	Large E	TF,D,MV	65−70	+	
EC−82	Large E	D	83−87	+	
T3M−1	E,C	TF,D	66−68	+	
TE−1			Hypotetraploid XY, with markers	+	
TE−2		D	Hypotetraploid XY	+	
HN−1	E,C,S	TF,D(few)	73 50−92 with markers	−	
HN−2			65 59−72	+	
HN−3	E,C		63 47−79	−	
HN−4			68 52−92 with markers	−	
HN−5	E,C,S			+	
HN−6				+	
HN−7					
HN−8					
HN−9					
HN−10					
SCC−4	E,C			+	
SCC−9	E,C			+	
SCC−12				+	
SCC−13	E,C			+	
SCC−15	E,C,ICD			+	
SCC−25				+	
UM−SCC−1	E,C,ICD	TF,MV		−	
UM−SCC−2	E,C	D,TF		+	
UM−SCC−3	E,C,S	MV,ICD		+	
SCL−1	E,C,S,ICD	TF,D,MV	Hypodiploid Hypotetraploid after P−10 with markers		

Cell line	Soluble markers[e]	Donor blood type	A or B blood group	HLA[f]	Pemphigus vulgaris	Bullous pemphigoid
				Antigen expression		
HeLa			−	$H^+\beta^+,DR^-$	−	−
ElCu						
HEp 1						
HEp 2						
HEp 3						
KB						
C−3 11						
C−4 1						
SiHa						
ME−180		A	A(57)	H^+,β^+,DR^-	+	+(24)
A−253						
A−388						
A−451						
HT−3		A	−			
COLO−16	CEA PTH					
SCaBER				5,7,9 2,5,W17		
	CEA			A2,B8		
COLO−227	PTH					
EC−50						
EC−82	HCG					
T3M−1	CSF					
TE−1	(CEA)					
TE−2	CEA					
HN−1	β-HCG PA					
HN−2	β-HCG PA,CEA					
HN−3	β-HCG PA,CEA					

[a] Morphological features as assessed by light microscopy are represented by the following: E − epithelioid shape; C − cohesiveness of cells to one another in culture; D − detached cells, do not cluster; F − fibroblast-like appearance; S − stratification, cells tend to pile up and may differentiate; ICC − intercellular connections; ICD − individual cell dyskeratosis; large E − large epithelioid (polygonal) cells.

[b] Ultrastructural features: TF − tonofilaments; D − desmosomes; MV − microvilli; ICD − individual cell dyskeratosis.

[c] Karyotype implies human chromosomes; XX − normal female karyotype with two X chromosomes; XY − normal male karyotype with one X and one Y chromosome. The range of chromosome numbers for individual cell lines is shown by the linked numbers. Mode indicates the number of chromosomes appearing in highest frequency of all metaphase cells counted. Numbers in parentheses indicate reference number if the karyotype was not reported in the original description of the cell line.

[d] Tumour production *in vivo* indicates the ability of the cell line to produce tumours in immunosuppressed laboratory animals Numbers in parentheses indicate reference numbers if this feature was not reported in the original report.

[e] Soluble markers: CEA − carcinoembryonic antigen; PTH − parathyroid hormone; HCG − human chorionic gonadotropin; CSF − colony stimulating factor; PA − plasminogen activator; β-HCG − β subunit of human chorionic gonadotropin.

[f] Expression of major histocompatability locus antigens was assessed with specific HLA typing sera (indicated b, numerals eg 5, 7, 9 or A2, B8), with antibodies to nonpolymorphic class-I HLA heavy chain determinants (indicated by H), antibodies to beta-2-microglobulin (indicated by β), or with a monoclonal antibody to nonpolymorphic class II (HLA-DR) determinants (indicated by DR). Commercial rabbit anti-β-2 microglobulin (Dako Immunoglobulins), rabbit anti HLA heavy chain (a gift from Dr. Tanagaki of Roswell Park Memorial Institute) and mouse monoclonal antibody to the HLA-DR common determinants (a gift from Dr. Ferrone of New York Medical College) were used in our laboratory. Numbers in parenthesis indicate reference number if antigen expression was not tested by originating laboratory.

TABLE 19.3 (Cont)

Cell line	Soluble markers[e]	Donor blood type	A or B blood group	HLA[f]	Pemphigus vulgaris	Bullous pemphigoid
HN−4	PA,CEA			.	.	
HN−5	β-HCG PA					
HN−6	β-HCG PA					
HN−7	β-HCG CEA		ᵃ			
HN−8	β-HCG CEA					
HN−9	β-HCG					
HN−10	β-HCG PA					
SCC−4	Keratin					
SCC−9						
SCC−12						
SCC−13						
SCC−15						
SCC−25						
UM−SCC−1		0	−	$H^+\beta^+$,DR^-	+	±
UM−SCC−2		0	−	$H^+\beta^+$,DR^-	+	±
UM−SCC−3		0	−	$H^+\beta^+$,DR^-	+	+
SCL−1	Keratins					

(2) that the specimens are not stored in growth medium which may allow overgrowth of organisms;

(3) that antibiotic solution be added to the specimen immediately after receipt; and

(4) that the tissue be kept cold until processed to reduce cellular damage and microbial growth.

Growth Medium and Support Substances

Plasma Clots

Early culture methods required the use of plasma clots to start cell cultures from tissue fragments.[8,9] In recent times Boukamp et al.[72] also used this method, although the authors did not suggest why. It is of interest to reflect that Carrel noted in 1909[8] that some human tumours were difficult to propagate in culture because of rapid dissolution of the clot in which the specimen was suspended. This fibrinolytic activity could be due to a fibrinolytic cascade begun by the production of plasminogen activator, such as the activator activity measured in the supernatant of SCC cultures by Easty et al.[69] Presumably the fibrin clot was initially selected empirically because these clots were a means of keeping the tissue covered with growth medium and because such clots may provide a growth-supporting matrix. Gey himself noted[18] that with improvements in the constitution of liquid media and the use of serum supplements, human cells would grow well on glass surfaces. In retrospect, our present knowledge of the existence of the platelet-derived growth factor which is released during the clotting process[78] may suggest still another reason why the early culturists had success with fibrin clots as growth-support substances. Fetal calf serum remains an important variable in tissue culture medium. In addition to being a source of lipids, trace elements, hormones, and so forth, it is presumed to supply growth factors.

TABLE 19.4   PEMPHIGUS SERUM REACTIVITY WITH CULTURED HUMAN CELL LINES

	Target cells								
	Normal	Carcinomas							
Antibodies[a]	Fibroblast WI-38	Breast ALAB	Ovary SK-OV-3	Colon HT-29	Bladder T-24	Melanoma SK-MEL-1	Squamous Cell		
							UM-SCC-1	UM-SCC-2	ME-180
Pemphigus Vulgaris	−	−	−	−	−	−	+	+	+
Rabbit $\alpha\beta_2$microglobulin	+	+	+	+	+	+	+	+	+

[a] Binding of antibodies in plasma from a patient with actue phase pemphigus vulgaris and antibodies to human β_2 microglobulin in commercial rabbit antisera ($\alpha\beta_2$M) (Dako, Accurate Scientific, Westbury, NY) to human cell lines was assessed using the protein-A haemadsorption assay.[24] Cells grown as monolayers in microtest plates were incubated with appropriate dilutions of sera, washed, incubated with protein A-coated erythrocytes, washed, and examined for erythrocyte binding under the light microscope. The UM-SCC-1 and 2 cell lines used in this experiment were established in this laboratory. The other lines were obtained from the Human Tumor Bank of Dr J. Fogh at the Sloan–Kettering Institute, Rye, NY.

Feeder Cell Method

Rheinwald and Beckett[70] cultured SCC cells on feeder layers of mitomycin C-treated mouse 3T3 cells. After washing their tumour specimens in antibiotic they used trypsin (0.2%) and collagenase (0.2%) to free viable tumour cells from tissue. Cell suspensions or the minced fragments were then plated on feeder cell monolayers. Medium in their experiments was DMEM (Dulbecco's modified Eagle's medium) supplemented with 20% selected fetal calf serum and hydrocortisone (0.4 µg/ml). In this method primary cultures were subcultured after about 2 weeks and after harvesting were recultured on new mitomycin C-treated feeder layers. With this method, six of 22 specimens gave rise to cell lines for an overall success rate of 26%. The authors found that one of their cell lines, SCC-13, was able to grow only on the feeder layer while other SCC lines derived in this manner could be subcultured directly on the plastic surface of tissue culture flasks.

Explant Method for Establishing Squamous Carcinoma Cell Lines

In our laboratory, at the time of processing each tissue specimen is vigorously agitated in three changes of triple antibiotic solution (penicillin, strepto-mycin, and amphoterian B) and transferred to a sterile plastic Petri dish where fat and necrotic tissue are trimmed away. The trimmed tissue is washed once more and placed into a fresh Petri dish where the tissue is finely minced using opposing scalpels. The use of scalpel blades is probably important since relatively little crushing damage is done to the tissue. In our experience tissue cut with scissors is less likely to produce good cell outgrowth. Three to 10 fragments are then carefully transferred to tissue culture flasks where they are allowed to adhere for several minutes before the addition of medium. If this procedure is not followed the fragments will float, and no cell outgrowth will occur. Growth medium is composed of Eagle's minimum essential medium (MEM) supplemented with 1% non-essential amino acid mixture (Gibco, Grand Island, NY), 20 mM glutamine, 100 µg/ml streptomycin, 100 iu/ml penicillin, and 15% fetal calf serum. Easty[69] reports that not more than 2.5 ml of medium should be used on explant cultures in T-30 culture flasks. We also use 2–3 ml for this size flask. The small amount of medium serves two purposes: it keeps the fragments from floating if they become dislodged, and it ensures that gas diffusion distances will be minimal. The flasks are then placed in the humidified chamber of a CO_2 incubator at 35–37 °C. The flasks are observed until medium has the proper colour (i.e. pH of 7.2–7.4), then the caps are tightly closed to prevent airborne contamination. Squamous cell outgrowth can usually be detected in 3–5 days and often occurs before significant fibroblast outgrowth is noted. Fibroblasts, if present, are removed at weekly or bi-weekly intervals with trypsin and EDTA. Trypsinization is monitored by observation under the microscope and stopped when most fibroblastic cells are loosened but before epithelial cells begin to round up and detach. We usually transfer the fibroblasts to new flasks for later use as control cultures and to observe for small islands of squamous cells which might have been successfully passaged. Each culture is observed and fed weekly until sufficient epithelial cells are present for sub-culturing. To subculture, the flask is rinsed with trypsin-EDTA twice and then incubated with fresh trypsin-EDTA until sufficient cells have been detached. The detached cells are washed in growth medium and transferred to new flasks at high density. All cultures are frozen in liquid nitrogen at several early passages and are tested for membrane phenotype as soon as practicable. All new cultures are also routinely tested by microbial culture methods for mycoplasma contamination.

Using the explant method we have had an overall culture success rate of 22% of all unselected tumour specimens over a 3-year period. Easty's group[69] had a success rate of 28% using this method.

ACKNOWLEDGEMENTS

I wish to acknowledge the excellent technical assistance of Russell Ott, Charles Hurbis, Donald Schwartz, and Diane Richter, each of whom helped to establish and serologically test new cell lines of squamous cell carcinoma. I also wish to thank my collaborators: Dr Luis Diaz, with whom the studies of pemphigus and pemphigoid antigen expression have been carried out; Dr Kenneth McClatchey, with whom histopathological studies have been carried out; Dr Joseph Regezi, with whom studies of the ultra-structural features of SCC cell lines were accomplished; and Dr Shan Baker, who has provided many specimens and who has participated in studies of human tumours in the nude mice. I am especially grateful to Dr Charles Krause, whose support and vision have made our studies possible. I appreciate the comments and suggestions for the manuscript given by Kathryn Kimmel and I am grateful to Judith Jacobs, who typed and re-typed the manuscript many times.

Support was provided by grant number CA-28564 from the National Cancer Institute, DHHS. T. E. Carey is the recipient of Research Career Development Award number CA-00621 awarded by the National Cancer Institute, DHHS.

REFERENCES

1. Kwan, T.H., and Mihm, M.C., Jr. (1979). In S.L. Robbins and R.S. Cotran (Eds), *Pathologic Basis of Disease*, W.B. Saunders Co., Philadelphia, p.1417.
2. Batsakis, J.G. (1979). *Tumors of the Head and Neck – Clinical and Pathological Considerations*, 2nd edn, Williams & Wilkins, Baltimore, p.144.
3. Matthews, M.J., and Gordon, P.R. (1977). In M.J. Straus (Ed.), *Lung Cancer – Clinical Diagnosis and Treatment*, Grune & Stratton, New York, p.49.
4. Bush, R.S. (1979). *Malignancies of the Ovary, Uterus and Cerivx*, Arnold, London, p.145.
5. Kaufman, R.H., Dreesman, G.R., Burek, J., Korhonen, M.O., Matson, D.O., Melnick, J.K., Powell, K.L., Purifoy, D.J.M., Courtney, R.J., and Adam, E. (1981). *N. Engl. J. Med.*, **305**, 483.
6. Hinds, M.W., Thomas, D.B., and O'Reilly, H.P. (1979). *Cancer*, **44**, 1114.
7. Penn, I. (1980). *Clin. Plas. Surg.*, **7**, 361.
8. Carrel, A., and Burrows, M.T. (1911). *J. Exp. Med.*, **13**, 571.
9. Gey, G.O., and Gey, M.K. (1936). *Am. J. Cancer*, **27**, 45.
10. Healy, G.M., Fisher, D.C., and Parker, R.C. (1954). *Canad. J. Biochem. Physiol.*, **32**, 327.
11. Waymouth, C. (1955). *Texas Rep. Biol. and Med.*, **13**, 522.
12. White, P.R. (1955). *JNCI*, **16**, 769.
13. Earle, W.R., Bryant, J.C., Schilling, E.L., and Evans, V.J. (1956). *Ann. NY Acad. Sci.*, **63**, 666.
14. Eagle, H. (1955). *J. Exp. Med.*, **102**, 595.
15. Gey, G.O., Coffman, W.D., and Kubicek, M.T. (1952). *Cancer Res.*, **12**, 265.
16. Leighton, J. (1957). *Cancer Res.*, **17**, 929.
17. Gey, G.O. (1954–55). *Harvey Lecture Series*, The Harvey Society, New York, p.154.
18. Gey, G.O., Bang, F.B., and Gey, M.K. (1954). *Texas Rep. Biol. Med.*, **12**, 805.
19. Owens, O.V.H., Gey, M.K., and Gey, G.O. (1954). *Ann. NY Acad. Sci.*, **58**, 1039.

20. Scherer, W.F., Syverton, J.T., and Gey, G.O. (1953). *J. Exp. Med.*, **97**, 695.

21. Schleich, A., Gey, M.K., and Gey, G.O. (1961). *Ann. NY Acad. Sci.*, **95**, 774.

22. Jones, H.W., Jr., McKusick, V.A., Harper, P.S., and Wuu, K-D. (1971). *Obstet. Gynecol.*, **38**, 945.

23. Krause, C.J., Carey, T.E., Ott, R.W., Hurbis, C., McClatchey, K.D., and Regezi, J.A. (1981). *Arch. Otolaryngol.*, **107**, 703.

24. Carey, T.E., Kimmel, K.A., Schwartz, D.R., Richter, D.E., and Krause, C.J. (1983). *Otolaryn. Head and Neck Surg*, **91**, 482.

25. Syverton, J.T., Scherer, W.F., and Elwood, P.M. (1954). *J. Lab. Clin. Med.*, **43**, 286.

26. Hsu, T.C. (1954). *Texas Rep. Biol. Med.*, **12**, 833.

27. Toolan, H.W. (1953). *Cancer Res.*, **13**, 389.

28. Toolan, H.W. (1954). *Cancer Res.*, **14**, 660.

29. Fjelde, A. (1955). *Cancer*, **8**, 845.

30. Moore, A.E., Sabachewsky, L., and Toolan, H.W. (1955). *Cancer Res.*, **15**, 598.

31. Eagle, H. (1955). *Science*, **122**, 501.

32. Eagle, H. (1955). *J. Exp. Med.*, **102**, 37.

33. Eagle, H. (1955). *Proc. Soc. Exp. Biol. Med.*, **89**, 362.

34. Chang, R. S-M. (1954). *Proc. Soc. Exp. Biol. Med.*, **87**, 440.

35. Berman, L., and Stulberg, C.S. (1956). *Proc. Soc. Exp. Biol. Med.*, **92**, 730.

36. Syverton, J.T., and McLaren, L.C. (1957). *Cancer Res.*, **17**, 923.

37. Reed, M.V., and Gey, G.O. (1962). *Lab. Invest.*, **11**, 638.

38. Gartlcr, S.M. (1967). *Natl. Cancer Inst. Monogr.*, **26**, 167.

39. Peterson, W.D., Jr., Stulberg, C.S., Swanborg, N.K., and Robinson, A.R. (1968). *Proc. Soc. Exp. Biol. Med.*, **128**, 772.

40. Peterson, W.D., Jr., Stulberg, C.S., and Simpson, W.F. (1971). *Proc. Soc. Exp. Biol. Med.*, **136**, 1187.

41. Nelson-Rees, W.A., Flandermeyer, R.R., Hawthorne, P.K. (1974). *Science*, **184**, 1093.

42. Rigby, C.C., and Franks, L.M. (1970). *Br. J. Cancer*, **24**, 746.

43. Franks, L.M., and Rigby, C. (1975). *Science*, **188**, 168.

44. Nelson-Rees, W.A., and Flandermeyer, R.R. (1976). *Science*, **191**, 96.

45. O'Brien, S.J., Kleiner, G., Olson, R., and Shannon, J.E. (1977). *Science*, **195**, 1345.

46. Pontes, J.E., Pierce, J.M., Jr., Choe, B-K., and Rose, N. (1979). *In Vitro*, **15**, 469.

47. Rafferty, K.A., Jr. (1975). In G. Klein and S. Weinhouse (Eds), *Advances in Cancer Research*, vol. 21, Academic Press, New York, p.249.

48. Norrby, K., Eriksson, O., and Mellgren, J. (1962). *Cancer Res.*, **22**, 147.

49. Auersperg, N., and Hawryluk, A.P. (1962). *JNCI*, **28**, 605.

50. Auersperg, N. (1964). *JNCI*, **32**, 135.

51. Auersperg, N. (1969). *JNCI*, **43**, 151.

52. Auersperg, N. (1969). *JNCI*, **43**, 175.

53. Auersperg, N. (1972). *JNCI*, **48**, 1589.

54. Herz, F., Miller, O.J., Miller, D.A., Auersperg, N., and Koss, L.G. (1977). *Cancer Res.*, **37**, 3209.

55. Friedl, F., Kinura, I., Osato, T., and Ito, Y. (1970). *Proc. Soc. Exp. Biol. Med.*, **135**, 543.

56. Sykes, J.A., Whitescarver, J., Jernstrom, P., Nolan, J.F., and Byatt, P. (1970). *JNCI*, **45**, 107.

57. Bloom, E.T., Fahey, J.L., Peterson, I.A., Geering, G., Bernhard, M., and Trempe, G. (1973). *Int. J. Cancer*, **12**, 21.

58. Fogh, J., Fogh, J.M., and Orfeo, T. (1977). *JNCI*, **59**, 221.

59. Giard, D.J., Aaronson, S.A., Todaro, G.J., Arnstein, P., Kersey, J.H., Dosik, H., and Parks, W.P. (1973). *JNCI*, **51**, 1417.

60. Moore, G.E., Merrick, S.B., Woods, L.K., and Arabasz, N.M. (1975). *Cancer Res.*, **35**, 2684.

61. Nelson-Rees, W.A. (1976). *Cancer Res.*, **36**, 1849.

62. Moore, G.E., Merrick, S.B., Woods, L.K., and Arabasz, N.M. (1976). *Cancer Res.*, **36**, 1849.

63. O'Toole, C., Nayak, S., Price, Z., Gilbert, W.H., and Waisman, J. (1976). *Int. J. Cancer*, **17**, 707.

64. Morgan, R.T., Quinn, L.A., Woods, L.K., and Moore, G.E. (1977). *Cancer Res.*, **37**, 2030.

65. Porter, J.C., Nalick, R.H., Vellios, F., Neaves, W.B., MacDonald, P.C. (1978). *Am. J. Obstet. Gynecol.*, **130**, 487.

66. Okabe, T., Sato, N., Kondo, Y., Asano, S., Ohsawa, N., Kosaka, K., and Ueyama, Y. (1978). *Cancer Res.*, **38**, 3910.

67. Nishihira, N., Kasai, M., Mori, S., Watanabe, T., Kuriya, Y., Suda, M., Kitamura, M., Hirayama, K., Akaishi, T., and Sasaki, T. (1979). *Gann*, **70**, 575.

68. Edwards, P.A.W., Easty, D.M., and Foster, C.S. (1980). *Cell Biol. Int. Rep.*, **4**, 917.

69. Easty, D.M., Easty, G.C., Carter, R.L., Monaghan, P., and Butler, L.J. (1981). *Br. J. Cancer*, **43**, 772.

70. Rheinwald, J.G., and Beckett, M.A. (1981). *Cancer Res.*, **41**, 1657.

71. Rheinwald, J.G., and Green, H. (1975). *Cell*, **6**, 331.

72. Boukamp, P., Tilgen, W., Dzarlieva, R.T.,

Breitkreutz, D., Haag, D., Riehl, R.K., Bohnert, A., and Fusenig, N.E. (1982). *JNCI*, **68**, 415.

73. Fogh, J., and Trempe, G. (1975). In J. Fogh (Ed.), *Human Tumor Cells in Vitro*, Plenum Press, New York, p.115.

74. Seman, G., and Dmochowski, L. (1975). In J. Fogh (Ed.), *Human Tumor Cells in Vitro*, Plenum Press, New York, p.395.

75. Beutner, E.H., and Jordan, R.E. (1964). *Proc. Soc. Exp. Biol. Med.*, **505**.

76. Diaz, L.A., and Marcelo, C.L. (1978). *Br. J. Dermatol.*, **98**, 631.

77. Carey, T.E., Diaz, L.A., Ott, R.W., Schwartz, D.R., and Krause, C.J. (1981). *Clin. Res.*, **29**, 281.

78. Ross, R., and Vogel, A. (1978). *Cell*, **14**, 203.

Chapter 20

Cloning of Malignant Cells from Epidermoid Head and Neck Cancer

Douglas E. Mattox* and
Daniel D. Von Hoff†
*Division of Otorhinolaryngology,
Department of Surgery*, and Division of
Oncology, Department of Medicine†,
University of Texas Health Science Center,
San Antonio, Texas.*

INTRODUCTION

The *raison d'être* of soft agar cloning assay is the rapid assessment of the chemosensitivity of individual tumours allowing a rational choice of chemotherapeutic drugs. In other tumours this assay correctly predicted sensitivity in 62% of patients and resistance in 96%.[1] Therefore, one of the major potential benefits of the assay is the avoidance of toxicity from drugs unlikely to produce a beneficial effect.

As will become evident in this discussion, the application of this technique to head and neck cancer has several limitations including a relatively low fraction of specimens which will grow in the assay, a high contamination rate, and a lack of effective drugs for the treatment of head and neck cancer. Potential applications of the technique include its use in new drug screening programmes and as a tool for investigation of the cell biology of head and neck cancer.

BACKGROUND

In every self-renewing tissue there is a subpopulation of stem cells which can produce both new stem cells (capacity for self-renewal) and mature differentiated cells.[2] Stem cells make up approximately 1% of the cell population of bone marrow, and cells in the base of the crypts of Lieberkuhn are the effective stem cells for the intestinal epithelium.

Tumours may also have a stem cell subpopulation and it is more likely they are derived from normal stem cells than from dedifferentiated mature cells.[3] In an attempt to identify and clone *in vitro* these tumour stem cells, the bilayer agar cloning system was developed by Hamburger and Salmon.[4-9] This technique used two layers of soft agar; a bottom feeder layer containing conditioned media and an upper layer containing a single cell suspension of tumour cells. This bilayer agar system inhibits the proliferation of fibroblasts by preventing the attachment to the sides of the vessel. The viable tumour cells (stem cells) form colonies (clones) which can be counted by hand or by electronic devices. Chemosensitivity testing may be performed by incubating the cells with chemotherapeutic agents before plating and comparing the number of colonies formed to control plates not exposed to drug.

Using this technique, Hamburger and Salmon were able to grow colonies from 53 (75%) of 70 patients with multiple myeloma and related disorders.[5,7] The important finding was that the number of colonies that grew was proportional to the number of viable cells plated, which made a quantitative evaluation of drug sensitivity possible. Appropriate morphological, biochemical, and functional tests demonstrated that the colonies formed were representative of the original tumour.

TECHNIQUE

Biopsy specimens were obtained from primary head and neck tumours at endoscopy and neck nodes at the time of definitive surgery. Where possible, 1 cm^3 of tumour was obtained. The tumour was minced into 1 mm cubes and immediately placed in McCoy's 5A with 10% heat inactivated fetal calf serum and 1% penicillin and streptomycin for transport to the laboratory.

Under aseptic conditions in laminar flow hoods, tumours were further minced and teased apart with needles. A single cell suspension was prepared mechanically by passing the tissue through 22- and 25-gauge needles. Enzymes were not used for dissociation of the tissue. The cells were then washed, centrifuged, and resuspended. The number of nucleated cells available for plating (exclusive of leucocytes) was determined on a

haemocytometer. Cells were cultured in a bilayer agar system as described by Hamburger and Salmon except that no conditioned media was used. The underlayer consisted of McCoy's 5A medium with 15% heat-inactivated fetal calf serum, tryptic soy broth, asparagine, DEAE dextran, and 0.5% agar. One millilitre of this medium was poured into 35 mm Petri dishes. Cells to be tested were suspended in a concentration of 500,000/ml in enriched CRML 1066 medium, supplemented with horse serum, penicillin G potassium, streptomycin sulphate, glutamine, insulin, and 0.3% agar. Just before plating, asparagine, DEAE dextran, and 2-mercaptoethanol were added to the cells. The resultant mixture was pipetted on top of the previously prepared feeder layer. After preparation of both the bottom and top layers, cultures were incubated at 37 °C in a humidified atmosphere of 7.5% carbon dioxide.

Drug sensitivity testing was performed on single-cell suspensions of one million cells per millilitre in Hanks' balanced salt solution and 10% fetal calf serum. Chemotherapeutic drugs were added so that the final concentration is equivalent to one-tenth of the clinically obtainable peak levels (methotrexate, 0.3 µg/ml; cisplatin 0.2 µg/ml; bleomycin 0.2 µg/ml) and incubated for 1 hour. Cells were then harvested, washed twice, and plated in triplicate at a concentration of 500,000 cells per plate.

Cultures were examined with a Zeiss inverted phase microscope at magnifications of 30 ×, 100 × and 200 ×. Colony counts were made between 14 and 21 days. Aggregates of 20 or more cells are considered colonies. Plates with six or more colonies were scored as positive cultures. The relative growth of specimens is expressed as the cloning efficiency: the number of colonies/number of cells plated × 100%. For chemosensitivity testing, treated and control cell suspensions were plated in triplicate. Chemosensitivity is expressed as 'percentage survival': colonies on treated plates/colonies on control plates × 100%.

RESULTS

Confirmation of *in vitro* Growth of Squamous Carcinoma

Colonies were plucked from the agar plates and processed for transmission electron microscopy. Numerous tonofilaments were contained in the cytoplasm of cultured cells, a finding which confirms their derivation from squamous carcinoma. Autoradiographs of colonies grown in the presence of tritiated thymidine showed silver grains throughout the colony, suggesting *in vitro* growth of the colony.

Success of *in vitro* Growth

In our first $2\frac{1}{2}$ years experience attempting to grow 158 specimens of head and neck squamous carcinoma in the soft agar cloning assay, 57 (36%) failed to grow. Positive cultures were obtained both from primary lesions of the aerodigestive tract and from metastatic lymph nodes, but bacterial contamination was less of a problem in specimens obtained from lymph nodes.

Success of Culture versus Demographic Factors

There was no statistical correlation between success of culture and age, sex, race, or site of primary lesion. Actively growing tumours after radiation therapy or chemotherapy had the same incidence of positive cultures as tumours not having prior treatment. We found no correlation between positive culture and the stage of disease, or any combination of initial disease and recurrent disease.[10]

Success of Culture versus Histological Differentiation

The histological appearance of all specimens was divided into 'well', 'moderate', and 'poorly' differentiated squamous carcinoma (contaminated cases were excluded). Although there appeared to be a trend for higher growth rates in poorly differentiated tumors, the difference was not statistically significant.

Success of Culture versus Patient Survival

Patient follow-up for at least 6 months after biopsy was available for 90 patients in the 'growth' and 'no-growth' categories (contaminated cultures excluded). Survival curves for both groups were calculated by the method of Kaplan and Meier[11] and tests of difference between the curves were made by using both the log rank test and the generalized Wilcoxin test for censored survival data.[12] There was no statistically significant difference between the survival curves for the 'growth' and 'no-growth' categories ($P = 0.50$) (Figure 20.1).

Culture of Non-malignant Lesions

In addition to the cases enumerated above, we have cultured specimens from a number of patients without a histological confirmation of malignancy. Some of these lesions were histologically benign, including salivary pleomorphic adenoma and lymph node follicular hyperplasia. In another case a maxillary sinus lesion had a high cloning efficiency (0.016%), but simultaneous biopsy showed only dysplasia. The high cloning efficiency prompted another biopsy which again failed to demonstrate malignancy. The patient was alive and well when last seen 1 year later. We have also observed colony formation in two patients with lymphadenopathy appearing after definitive treatment of head and neck cancer. In both of these instances the nodes showed histologically only radiation changes and lymphoid hypertrophy. These two patients are alive without clinical disease 12–24 months after culture. Unfortunately electron microscopic confirmation of the cell type of the colonies is not available.

We also have several instances in which the specimen grew *in vitro*, pathological examination of the biopsy specimen failed to show

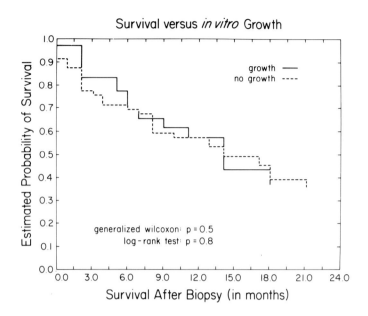

Figure 20.1 Kaplan–Meier survival curves for patients with positive growth (six or more colonies per plate) and no growth *in vitro*. There is no significant difference between the two curves (*P* = 0.50).
(Republished with permission from *Cancer*, (Mattox *et al.*, 1984).

tumour, but the subsequent clinical course was consistent with squamous carcinoma at the site of the biopsy. Again histological confirmation of the cell type growing *in vitro* is lacking. The question of whether all tumour was sent to the cloning laboratory and only reactive tissue sent for pathological examination remains unresolvable.

Chemosensitivity Testing

Fifty-four per cent of the specimens which grew *in vitro* (27% of the total series) had sufficient cells to perform chemosensitivity testing. However, only 16, or 10%, of all specimens obtained had enough cells to test three or more drugs.

A percentage survival less than 30% is generally required in other tumour systems before clinical response can be predicted *in vivo*. A total of 81 separate chemosensitivity tests were performed and six (6%) had percentage survival less than 30% (2-cisplatin,

1-methotrexate, 1-bleomycin, 1-mitoxantrone). Chemosensitivity testing was not done in a prospective manner with respect to treatment; therefore *in vitro – in vivo* correlations are not available.

The chemosensitivity of individual tumours to multiple drugs was highly variable and the sensitivity of the tumour to one drug did not predict sensitivity to others, nor did the response of one patient's tumour predict the sensitivity of another tumour (Table 20.1).

DISCUSSION

Limitations

The application of the soft agar cloning assay to head and neck cancer is still in its developmental stages and faces several limitations. The success rate of culture has been disappointing; only 36% of specimens were successfully cultured and we suffered a 29%

TABLE 20.1   INDIVIDUAL *IN VITRO*
CHEMOSENSITIVITY

Case No.	Cisplatin	Methotrexate	Bleomycin
4	12 %	36 %	99 %
5	45	48	75
10	52	26	17
15	52	105	102
18	—	30	80
22	63	42	48

Representative *in vitro* sensitivities (percentage survival)
of head and neck squamous carcinomas after a 1 hour
incubation with chemotherapeutic drugs. Individual
tumours are extremely variable in their individual sen-
sitivies, and sensitivity to one drug does not predict the
sensitivity to other drugs.

contamination rate. These statistics could
probably be improved by selective culture of
patients with large tumours or by only culturing lymph nodes, but our interest has been to
evaluate the applicability of the technique to
unselected patients. Therefore, we have
reported our results based on the number of
specimens which actually arrived at the cloning laboratory.

Ideally 1 cm³ of tumour should be obtained
to have sufficient cells for multiple drug sensitivity testing. Despite the large appearance of
oropharyngeal carcinomas in relationship to
adjacent normal anatomical structures, frequently these tumours are thin, superficially
spreading, and have necrotic surfaces.
Therefore the amount of tumour which can be
removed without endangering neurovascular
structures or violating salivary barriers is
limited. Furthermore, a substantial amount of
the tumour mass is not tumour cells, but blood
vessels, fibrous elements, and inflammatory
reaction. All of these factors unfavourably influence the number of cells available for
culture and contribute to the inaccuracy of
establishing the initial cell concentration
because these elements cannot be distinguished
from tumour cells in suspension. Methods to
increase the cell yield from biopsy specimens
need to be developed. The number of cells in
suspension can be increased by using enzy-
matic disaggregation but we have refrained
from using these techniques because of pos-

sible effects on chemosensitivity testing. It is
likely that further modifications in the media
with specific requirements for each histological
type of tumour may also increase cloning
efficiency.

We have observed that the colony yield can
also be increased by growth factors such as
epidermal growth factor, but again the effects
on chemosensitivity are unknown. The
possibility of growing the tumours in an
animal host (nude mouse) has been explored,
but the time delay in growing the tumour *in
vivo* makes the assay impractical for clinical
use. A preliminary report by Schiff *et al.*[13]
demonstrated an improved cloning efficiency
if agarose is substituted for agar in the culture
plate.

Bacterial and fungal contamination rates of
22–29% restrict the number of evaluable
plates. Johns reports a contamination rate of
only 14% but a larger population of his
specimens were taken from lymph nodes.[14]
Our specimens are transported and cultured in
penicillin and streptomycin and we have
recently added amphotericin B to the transport
media but do not have enough experience to
evaluate its effect.

All of these factors combined substantially
limit the usefulness of the soft agar assay as a
chemosensitivity test in head and neck cancer.
The combined experience of our laboratory,
and that of Johns, is that 10% of specimens
have sufficient cells to perform sensitivity
testing on three drugs.[10,14] Ideally nine drugs
should be tested in order to obtain a high probability of finding one with significant
activity.[15]

Another unsolved problem is how to quantify the results of the assay. Expressions of both
number of colonies and cloning efficiency
depend upon the plating of a known number of
viable cells. Unfortunately the dye exclusion
(trypan blue) test is not a reliable means of
determining the number of viable cells in the
initial suspension and we have discontinued its
use.[16] Furthermore, the histological type of individual cells (e.g. tumour versus fibroblast) in
the single cell suspension cannot be deter-

mined in the fresh suspension. Thus, the actual number of viable tumour cells plated is unknown. We are currently developing cytological techniques to enable us to determine, at least retrospectively, what proportion of the cell suspension was tumour.

We have attempted to correlate a number of factors with both success of *in vitro* growth and cloning efficiency. There is no correlation with age, sex, site of primary disease, previous radiation, or chemotherapy. Johns reported a correlation of *in vitro* growth with the N-stage of the tumour.[14]

Early in our experience it appeared as if there was a correlation between high cloning efficiency and shortened survival which has also been reported by Johns; subsequent experience, however, has not borne out this trend.[10,17]

The results of chemotherapy testing all point to the highly heterogeneous nature of head and neck squamous carcinoma. The *in vitro* sensitivity to one drug was not predictive of the response of the same tumour to different drugs or of different tumours to the same drug. Perhaps the most important information to come from this study is the relationship between tumour sensitivity and drug concentration. A failure to produce increased cell kill with increasing concentration of drug was the rule rather than the exception. This finding has significant implications to the fields of intra-arterial chemotherapy and high-dose chemotherapy with bone marrow transplantation. The frequent short duration of clinical response to chemotherapy further suggests that resistant subpopulations of the tumour are being selected.[18] The ultimate limitation of the chemosensitivity assay as a clinically useful tool is the need for more drugs with higher response rates and longer durations of response.

The colony formation by benign lesions also deserves further comment. It is clear that *in vitro* growth is not pathognomonic for malignancy. *In vitro* growth of benign lesions has been observed by us and reported by Johns.[14] The significance of the positive

cultures in patients suspected of having a malignancy but having negative histology is as yet unknown. It is possible that in several of our cases the part of the biopsy containing malignant cells was sent to the cloning laboratory and the pathologist had only tissue without tumour cells to observe. However, there are well-documented instances in which bone marrow biopsies were read as negative but simultaneous cloning grew electron-microscopically confirmed malignancy.[19] Thus the cloning assay may become an adjunct to the identification of recurrent or metastatic carcinoma. One critical application is the early identification of recurrent carcinoma after radiation therapy. We have shown that previous radiation therapy has no effect on the *in vitro* culture rate of actively growing tumour.[17] However, in the first weeks after radiation therapy the pathologist may have difficulty determining if the biopsy contains residual but lethally damaged tumour cells or cells capable of growth, proliferation, and invasion. Positive cloning during this critical period would argue for early therapeutic intervention in these patients.

New Applications

New potential applications for the cloning assay are being explored along with the conventional uses. We have been using the assay as an integral part of a new drug development programme. Although enough different drugs cannot be tested to be beneficial to an individual patient, we have been testing individual tumours against new agents. This information may provide data on which histological types of tumour are likely to be sensitive *in vivo* to a given drug. In addition, the cloning assay is also potentially an important tool for the study of tumour biology, for instance the heterogeneity of the cell populations in a squamous cell carcinoma.

ACKNOWLEDGEMENT

This work was supported by the Medical Oncology Program Project Grant, (#CA

30195). We wish to acknowledge the assistance of Darlene J. Langfeld in preparation of the manuscript.

REFERENCES

1. Salmon, S.E. *et al.* (1980) in Mathé, G., and Muggia, F.M. (Eds) Factors that Influence Growth of Head and Neck Squamous Carcinoma in the Soft Agar Assay. *Recent Results in Cancer Research*, **74**, 300–305. Springer-Verlag, Berlin.

2. Steel, C.G. (1975). In K. Bagshane (Ed.), *Oncology: Medical Aspects of Malignant Disease*, Oxford, p.49.

3. Pierce, G.B. (1974). *Am. J. Pathol.*, **77**, 103–113.

4. Hamburger, A.W., and Salmon, S.E. (1977). *Science*, **197**, 461–463.

5. Hamburger, A.W., and Salmon, S.E. (1977). *J. Clin. Invest.*, **60**, 846–854.

6. Hamburger, A.W., Salmon, S.E., Kim, M.B. *et al.* (1978). *Cancer Res.*, **38**, 3438–3444.

7. Hamburger, A.W., Kim, M.B., and Salmon, S.E. (1979). *J. Cell Physiol.*, **98**, 371–376.

8. Salmon, S.E., Hamburger, A.W., Soehnlen, B. *et al.* (1978). *N. Engl. J. Med.*, **298**, 1321–1327.

9. Salmon, S.E., Soehnlen, B., Durie, B.G.M. *et al.* (1979). *Proc. Am. Assoc. Cancer Res. A.S.C.O.*, **20**, 340.

10. Mattox, D.E., Von Hoff, D.D., Clark, G.M. (1983). *Cancer*, **53**, 1736–1740.

11. Kaplan, E.L., Meier, P. (1958). *J. Am. Stat. Assoc.*, **53**, 457–481.

12. Mantel, N. (1966). *Cancer Chemother. Rep.*, 163–170.

13. Schiff, L.J. *et al.* (1982). *In Vitro*, **18**, 284.

14. Johns, M.E. (1982). *Laryngoscope*, **92**, Supp. 28, 1–26.

15. Von Hoff, D.D. *et al.* (1983). *Cancer Res.*, **43**, 1926–1931.

16. Mattox, D.E., and Von Hoff, D.D. (1980). *Arch. Otolaryngol.*, **106**, 672–674.

17. Mattox, D.E., and Von Hoff, D.D. (1980). *Am. J. Surg.*, **140**, 527–530.

18. Von Hoff, D.D. *et al.* (1981). *Cancer Clin. Trials*, **4**, 215–218.

19. Von Hoff, D.D., *et al.* (1980). *Cancer Res.*, **40**, 3591–3597.

E
METHODOLOGY

Chapter 21

Planning and Execution of Large-Scale Multicentre Comparative Trials

Robert W. Makuch
Biostatistics and Data Management Section, National Cancer Institute, Bethesda, Maryland, USA

INTRODUCTION

Multicentre cancer clinical trials are recognized as a major research tool in the search for new, effective treatments. They provide the opportunity to evaluate treatment efficacy over shorter time periods than single-institution studies, and the conduct of investigations in a variety of settings broadens the scope of scientific inferences. Such studies are a complex undertaking which requires the effective collaboration of clinicians, biostatisticians, data managers, and computer programmers over a prolonged period of time. Because of the multiplicity of investigators in geographically diverse regions, all the procedures involved in the planning and execution of a multicentre clinical trial must be outlined in detail. This chapter describes some of the basic components required in the planning and conduct of comparative, multicentre cancer clinical trials in head and neck cancer.

PROTOCOL COMPONENTS

A protocol is a written document that should describe completely the proposed study. A clear explanation of the scientific underpinnings and rationale for the study is required as well as the hypotheses of interest. Literature reviews are needed to help focus on the current state-of-the-art in regard to treatment and the most important future studies to be undertaken. This initial process increases the likelihood that the study will have a major impact on general medical practice. Once an important hypothesis has been established, the protocol development process follows. The primary responsibility for writing a protocol for a multicentre clinical trial should rest with a few experts who will be involved in the study. Upon its completion, and prior to commencement of patient accrual, the protocol should be evaluated by a review body.

The protocol should be as specific as possible

in describing the patient population to be studied, the objectives of the study, the experimental design, the therapies under investigation, major and minor endpoints, data management and collection procedures, and scheduling and follow-up. All investigators and data managers should be identified. A typical outline for a comparative multicentre clinical trial is given in Table 21.1.

TABLE 21.1   EXAMPLE OF PROTOCOL OUTLINE

1. Introduction
2. Objectives
3. Patient selection
4. Pretreatment evaluation
5. Patient registration and randomization
6. Treatment plans
7. Post-treatment evaluation and follow-up (for all patients)
8. Pathological evaluation
9. Summary of study parameters
10. End-results evaluation
11. Statistical considerations
12. Data forms submission requirements
13. References
14. List of investigators and support personnel

A good protocol is a clear, self-contained unit whose components comprise a consistent theme of scientific thought as well as a guideline for clinical management. This implies, for example, that sample sizes based on the study's endpoints are large enough to reach definitive conclusions regarding the main hypotheses within a reasonable period of time. The protocol also should indicate that all patients be treated and followed as uniformly as possible, in accordance with the treatment regimen to which they were assigned. Although some flexibility in the protocol consistent with sound medical judgement may be required, important decisions should not be left to the discretion of the investigator; otherwise, one may be left with a number of case reports that contribute little to testing the initial hypotheses.

STUDY OBJECTIVES

The objectives of a study should be stated carefully, for they serve as a basis for the hypotheses to be addressed. Clearly stated objectives help the study planners develop a protocol that represents a coherent scientific research plan. P.B. Medawar stated: 'It is a truism to say that a good experiment is precisely that which spares us the exertion of thinking: the better it is, the less we have to worry about its interpretations, about what it really means'.[1] A major strength of prospective clinical trials is that the objectives are defined in advance so that the patients can be selected, treated, and evaluated in accordance with standardized procedures and the data can be recorded in a careful manner. This permits an immediate and straightforward interpretation of the study results. In general, it is best to specify at most two or three major questions since sample sizes place an upper limit on the number of questions that can be validly addressed in one trial.

Detailed specification of the objectives is also useful to direct the type of analyses that will be performed upon completion of the study. To some investigators it is attractive to provide less specific study objectives in advance, and perform exhaustive data analyses at the end of the study. But these less structured investigations are more likely to lead to erroneous conclusions because of the multiplicity of questions asked. 'Just as the Sphinx winks if you look at it long enough, so, if you perform enough significance tests, you are sure to find significance even if none exists'.[2] For example, if 2 treatment groups known to be equivalent are compared in 10 independent subgroups defined by age, sex, and disease state, the probability is approximately 40% that at least 1 of the 10 subgroups would turn up a significant treatment difference at the 0.05 significance level. In the interpretation of clinical trial results, the distinction often is not appreciated between reaching conclusions from analyses performed to test a few hypotheses specified in advance, versus exploratory data analyses used to generate new hypotheses. Results derived from exploratory data analyses should not become the cornerstone of a report in which definitive conclusions are made.[3]

Finally, the objectives should be structured so that important medical questions are addressed, and answers can be obtained within a reasonable time period. For most studies the accrual period should be completed within 4 years since new therapies may be developed or participants in the trial may lose interest. The objectives should be formulated so that the study outcome will expand on previous medical knowledge, and useful information for patient management and development of better treatments will result whether the trial is positive or negative.

PATIENT POPULATION

The types of patients to be studied are indicated by the protocol inclusion and exclusion criteria. A well-defined, uniform set of criteria should be specified. For randomized studies, patients who can tolerate some, but not all, treatment schedules should be excluded before randomization. Generally the on-study patient population should be composed of a relatively homogeneous group of patients unless the study is sufficiently large that valid analysis of subgroups is possible. A coherent statement can then be made as to whom the study results apply. Othewise, incorrect conclusions may be reached regarding comparative treatment efficacy because of an excess of variability in the endpoint evaluated or a differential effect of treatment among patient subgroups.

To illustrate this point, suppose that head and neck cancer patients with $T_2 - T_4$ lesions are randomized to receive or not receive chemotherapy prior to surgery; survival time is the endpoint. Further assume that most patients with T_2 or T_3 primary tumours obtain a complete response with chemotherapy, and that this event translates into prolonged survival relative to patients who receive surgery alone. Patients with T_4 tumours tend to show less frequent complete response to chemotherapy and have a similar survival experience to those receiving surgery alone. For most studies the major treatment comparison will be based on all patients. Thus, no matter what overall conclusion is drawn regarding treatment efficacy in this example, it could not correctly apply to both T-class subsets. Sir A. Bradford Hill recognized this issue in discussing a Medical Research Council trial of streptomycin for respiratory tuberculosis:[4] '. . . for it was realized that no two patients have an identical form of the disease and it was desired to eliminate as many of the obvious variations as possible. This planning . . . is a fundamental feature of the successful trial. To start out upon a trial with all and sundry included, and with the hope that the results can be sorted out statistically in the end, is to court disaster.'

Only if the trial is very large, and there exist sufficient numbers of patients for valid analysis within each major patient subset should broad eligibility criteria be considered. Even with large patient numbers, however, cautious interpretation is required in drawing conclusions based on treatment differences within subgroups of the originally randomized sample. In most instances these subset analyses should be considered heuristic in that they generate hypotheses to be tested in future experiments.[5] Some contend that the introduction of life-table regression models and other methods of stratified analysis provides a way to deal with heterogeneous subgroups even when the number of patients in each subgroup is very small. But such analyses are model-dependent, and require more subjectivity on part of the data analyst than many seem aware. In short, patient eligibility criteria should focus closely on the patient population of particular clinical interest to ensure that definitive answers regarding comparative treatment efficacy can be obtained.

ENDPOINTS

The term endpoint refers to a specified measure by which a therapy is evaluated. Explicit definitions of the endpoints are required *a priori* in order to provide appropriate sample size calculations, develop concise data forms and data collection procedures, specify unbiased follow-up evaluations for all patients, and eliminate potential questions regarding the statistical analysis and interpretation of results.[6] In comparative studies a common endpoint is survival time, since it is often a meaningful and unequivocal measure of treatment efficacy. However, head and neck cancer may be one disease where other endpoints may be useful since many patients are old and in generally poor health; a relatively higher incidence of deaths, therefore, may arise from causes unrelated to the treatment or the cancer. For example, one might indicate whether patients who die of causes unrelated to the treatment or malignancy are considered failures or not. If disease-free interval is used as an endpoint, one should state whether or not patients who die disease-free are considered failures.

Regular patient follow-up schedules and guidelines for evaluation of all patients are recommended to avoid bias. Decisions as to when to perform procedures such as bone or CT scans should not be left totally to the discretion of the investigators. They should be done at regular intervals, or in well-defined situations, in addition to investigator-initiated requests. If more than one treatment modality is used in the study, a team approach including an investigator representing each modality is useful for patient follow-up.

To illustrate the rationale for these guidelines, consider the following hypothetical trial. All patients receive surgery, and if they are rendered free of disease they are randomized to receive or not receive monthly adjuvant chemotherapy for 12 months. The study is designed so that the patients who received surgery alone are seen once every 6 months by the surgical oncologist. The chemotherapy-treated group of patients is seen monthly by the medical oncologist, and by the surgeon only if surgical complications arise. Since this latter group of patients is seen more frequently in the first year, recurrent disease may be detected sooner in this group even if there is, in fact, no real difference between the two groups. Moreover, the differing views about follow-up procedures by surgical and medical oncologists may confound the comparison of the treatments. Thus it becomes apparent that all patients must be seen at similar time points and examined in a standardized fashion to ensure that the study is not jeopardized by biased evaluation of the endpoints of interest.

Every effort should be made to obtain the required endpoint information for each patient since difficulties can arise in the interpretation of results when follow-up procedures are lax. The need for complete ascertainment of endpoint data is particularly acute when missing data or losses to follow-up cause the endpoint of interest to be unobserved. As an example, suppose that survival time is the endpoint of interest, and patients in a particular treatment group tend not to return for their scheduled follow-up visit when they are very ill and likely to die soon thereafter. Such patients who prematurely drop out of the study are considered to be censored observations in a survival analysis, i.e. they are analysed as being alive at their most recent follow-up date. Because the censoring event carried prognostic information about subsequent survival time, the censoring event and survival are associated. This violates a major assumption of most survival analysis techniques. Such an analysis would provide an overly optimistic assessment of treatment efficacy in this situation.

CONTROL GROUPS

The primary objective of a comparative clinical trial is 'both to ensure a high probability of identifying the better treatment (if there is one) and to convince others of the validity of the conclusions'.[7] This is achieved by carefully considering alternative experimental designs and selecting one which will answer the primary questions of interest. A basic component of the experimental approach in comparative trials is the use of controls against which one or more new treatment groups will be compared. For some diseases in which death is inevitable within a relatively short period of time, historical controls may represent an appropriate control group. Any new treatment that prolongs survival can be recognized quickly as a clinical advance. No one can argue rationally that selection bias or other unknown patient features led to the survival enhancement since the patient group is homogeneous in regard to their outcome. But this ideal situation is extremely infrequent in practice. For patients with head and neck cancer the disease course is highly variable and influenced by many treatment and non-treatment factors.

Gehan and Freireich assert that historical controls can be used, particularly when there has been a sequence of studies in which the eligibility requirements, criteria for evaluating response, patient work-up and follow-up, and referral patterns remain constant.[8] But even under these ideal conditions one is still not protected from possible biases produced by changes over time in diagnostic methods, staging criteria, supportive care, patient referral patterns and effects of unmeasured or unknown prognostic factors. Pocock reported that in 19 unselected instances where a collaborative group carried the same treatment over two successive studies, four of the 19 pairs of trials had differences in outcome which were significant at the $P < 0.02$ level.[9] Farewell and D'Angio also demonstrated the instability of results with the same treatment in ostensibly similar situations. They discussed an actual clinical trial in which historical controls could have been used instead of randomized controls, and showed that the conclusions of the study based on the historical control group differed materially from those based on concurrent controls.[10] Although Freireich has stated that 'science requires creativity and open-mindedness' and that one should not worship at the altar of randomization, the issues mentioned above indicate that historical controls are rarely an adequate substitute for concurrently randomized controls.

The randomization process offers many advantages.[7] It guards against systematic selection bias in the assignment of treatment. Consequently if treatment differences are detected, one can likely attribute these dif-

ferences to the effect of treatment. Without randomized treatment allocation a 'statistically significant treatment difference' may be due to differences in the distribution of prognostic factors introduced consciously or unconsciously by the physician. For example, biased treatment assignment may occur in a non-randomized study of adjuvant maintenance chemotherapy in head and neck cancer patients rendered disease-free by surgery and radiotherapy. Patients assigned to receive adjuvant chemotherapy may represent a better prognostic group of patients compared to those not assigned to receive such therapy. The possible conclusion that maintenance chemotherapy is superior could be due merely to the fact that the patients receiving the therapy were more likely to live longer anyway.

The second major advantage of randomization is that the treatment groups will tend to be balanced in regard to prognostic factors, whether they are known or unknown. Statistical adjustment procedures are often proposed as a way to account for any known differences among the groups. But many investigators question the ability of such procedures to perform this task adequately. In addition one can obviously not adjust for imbalances in important, but currently unrecognized, prognostic factors. Randomization ensures that the unknown biasing factors are distributed according to a known random distribution. This guarantees the validity of the statistical tests of significance that are used to compare the treatments.[11]

The principle of randomization can be abused if some systematic procedure is used whereby the physician knows what the next treatment assignment will be prior to the time of patient registration on-study. Examples include basing the patient's treatment assignment on the day of hospital admission, the patient's birth date, or alternating the treatment assignment in a deterministic manner. This information can be used consciously or unconsciously in deciding whether to enter the patient onto the study. Randomization should be performed in such a way that the treatment assignment is unknown to the physician until the patient is declared eligible and treatment is to commence. In addition, randomization should take place just prior to the time when the different treatment groups diverge in terms of patient therapy.

A compromise between the use of historical controls and randomized concurrent controls has been proposed by Pocock using an imbalanced randomization.[12] The pool of historical controls is utilized by randomizing new patients to the new and standard treatments in a 2 : 1 or 3 : 1 ratio. The concurrent controls are compared to the historical controls, and both control groups are combined and compared to the new treatment if there are no significant or important differences between them. However, it is very likely that an insufficient number of concurrent controls will be available to demonstrate comparability to the historical controls since: (1) the purpose of this type of design is to minimize the number of concurrent controls, and (2) Makuch and Simon have shown that substantial numbers of patients (usually more than 150 patients per group) are needed to demonstrate comparability with a high degree of certainty.[13] Using data from an actual clinical trial, Farewell and D'Angio showed that dramatically different conclusions can be drawn if a 2 : 1 randomization including historical controls is used rather than a 1 : 1 randomization using concurrent controls only.[10] Thus the view that an imbalanced randomization incorporating historical controls will provide valid treatment comparisons at the end of the study is not always justified.

METHODS OF PATIENT ALLOCATION

Simple, unrestricted randomization is the most elementary kind of randomization and is recommended by some for large multicentre clinical trials.[14] As the total number of patients entered on study increases, the number of patients randomized to each treatment group will tend towards equality. However, this final outcome provides little consolation if interim analyses must be performed on widely discrepant patient numbers among the treatment groups.[15] Simple randomization may also result in serious imbalances in treatment assignments within an institution; this may make some investigators question the randomization process itself. Finally, simple randomization does not guarantee that the treatment groups will be comparable in regard to known prognostic factors, either during or at the end of the study. It is unfortunate if imbalances exist and statistical analyses used to adjust for this lack of comparability are challenged. Prospective stratified randomization can alleviate these problems, by insuring against low probability events of severe imbalance that can ruin a study.[16]

A stratified randomization is 'blocked' so that after every b T treatment assignments, each of the T treatment groups has been assigned to b patients. This process ensures protection against unknown time trends in the characteristics of arriving patients as well as comparability of the treatment groups in regard to the stratification factors. For each combination of stratification factors a separate randomization list is derived, and each patient is randomized using the list corresponding to his particular set of stratification features.

To illustrate, assume that two treatments (A and B) will be compared for Stage III and IV patients with squamous cell carcinoma of the oral cavity. Two prognostic factors of survival are stage (Stage III vs Stage IV) and site of the primary (anterior tongue, floor of mouth, and retromolar trigone/anterior tonsillar pillar). Thus a total of $2 \times 3 = 6$ strata are present into which any patient will belong, as shown in Table 21.2. Assume that we wish to have two treatment A's and two treatment B's in each stratum after every four treatment assignments. For this permuted block of size $b = 2$, only one of the six following combinations of two A's and two B's is possible: AABB ABAB ABBA BBAA BABA BAAB. To avoid the possibility of selection bias, the generation of the particular sequence of treatment

TABLE 21.2   PATIENT STRATA BASED ON
STAGE AND SITE

	Stage	
Site of Primary Disease	III	IV
Anterior tongue Floor of mouth Retromolar trigone/anterior tonsillar pillar		

assignments is best left to the study statistician or some other individual not involved directly in the patient selection process. The treatment assignments for each stratum are then transferred to a list or sealed envelopes. A central operations office should be responsible for treatment assignment, which is given to the investigator only after the patient is willing and eligible to be entered on study, and has signed an informed consent.

Although it is important to account for major prognostic factors in the randomization process, overstratification can destroy the desired goal of patient comparability among the treatment groups.[17] The number of strata increases multiplicatively as the product of the number of levels in each stratification factor. Thus gross overall treatment imbalances may result if many strata do not contain enough patients to fill the first permuted block. It is best to select only those few stratification factors that have an important and independent association with a major study endpoint (e.g. survival time).

For multi-institution studies one may wish to include institution as a stratification factor so that serious treatment imbalances will not occur within each institution. Consistency of comparative treatment efficacy can thus be examined across the institutions during interim and final analyses. More importantly, the possibility is minimized that treatment and institution are confounded with one another, in which case it is difficult to determine which of these two factors is more important in effecting differences in patient outcome. But it may be difficult to formally include 'institution' in a stratified randomization procedure if the number of institutions is large.

Zelen provides a solution to this problem when a randomization is carried out by a central operations office.[15] A randomization list is produced for each prognostic stratum, ignoring institution. The randomization procedure consists of an investigator phoning the randomization office and giving the required stratification features. A tentative treatment assignment is determined by taking the next treatment assignment in the stratum defined by the patient's characteristics. An individual at the operations office then calculates for that institution the difference, DF, between the number of cases on the selected treatment (including the tentative assignment) minus the number of cases for that treatment with the minimum number of cases. If DF is less than or equal to some preassigned integer, n, then the tentative assignment is the one given to the investigator. If $DF > n$, the tentative assignment is not given and the next treatment allocation on the randomization list is selected as the tentative assignment. The procedure is repeated until the investigator is provided a treatment assignment such that $DF \leqslant n$. Efron[18] and Wei[19] provide two general alternatives to Zelen's procedure. These designs require more extensive computer programming to produce the list of treatment assignments. This list is, however, produced once at the start of the study, and is used thereafter in a straightforward way.

SIZE OF THE STUDY

An important aspect of the planning of a clinical trial is determination of sample size. Sample size estimates are essential in order to ensure that sufficient numbers of patients can be accrued over a reasonable time period while the primary question is still of interest. Insufficient numbers of patients can lead to ambiguous or erroneous conclusions, with the consequence that beneficial treatments are discarded without sufficient testing.[20] The determination of sample size should be based on the specific study objectives and endpoints used. For example, a multicentre National Cancer Institute clinical trial comparing three treatments was instituted for Stage III and Stage IV head and neck cancer patients whose primary tumour was located either in the larynx/hypopharynx or oral cavity. For these two distinct subsets of patients, survival was the major endpoint. It was anticipated that these two subgroups of patients would be analysed separately since they were likely to differ substantially in regard to survival. Thus the overall study sample size was planned so that adequate numbers of patients were available for each major subgroup.

For the situation where two treatments are compared, an extensive literature is available on sample size requirements. The approaches are based on normal theory and can be classified broadly according to the type of endpoint considered. Two of the most common endpoints involve a dichotomous response (i.e. alive or dead),[21] or time to some critical event (e.g. tumour recurrence or death).[22] The approach taken to calculate sample size is that one specifies the treatment difference, D, which is considered important to detect together with the Type-I and Type-II error rates associated with the statistical test to be used.

More specifically, consider the dichotomous response situation and assume the true (unknown) proportion of 'success' patients (e.g. alive at 2 years) is p_T in the new treatment group. The proportion of control patients is p_c. The clinical trial provides estimates of these true proportions, denoted as $\hat{p}_T$ and $\hat{p}_c$ respectively. Since only these estimates are observed, it may occur that the observed difference $(\hat{p}_T - \hat{p}_c)$ is significantly different from 0 even though the null hypothesis, $H_0 = (p_T - p_c) = 0$, is true. This kind of error is called Type I error, and represents the event of falsely rejecting the null hypothesis. The probability of making this error is called the significance level and is denoted α. On the other hand it may happen that $(\hat{p}_T - \hat{p}_c)$ is not significantly different from 0 and H_0 is not rejected although the alternative hypothesis, $H_A : (p_T - p_c) = D \neq 0$, is in fact true (indicating that a true difference exists between the treatment groups).

This type of decision-making error is called Type-II error, and the probability of making this type of error is denoted β. Thus the probability of correctly rejecting H_0 is $(1 - \beta)$. This quantity is referred to as power, and describes the ability of the study to detect true differences of magnitude D. While theoretically any value of α and β can be selected between 0 and 1, it is traditional in sample size determination to select α as 0.01 or 0.05, and to select β as 0.10 or 0.20. Two-sided significance tests should be used for planning purposes unless a strong justification exists for expecting a difference in only one direction between the two treatments.

Table 21.3 indicates the number of patients required per group in order to achieve a specified power and significance level as a function of the true success rates. These values were obtained using the method of Casagrande et al.[21] To illustrate how to use the table, assume that we wish to have power 0.80 of detecting a difference $D = 0.20$ in the 3-year survival rate between a new and standard therapy. Although one expects patients receiving the new experimental therapy to do better than those treated with the standard therapy, unexpected morbidity and mortality may arise in the new therapy group and therefore a two-sided significance level is chosen. Table 21.3 shows that 82 patients are needed in each treatment group if the proportion of 3-year survivors in the standard treatment group is 0.15 and a two-sided 0.05 significance level is desired. When the smaller success rate exceeds 0.50 the table is used by considering the failure rate and entering the table with 1 − (success rate).

One can see from this table that the number of patients increases as the expected magnitude of the treatment difference decreases between the two treatment groups. Thus some investigators may find it attractive to specify a larger treatment difference for planning purposes than may be realistic. One must guard against such optimism during the planning stages of a clinical trial, since the power of the study will be very low for detecting differences of moderate but still clinically

TABLE 21.3 NUMBER OF PATIENTS IN EACH OF TWO TREATMENT GROUPS (TWO-SIDED TEST)

Smaller success rate	Larger minus smaller success rate									
	0.05	0.10	0.15	0.20	0.25	0.30	0.35	0.40	0.45	0.50
0.05	620*	206	113	74	54	42	33	27	23	19
	473†	159	88	58	43	33	27	22	18	16
0.10	956	285	146	92	64	48	38	30	25	21
	724	218	112	71	50	38	30	24	20	17
0.15	1250	354	174	106	73	53	41	33	26	22
	944	269	133	82	57	42	32	26	21	18
0.20	1502	411	197	118	79	57	44	34	27	22
	1132	313	151	91	62	45	34	27	22	18
0.25	1712	459	216	127	84	60	45	35	28	23
	1289	348	165	98	65	47	36	28	22	18
0.30	1880	495	230	134	88	62	46	36	28	22
	1414	375	175	103	68	48	36	28	22	18
0.35	2006	522	239	138	89	63	46	35	27	22
	1509	395	182	106	69	49	36	28	22	18
0.40	2090	537	244	139	89	62	45	34	26	21
	1571	407	186	107	69	48	36	27	21	17
0.45	2132	543	244	138	88	60	44	33	25	19
	1603	411	186	106	68	47	34	26	20	16
0.50	2132	537	239	134	84	57	41	30	23	17
	1603	407	182	103	65	45	32	24	18	14

* Upper figure: significance level 0.05, power 0.90.
† Lower figure: significance level 0.05, power 0.80.

important magnitude. With such experimental design characteristics a new experimental treatment may be found not to differ significantly from the standard therapy. As a consequence the new treatment may receive a very low priority for further testing although it represents a true therapeutic advance.

Final analyses of cancer clinical trials often include the comparative evaluation of entire survival curves, not just the proportion alive at some fixed time-point. Sample size methods are available for this situation if one is willing to assume some mathematical form for the survival distribution. George and Desu developed sample size requirements for the case where the survival distribution is assumed to be exponential.[22] Their tables indicate the required numbers of deaths that must be observed in each of two treatment groups for a specified α, β, and ratio of median survival times. Rubinstein et al.[23] have generalized the work of George and Desu, and allow both for

loss to follow-up and a continuation period. The continuation period is the length of time after accrual has stopped before the analysis is performed. This mimics more closely an actual clinical trial setting. They show that the number of patients required for a specified α, β, and ratio of median survival times can be reduced if one is willing to have a continuation period. This holds since the statistical power of the comparison depends on the number of deaths observed. Continued observation can decrease substantially the required number of patients, especially if accrual is rapid. When the accrual rate is 200 per year, and the ratio of median survival times is between two and three, the accrual time (and hence the required number of patients) can be reduced by 50% or more. If the entry rate is 40 per year the benefits of a continuation period are less noticeable. Thus some knowledge of accrual rate patterns can prove quite useful during the planning stages of a study.

Finally, there are a number of clinical trials in which three or more treatments are compared. The straightforward application of the above two-treatment methods is inappropriate unless the α-level at which sample sizes are calculated is adjusted downward. If every pairwise comparison is performed at the α-significance level then the overall probability of finding a significant difference when all the treatments are the same is much higher than α; this is known as the multiple comparisons problem.[5] Thus one has a higher chance of false-positive results than expected. Lachin[24] and Makuch and Simon[25] have generalized the two-treatment group situation to k-treatment groups $(k > 2)$ for the dichotomous response and exponential survival times situation, respectively.

CONDUCTING A CLINICAL TRIAL

Once a protocol has been written and accepted by all the investigators the plan must be implemented. This includes a diverse number of activities including patient registration, development of data forms, data management, computer services, and quality control. The proper integration of these tasks can contribute significantly to the success of a multicentre trial. Daily activities needed to perform these tasks require the same planning and professional expertise utilized in the other aspects of the study. Their effective execution can enhance the accrual rate, quality of the data, and investigators' interest in maintaining the scientific integrity of the study. Thus, the individuals who take on these responsibilities should be included early on during the protocol writing process so that they are familiar with the letter and intent of the protocol.

Patient registration refers to the process in which a patient is diagnosed at a member institution with the disease under investigation and, when appropriate, is entered on study and issued a treatment assignment. Objectives of patient registration include: (1) initiating data collection, (2) providing a treatment assignment, and (3) improving quality control

aspects of the study. For randomized multicentre studies an extended telephone registration from a central office is recommended to initiate data collection.[26] This strategy involves the investigator's calling the central office to register the patient. During the conversation the registrar determines whether the patient is eligible for the study based on the protocol specifications. If so, then a random treatment assignment is provided and an eligibility form is completed. Ideally, every randomized patient should be included in the primary endpoint analyses of a clinical trial.[14] Randomized patients who are subsequently excluded inevitably raise questions of bias and may cause problems in interpreting the final results. The extended telephone registration alleviates such difficulties.

After providing a treatment assignment at the time of randomization, the central office personnel can set a timetable when future data forms are expected. In addition, these personnel can play an active role in enhancing data quality. For example, if a treatment regimen involves radiotherapy following surgery, the investigator's radiotherapy plan for each patient can be routed through the central office to a central radiotherapy quality review board to insure that the investigator plans the therapy per protocol specifications. The central office can then communicate any treatment changes recommended by the review board to the investigator prior to the start of radiotherapy. By monitoring the flow of information the central office can ensure that all required review material is received promptly from the investigator, and that the requests of the review board are satisfied, with minimal administrative burden placed on the investigators.

Once a patient has been entered onto the study the data collection process begins. Although it is mandatory that sufficient information is collected to address all the objectives of the study stated in the protocol, it is usually the case that more extensive data collection is undertaken than is required. This results in unnecessary complexity in the conduct of the study, and the quality of all the data collected usually suffers. For multicentre studies, data management is very complex and time-consuming. One solution is to collect a large amount of initial on-study patient data and only the most essential endpoint and complications data thereafter.[14]

The development of good data forms and procedures for handling these forms are important to the success of a clinical trial. The forms should be as unambiguous as possible. For instance, it may be undesirable to ask whether a liver is normal or abnormal without further specification that abnormal is interpreted as a liver with metastases, not merely cirrhotic changes. Since many individuals with different backgrounds will complete the forms, it is advisable that a manual be provided which explains the intent underlying the request for a given piece of information. The forms also should be designed so that they are convenient for data entry. Where possible, multiple-choice items with responses to be checked, circled, or filled out in an appropriate box are recommended rather than free-form replies. It is usually wise to have a specific entry for 'unknown' to distinguish an unobtainable answer from one inadvertently left blank.

Wright and Haybittle[27] give specific suggestions for the design of data forms. Before the forms are finalized and distributed to the study participants they should be pretested and given to some individuals to complete, verify, code, and keypunch.

One general proposal for handling the data forms involves mailing the forms to a central office at appropriate times specified in the protocol. These forms are logged in and visually checked for gross errors. If any gross errors are detected then the form originator is contacted and the error is corrected prior to keystroking. The forms are then keystroked and data are entered onto the computer. Computer-driven single-field edits and cross-field logical edits are performed to ascertain whether a field contains a valid entry, and whether the entries are logically consistent with one another. Any errors detected at this step are again corrected by contacting the form originator. The dataset resulting from this process is then integrated with the data previously stored in the computer; the forms are filed for safe keeping. Great care should be taken to ensure the integrity of the data, and that adequate procedures exist so that the data will not be lost.

From this database, reports are sent to

TABLE 21.4   EXAMPLE OF FORMS STATUS REPORT FOR MULTI-MODALITY STUDY IN HEAD AND NECK CANCER

Institution	Case number	Patient initials	Randomization date	Treatment assignment*	On study	Induction chemotherapy summary
A	1003	WTW	5/12/78	1	Received	Received
A	1021	KAH	31/ 1/79	2	Received	Received
A	1086	CTS	16/ 3/79	1		
A	1215	CS	27/ 3/79	3	Received	Received

Surgery summary	Post-operative	Radio-therapy	Maintenance chemotherapy summary	Latest progress report
Received	Received	Received		29/ 8/79
Received	Received	Received		19/11/79
Received	Received	Received		10/ 1/80
Received	Received	Received	Received	22/10/79

* 1 = Surgery and radiotherapy.
  2 = Induction chemotherapy and surgery and radiotherapy.
  3 = Induction chemotherapy and surgery and radiotherapy and maintenance chemotherapy.

member institutions at regular intervals which may, for example, list all overdue forms and identify all patients entered on study from that institution, as shown in Table 21.4. Each row summarizes the entire treatment course and follow-up period for each patient. The headings identify the institution, patient, his date of randomization and treatment assignment, and types of data forms used to gather study information. From the time a patient is entered on study through his most recent follow-up status, data forms and patient status information are available. This type of information helps to maintain investigator interest,[28] as well as providing a check that all information sent to the central office has indeed been received and processed.

To summarize, the execution of a comparative, multicentre clinical trial is the culmination of efforts made by a large group of individuals representing many specialties. All aspects of the study require proper planning, from the initial focus on developing hypotheses of interest, to the conduct of properly carrying out the trial. Specific features of new studies in head and neck cancer will naturally evolve to accommodate advances in cancer treatment techniques as well as clinical trial methodology. Nevertheless, the major points set out in this chapter should provide a useful, general framework for the design and conduct of these important, large-scale clinical trials.

REFERENCES

1. Medawar, P.B. (1969). *Induction and Intuition in Scientific Thought*, American Philosophical Society, Philadelphia.
2. Cornfield, J. (1976). *Am. J. Epidemiol.*, **104**, 408.
3. Tukey, J.W. (1977). *Science*, **198**, 679.
4. Hill, A.B. (1951). *Br. Med. Bull.*, **7**, 278.
5. Byar, D.P., and Corle, D.K. (1977). *J. Chron. Dis.*, **30**, 445.
6. Makuch, R.W. (1982). *Cancer Treat. Rep.*, **66**, 217.
7. Byar, D.P., Simon, R.M., Friedewald, W.T., Schlesselman, J.J., DeMets, D.L., Ellenberg, J.H., Gail, M.H., and Ware, J.H. (1976). *N. Engl. J. Med.*, **295**, 74.
8. Gehan, E.A., and Freireich, E.J. (1974). *N. Engl. J. Med.*, **290**, 198.
9. Pocock, S.J. (1977). *Br. Med. J.*, **1**, 1661.
10. Farewell, V.T., and D'Angio, G.J. (1981). *Biometrics*, **37**, 169.
11. Fisher, R.A. (1966). *The Design of Experiments*, 8th edn, Oliver & Boyd, Edinburgh.
12. Pocock, S.J. (1976). *J. Chron. Dis.*, **29**, 175.
13. Makuch, R., and Simon, R. (1978). *Cancer Treat. Rep.*, **62**, 1037.
14. Peto, R., Pike, M.C., Armitage, P., Breslow, N.E., Cox, D.R., Howard, S.V., Mantel, N., McPherson, K., Peto, J., and Smith, P.G. (1976). *Br. J. Cancer*, **34**, and **35**, 585.
15. Zelen, M., *J. Chron. Dis.*, **27**, 365.
16. Lasagna, L. (1976). *N. Engl. J. Med.*, **295**, 1086.
17. Pocock, S.J., and Simon, R. (1975). *Biometrics*, **31**, 103.
18. Efron, B. (1971). *Biometrika*, **58**, 403.
19. Wei, L.J. (1978). *J. Am. Stat. Assn.*, **73**, 559.
20. Freiman, J.A., Chalmers, T.C., Smith, H., Jr., and Kuebler, R.R. (1978). *N. Engl. J. Med.*, **299**, 690.
21. Casagrande, J.T., Pike, M.C., and Smith, P.G. (1978). *Biometrics*, **34**, 483.
22. George, S.L., and Desu, M.M., *J. Chron. Dis.*, **27**, 15.
23. Rubinstein, L.V., Gail, M.H., and Santner, T.J. *J. Chron. Dis.*, **34**, 469.
24. Lachin, J.M. *Biometrics*, **33**, 315.
25. Makuch, R.W., and Simon, R.M. (1982). *J. Chron. Dis.*, **35**, 861.
26. Herson, J. (1980). *Controlled Clin. Trials*, **1**, 101.
27. Wright, P., and Haybittle, J. (1979). *Br. Med. J.*, **2**, 529, 590, 650.
28. Prescott, R.J. (1979). In H.J. Tagnon and M.J. Staquet (Eds), *Controversies in Cancer: Design of Trials and Treatment*, Masson, New York, p.55.

Chapter **22**

The Problem of Accrual to Clinical Trials

Robert E. Wittes and
Patricia W. Sellers
*Cancer Therapy Evaluation Program,
Division of Cancer Treatment, National
Cancer Institute, Bethesda, Maryland,
USA and Department of Surgery,
Memorial Sloan – Kettering Cancer Center,
New York, NY, USA*

The enlistment of adequate numbers of patients on experimental treatment protocols is a necessary condition for a successful trial. It is ironic, therefore, that in the process of protocol planning, while certain less critical features of the clinical experiment may be specified in excruciating detail, estimates of accrual rates are often no more than semi-educated guesses.

The reason for this state of affairs is clear – the patient database of most institutions, even university hospitals and cancer centres, is not set up to meet the needs of clinical research. One can usually ascertain from a hospital's record room or cancer registry how many patients with a certain type of malignancy were admitted over a specified time interval, and it is usually possible to find out certain elementary demographic facts about these patients without a formal review of individual medical records. It is rarely possible, however, to fix the percentage of this total which satisfies the detailed eligibility requirements of most

experimental treatment programmes; these generally involve medical and psychosocial criteria that are simply impossible to ascertain from computer printouts.

The imprecision in accrual estimates resulting from such incomplete databases depends very much on the type of cancer under study, as well as the therapy. Since testicular cancer occurs predominantly in young otherwise healthy men, a large majority of patients with the correct histological diagnosis, stage, and prior therapy characteristics will turn out to be eligible for most treatment programmes, even those which have quite restrictive requirements. Similarly, therapies which are very radical or aggressive will necessarily result in a higher rate of ineligibility than less toxic or mutilating procedures.

The head and neck cancers tend to occur in an older population with a high prevalence of alcohol and tobacco abuse. One can confidently anticipate that a significant proportion of cases will not be eligible for a study which has anything more than the most relaxed eligibility criteria.

From 1 December 1979 until 30 April 1982 the Memorial Sloan–Kettering Cancer Center participated with other institutions in a prospective randomized trial to evaluate the efficacy of chemotherapy as an adjuvant to local treatment.[1] Patients with operable, previously untreated epidermoid carcinoma, Stage III or IV, with primary site in the anterior tongue, floor of mouth, retromolar trigone/anterior tonsillar pillar, supraglottic or glottic larynx, or pyriform fossa were eligible for entry. The three study arms included: (1) local therapy only (surgery and postoperative irradiation); (2) initial chemotherapy with one cycle of cisplatin and bleomycin, followed by local therapy; (3) initial chemotherapy, followed by local therapy, followed in turn by six treatments at monthly intervals with 24-hour cisplatin infusions.

Because of the nature of the therapy and the goals of the trial, the eligibility requirements were strict. Patients had to exhibit normal renal, haematological, and auditory function according to standard laboratory criteria; they also had to have clinically normal cardiac and pulmonary function. Patients with prior or synchronous second cancers other than non-melanoma skin cancer were excluded, as were those with evidence of metastatic disease after a prescribed extent-of-disease work-up. Karnofsky performance status (PS) had to be at least 50. Patients younger than 30 or older than 78 could not enter the trial, nor could those whose psychosocial characteristics or geographical distance from the hospital made good compliance with treatment and reliable long-term follow-up questionable. All patients had to be capable of giving a meaningful informed consent, and had to accept the possibility of entry into any of the three study arms, as well as the process of randomization itself.

During the 41 months of accrual, one of us (P.S.) screened all admissions to the Head and Neck Service, MSKCC. Of a total of 3774

admissions, 183 patients presented with previously untreated epidermoid cancer of the appropriate site and stage. Information on histology, prior therapy, site, and stage was gleaned from the medical record on the day following admission and was usually found in the attending surgeon's or fellow's admitting note, generally written 2–14 days prior to admission.

Of these, 40 could be recognized immediately as ineligible based on either age (16) or geography (24). A history and physical examination, together with the baseline staging work-up, served to eliminate another 33 patients from entry. Nine of the 33 had inadequate PS scores; as one might expect in this patient population, several of these cases had unstable cardiac, pulmonary, or metabolic problems on admission. One patient developed sudden bleeding at the primary site and required immediate surgery. Six patients had had previous malignancies. These included quite a diverse group of histologies and sites (breast (2), cervix (1), bladder (1), rectum (1), and Hodgkin's disease (1)), all but one of which share no common aetiological associations with head and neck cancer. Four patients had separate synchronous primary cancers; three of these were at other upper aerodigestive sites and one was in the lung. One patient, apparently an excellent candidate for the trial, died suddenly during the work-up, of no apparent cause. Three were unable to give a legitimate informed consent because of either disabling psychiatric illness (2) or mental retardation (1). After the full extent of disease evaluation was completed, 13 patients turned out to have inoperable disease, because of either locoregional spread (11) or metastases to the liver (1) or lungs (1).

Studies of kidney function and auditory acuity eliminated another 11 and seven patients respectively. Only a minority of those failing the audiogram, and none of those with insufficient creatinine clearances, could have been identified clinically prior to performance of these tests. An additional patient was ineligible for unknown reasons.

Thus, of 183 previously untreated patients with the appropriate site, apparent stage, and histology, a total of 88 remained for consideration. Of these, only half actually entered the trial. The 44 who did not failed to do so for a variety of reasons.

(1) Patient refusals – 32. Of these 12 declined chemotherapy without further clarification; two additional patients gave fear of toxic side-effects as the explicit reason for refusal. Four patients did not want the necessary surgery to be delayed by chemotherapy. Four refusals had to do with the nature and/or consequences of the randomization process; of these two did not want to risk the chance of being allocated to 6 months of maintenance chemotherapy. One could not understand why the physician did not simply choose the treatment that was best for him, and one patient insisted on receiving the chemotherapy. Another four patients refused participation because the treatment was experimental. Two patients declined the necessary surgery. One refused because of inadequate insurance, another patient refused to have radiation therapy at a participating institution, and two patients simply said 'no' without any explanation.

(2) Surgeon refusals. On 12 occasions the attending surgeon did not propose enlistment on study to an eligible patient. Several of these episodes occurred during the initial phases of the trial and may have been due to lack of awareness of eligibility criteria. In the other instances, however, the attending surgeon actively declined to involve the patient, and usually cited psychological factors as the main reason.

In summary, our experience attempting to accrue head and neck cancer patients to a large, multi-institutional, multimodality study has important implications for the design of future trials. Of the total group eligible on the basis of histology, stage, and site, about half turned out to be ineligible for a wide variety of reasons (Table 22.1). A referral centre such as MSKCC may have more of a problem with geographical inaccessibility of its patients than other institutions. Only 18 of the 95 ineligible cases were ineligible because of physiological requirements dictated by the properties of cisplatin (renal and auditory); if methotrexate had been used instead of cisplatin, prudence would probably have dictated similar critera for adequate kidney function.

Of the eligible patients, only half were entered on study. Patient refusals outnumbered physician non-compliance by nearly 3 to 1. These data show that the randomization procedure itself is an unimportant stated cause of patient refusal. Though we cannot rule out that randomization may have played some role in the negative decision of some of the patients who refused ostensibly for other reasons, our impression is that other considerations, notably the fear of chemotherapy toxicity, were much more important. The low rate of refusal for fear of radical surgery is probably a function of selection; patients referred to MSKCC, an institution with a reputation for aggressive treatment approaches, may be less likely to refuse such surgery than those at other institutions.

The problem of adequate patient recruitment to clinical trials is certainly not new, nor is it peculiar to cancer trials. Considerable efforts have been devoted to this area[2] and to developing strategies to deal with accrual problems in ongoing trials.[3] For a trial such as the head and neck cancer adjuvant study described here, the problem is a complex one; several aspects should be dealt with separately.

Eligibility

It is obvious that the more stringent the on-study requirements, the fewer patients will be eligible and the less generalizable the results will be to the population as a whole. Eligibility requirements which promote patient safety are necessary for an ethical study. Requirements which limit the primary site, stage, and histology are frequently necessary to ensure that the results will be interpretable.

TABLE 22.1

Total	183	% of Total 100%
Ineligible 95		52%
Geography	24	
Age	16	
Inoperable	13	
Renal	11	
Poor PS	9	
Auditory	7	
Prior cancers	6	
Double 1°'s	4	
Informed consent	3	
Unknown reason	1	
Sudden death	1	
Eligible 88		48%
Patient refusals	32	
Surgeon refusals	12	
Entered 44		24%

Psychosocial and geographical restrictions similarly seem reasonable ways of minimizing losses to follow-up. The only point here is that eligibility requirements should be very carefully considered and should probably be the minimal number that will ensure the goals set forth above. In addition, much more effort should be devoted to ascertainment of the number of patients within each participating institution which actually *meet* the requirements. This will mean the abandonment of the assumption that figures from a hospital record room are an accurate reflection of what will actually take place. Most record rooms are organized with the administrative, and not the research, needs of the hospital in mind. It may be that for the planning of some studies a manual review of (a sample of) patient records will be required to establish likely accrual. Even this dreary task, however, is simpler and certainly cheaper than mounting a clinical trial whose accrual goals, and hence research objectives, cannot be possibly met.

Patient Acceptance

Most noteworthy here is the apparently small impact of the randomization procedure on patient unwillingness to enter the trial. That physicians and surgeons are often less than enthusiastic about participation in randomized clinical trials is well known; our experience here, however, suggests that patients (at least those patients who were approached to enter the study) do not have the level of concern about coin-flipping that is often attributed to them. A survey by Greco and Perry has suggested similar conclusions.[4]

On the other hand, patients obviously care very much about the content of the study arms. Concern about toxic side-effects, the experimental nature of the treatment, and the effect of a 6-month commitment to a maintenance regimen on quality of life or personal finances account for at least 21 of the 32 refusals. It may also be that a patient's own perception about the value (or lack of value) of the experimental treatment played a role in rejection of study entry. In a retrospective evaluation of this kind, such factors are impossible to evaluate. Our experience here is in general agreement with that of Barofsky and Sugarbaker.[5] In an examination of factors determining patient non-participation in sarcoma treatment trials, they concluded that the most significant determinants were the patient's perception of differences between the various treatment options on quality of life (e.g. amputation vs. limb-sparing surgery + irradiation; or surgery + irradiation + chemotherapy versus the same treatment plus intravenous *C. parvum*, which was associated with four additional hospital days per month and febrile episodes with *C. parvum* administration).

Surgeon Attitudes

Several failures to recruit eligible patients occurred during the first few months of the study. Increasing accrual rates during the initial phases of a trial are a familiar occurrence. Certainly the ultimate decision about the appropriateness of study entry for a particular patient must always rest with the treating physician or surgeon. We made no effort here to establish retrospectively whether these exclusions were 'justifiable', since most of them were based on assessments of the patients' personality characteristics that could not in any case be evaluated by a chart review. It goes without saying, but is often forgotten, that no study should be mounted without a firm commitment on the part of the participating investigators. How to assess such a commitment may not be so simple. Good participation in previous similar trials is probably the most reliable indication. Pious assurances of support by themselves have a way of evaporating when competing priorities, such as a bed shortage, operating room scheduling difficulties, or an anxious patient appear on the scene.

The fact that MSKCC surgeons were as a group committed to this trial places this experience in contrast to that reported by Lee *et al.*[6] who examined the reasons why only 41 of 77 cases eligible for a cooperative group lung cancer trial were actually entered; they found that lack of physician enthusiasm was the major problem.

This chapter has dealt with intra-institutional factors. We did not attempt in a planned, systematic way to increase accrual to this trial by extensive publicity in lay publications or by approaching potential referring physicians and surgeons outside MSKCC. Such a strategy is an obvious one when dealing with interventions in a healthy population of outpatients and has been done successfully, for example, in the Coronary Prevention Trial.[7] In the present setting, however, one is dealing

with a sick patient population requiring a highly integrated and complex treatment and the commitment of present and future hospital resources. A decision to increase the referral rate from outside the institution has to be made only in the setting of overall institutional goals. In addition, such an effort might well strain relations between a centre and the community, since a shift in referral patterns for patients with certain operable head and neck cancers would have economic and professional implications for community-based oncologists of all disciplines. One may hope that the increased integration between community care and the cancer centres evolving from such efforts as the Community Clinical Oncology Program of the National Cancer Institute may lead to a solution of this problem.

REFERENCES

1. Baker, S.R., Makuch, R.W., and Wolf, G.T. (1980). *Proc. Int. Head and Neck Oncol. Conf.*, Abstract 5:12, National Cancer Institute.
2. Roth, H.P. and Gordon, R.S. (Eds) (1979). *Clin. Pharmacol. Ther.* **25**, 629.
3. Collins, J.F., Bingham, S.F., Weiss, D.G., Willifred, W.O., and Kuhn, R.M. (1980). *Controlled Clin. Trials*, **1**, 227.
4. Greco, A.O., and Perry, M.C. (1980). *Proc. Am. Soc. Clin. Oncol.* Abstract C 146.
5. Barofsky, I., and Sugarbaker, P.H. (1979). *Cancer Clin. Trials*, **2**, 237.
6. Lee, J.Y., Marks, J.E., and Simpson, J.R. (1980). *Cancer Clin. Trials*, **3**, 381.
7. Prout, T.E. (1981). *Controlled Clin. Trials*, **1**, 313.

Chapter 23

Current Trends in Therapeutic Research

Robert E. Wittes
*Cancer Therapy Evaluation Program,
Division of Cancer Treatment, National
Cancer Institute, Bethesda, Maryland,
USA*

As a multidisciplinary endeavour, the treatment of head and neck cancer has clearly come of age. Since the direction of future progress with these tumours will depend on the paths investigators elect to follow, it seems of interest to consider what the current paths actually are. From such a survey it should be possible to draw conclusions about what specific issues investigators deem most urgent, as well as to establish what type of methodologies are being used to answer these questions.

Under the headings Head and Neck Neoplasms, Mouth Neoplasms, Pharyngeal Neoplasms, and Laryngeal Neoplasms, the 1981 Index Medicus lists a total of 94 articles whose principal orientation appears to be with therapy. It should be recognized that the composition of the published literature in any one year is really a summation of the cumulative concerns of the head and neck oncology community for probably the past 2–15 years. These 94 papers may be divided into a few broad categories, according to the major issues they address:

Total – 94
Surgery – 43

Radiotherapy – 13
Surgery and radiotherapy – 26
Chemotherapy plus local therapy (surgery and/or radiotherapy) – 11
Immunotherapy plus local therapy – 1

SURGERY

As shown in Table 23.1, the largest single concern in the surgery literature is with problems of reconstruction. Twenty-four papers deal with a variety of approaches, of which the most popular is the development of various flaps. Jejunal grafts, larynx reconstruction, and the use of irradiated autogenous mandible also received attention. Six publications discussed

TABLE 23.1 ARTICLES IN SURGERY

Reconstruction	24
Technical issues in cancer surgery	6
Treatment of the neck	5
Review of overall treatment policies for defined group of patients	3
CO_2 Laser	2
Prophylactic antibiotics	2
Nutrition	1
Total	43

technical problems in ablative cancer surgery; these included problems of access (mandibular swing), adequacy of margins (frozen section control), carotid protection (dermis grafting), or issues surrounding the scope of certain operations (extended hemilaryngectomy for T_3 glottic cancer, treatment of the patient with carotid invasion, extended resection for tracheal involvement). The treatment of the neck was the subject of five papers; questions addressed included the clinical evolution of the N0 neck, the performance of simultaneous or staged bilateral neck dissections, and modifications of the classical neck dissection. The use of the CO_2 laser, the utility of prophylactic antibiotics and surveillance skin cultures, and a study of parenteral nutrition accounted for five papers. The remaining three articles dealt with reviews of past treatment policies in a patient population usually defined by primary site and/or demographic variables (e.g. experience with surgery in patients with larynx cancer who are older than 70 years).

Of these 43 papers only four were prospective studies. The 39 retrospective reports varied greatly in type, from a report of a reconstructive technique in a handful of patients to a review of the experience of a major cancer centre with hundreds of patients in a certain disease category. Of the four prospective studies, only one involved surgical technique; the other three related to nutrition or prophylaxis of infection with antibiotics. All but two of the 43 papers were single-institution studies.

RADIOTHERAPY

The 13 publications whose major focus was radiotherapy also had diverse areas of concern. Radiotherapists are attempting to explore strategies aimed at optimizing treatment with simultaneous use of sensitizers. Therapy with neutrons, mixed beams of neutron and photons, and pions was the subject of four. Three other articles were reviews of treatment policies in defined populations.

Of the 13 papers or trials listed in Table

TABLE 23.2   RADIOTHERAPY

Misonidazole	1
Hyperfractionation	2
Brachytherapy and sensitizers	1
Review of therapy policies	3
Neutrons	3
Therapy of T_2 by ERT	1
Hypofractionation	1
Pions	1
Total	13

23.2, nine appeared to be prospective. Of these, only one was randomized. All but one of the 13 were studies from single institutions.

SURGERY AND RADIOTHERAPY

In view of the currently prevailing view that combined-modality local therapy is superior to the single-modality treatment of advanced epidermoid head and neck cancer, it is not surprising that articles on this subject greatly outnumber those dealing with radiotherapy or ablative surgery alone. Of the 26 publications on combined therapy, the majority consist of retrospective reviews of treatment policies in defined populations (17/26). Seven papers deal with the use of radiotherapy as an adjuvant to surgery. In one of these, preoperative radiation is compared to postoperative; in another, preoperative radiation and surgery are compared to surgery alone; and in the third, surgery and postoperative radiation are compared to surgery alone.

Of these 26 reports, four are prospective and three are randomized. Two (one randomized, one not) are multi-institutional.

TABLE 23.3   SURGERY AND RADIOTHERAPY

Review of past treatment policies	17
Radiotherapy as adjuvant to surgery	7
Tolerance to surgery after radiotherapy	1
Case report	1
Total	26

CHEMOTHERAPY

In applying the systemic use of drugs to the head and neck cancer problem, the literature indexed during 1981 reflects a preoccupation with chemotherapy in a combined modality context. All 11 papers deal with combinations of drugs and local therapy. In a group of conditions for which chemotherapy is such a manifestly inadequate modality in advanced disease, the paucity of Phase II studies is surprising.

The 11 trials are split between the simultaneous and sequential application of systemic and local therapy. In five trials the radiosensitizing properties of bleomycin, or cisplatin, or a combination of fluorouracil, doxorubicin, and bleomycin were explored. The six remaining studies looked at various sequential combinations of chemotherapy and local treatment.

Of these 11 studies, two were large randomized trials, the remainder were single-arm studies. All 11 were prospective.

One additional study attempted to examine the role of the immunopotentiator levamisole in a randomized trial from which no conclusions could be drawn. This study is the only one utilizing a biological response modifier indexed during 1981.

The 29 prospective trials indexed in 1981 varied widely in the numbers of patients entered (Table 23.4). Four of the 11 randomized trials had sample sizes less than 30 patients per arm, numbers which are far too small to detect any but the grossest differences between treatments. On the other hand, five of the

trials, each with a total accrual greater than 150, appeared to have been designed realistically and were adequate to answer the questions originally posed by the investigators.

PROCEEDINGS OF NATIONAL MEETINGS

Perhaps a more accurate picture of the current concerns of the community of clinical investigators is reflected in proceedings of the annual meetings of professional societies. For medical oncology, the largest and most representative one is clearly the American Society of Clinical Oncology (ASCO). An examination of the *Proceedings* of these meetings over the past 9 years (Table 23.5) shows that the number of abstracts dealing with head and neck cancer have gone from negligible (three in 1974) to appreciable (39 in 1982). This 13-fold increase over the past 8 years is obviously greater than can be explained by the general increase in the total number of abstracts, and is also somewhat greater than the relative increase for breast, lung, and colorectal cancers.

Of the 60 abstracts appearing in the *ASCO Proceedings* for 1980 and 1982, 56 deal with therapeutic trials (Table 23.6). Chemotherapy trials are the commonest; most of these, in turn, were conducted in patients who had already failed radiotherapy and/or surgery. Of the 18 trials dealing largely or completely with previously untreated patients, all but one are non-randomized pilot or feasibility studies, though some of these have rather impressive accrual figures and, at least in retrospect,

TABLE 23.4   ACCRUAL TO PROSPECTIVE TRIALS

Modalities	No. of trials	Median accrual	Range	Accrual to randomized trials
Surgery	4	53	24–69	51, 56, 69
Radiation	9	38	9–250	73
S + R	4	200	52–354	152, 248, 354
Chemo + local	11	40	3–712	23, 157, 72
Immunotherapy	1	24	—	24

TABLE 23.5   ASCO ENTRIES

	Total	H & N (%)	Breast(%)	Lung (%)	Colon(%)
1974	145	3 (2.1)	12 (8.3)	8 (5.5)	4 (2.8)
1976	299	3 (1.0)	35 (11.7)	24 (8.0)	8 (2.7
1978	449	19 (4.2)	54 (12.0)	36 (8.0)	12 (2.7)
1980	638	21 (3.3)	55 (8.6)	80 (12.5)	17 (2.7)
1982	788	39 (4.9)	81 (10.3)	78 (9.9)	32 (4.1)
Relative increase since 1974	5.4	13	6.8	9.8	8

TABLE 23.6   ASCO ABSTRACTS IN HEAD AND NECK CANCER 1980 AND 1982

Total	60
Therapeutic trials	56
Chemotherapy	53
Combination chemotherapy	39
Single agent Phase II	7
Intra-arterial therapy	2
Trials in predominantly previously untreated patients	18
BRMs	3
Adjuvant	2
Advanced disease	1
Randomized	10

might more profitably have been designed as definitive comparative studies. Over these 2 years, seven Phase II studies were reported; these have examined the activity of bleomycin by continuous intravenous infusion, vindesine, vindesine by continuous intravenous infusion, cisplatin, guanazole, and 4'epidoxorubicin. Two adjuvant studies with BCG and one Phase II study with interferon in nasopharynx cancer constitute the effort with biological response modifiers.

The contents of the 1980 *Proceedings of the American Society of Therapeutic Radiology* show that 18 of the 187 abstracts deal with aspects of head and neck cancer radiotherapy. The pattern of issues and methodologies is very similar to that of the completed and published papers already discussed (Table 23.2).

Similarly the *Proceedings of the Joint Meeting of the Society of Head and Neck Surgeons and the American society for Head and Neck Surgery* (1981) yields few surprises. Although several papers

on biomarkers, immunological factors, and chemotherapy were presented, the major focus of the meeting was on issues of ablative or reconstructive surgical technique (17/41) or questions involving natural history (11/41); in both areas virtually all the information presented was retrospectively derived and not the result of prospective clinical trials.

COMMENTS

Certainly a survey such as this has many inherent limitations. Chief aong these are the relatively small number of articles and abstracts examined. Nevertheless, the published literature indexed over a 12-month period, together with the *Proceedings* of professional societies, are an accurate reflection of the research activities of the head and neck oncology community. From this survey certain broad generalizations seem valid.

Of the 82 published papers involving surgery and/or radiotherapy, only 17 were prospective studies. The vast majority of the retrospective reports were either descriptions of surgical procedures, or broad surveys of the characteristics of certain disease entities in institutions bearing large population bases. The latter type of paper ('The experience with Disease X in Institution Y from 1945 to 1975') has a long and proud history in oncology generally, and such surveys often are the source of valuable information on the clinical behaviour of cancers as modified (or unmodified) by various forms of treatment. Such reviews are, however, a very specious way of developing notions about the comparative efficacy of treatment policies, chiefly because treatment selection is not made in an unbiased fashion. If the 1981 *Index Medicus* is representative of the head and neck cancer literature generally (and on the basis of prior experience it certainly seems to be), it seems quite clear that most of our ideas on how head and neck cancer is best managed come from retrospective reviews rather than carefully designed prospective trials.

In apparent contrast, all the 11 studies involving chemotherapy, as well as all the ASCO abstracts in which chemotherapy trials were reported, appeared to be prospective. This may simply reflect the fact that, in the US, current regulations on the use of experimental drugs naturally compel that they be used in prospective studies only, simply by the very nature of the approval process and the reporting requirements. it is probably also true, however, that there is a longer tradition of prospective study in the medical subspecialties than in either radiotherapy or surgery.

It is also clear than randomization is not a favourite procedure with any of the modalities. The low proportion of trials using a randomized design (11/29 prospective studies in the published papers and 10/56 in the ASCO abstracts) is not automatically a criticism. Many trials, such as Phase II activity studies and feasibility trials of various kinds, are probably best done in an uncontrolled way. Nevertheless, one comes away from this literature with the clear impression that most often the uncontrolled feasibility study is motivated by considerations other than the desire to ascertain the feasibility of a regimen. The chemotherapy trials, in particular, are often empirically combinations of two or more drugs, selected without reference to an obvious

standard. Even if there is a logical standard the investigator may doubt that he has access to a sufficient number of patients to perform a prospective randomized trial; hence he compromises, performs a single arm study and calls it a 'pilot' to make it respectable. What he secretly hopes, of course, is that he will strike gold and end up with results so good that the need for a controlled study may itself be doubtful. Such an investigator needs to be gently reminded that this sort of result has not yet occurred in head and neck cancer.

For this reason, the choice of an uncontrolled design over a controlled one because of a small anticipated accrual is self-defeating. Since an unambiguously wonderful result is not at all likely to occur, the investigator will be left with a more or less promising result which then has to be related to a large number of similar studies going on elsewhere or to some historical experience. The issue of comparative efficacy, therefore, *always* comes up, unless one is doing a true pilot study in a Phase I sense.

Since the head and neck cancers are relatively rare, no single institution has the resources to execute large-scale controlled trials as definitive tests of efficacy within a reasonable period of time. Naturally, of course, the resources do exist, and a few large cooperative trials done over the past few years, notably in the RTOG and in the Head and Neck Contracts Program of the National Cancer Institute, show that under the proper conditions, and with the proper support, they can be mobilized. Increasing the extent of interinstitutional cooperation will be very important over the next few years; if this can be accomplished, at least a few important questions can be dealt with definitively, rather than inconclusively.

Subject Index